Management of Pain in the Hand and Wrist

Editorial Advisory Board

Chairman:
Douglas W. Lamb FRCS
Princess Margaret Rose Orthopaedic Hospital, Edinburgh, UK

W. Bruce Conolly FRCS FRACS FACS
Hand Unit, Sydney Hospital, Sydney, New South Wales, Australia

Nicholas Barton FRCS
Department of Hand Surgery, University Hospital,
Queen's Medical Centre,
Nottingham, UK

Lee W. Milford Jr BS MS MD
The Campbell Clinic, Memphis, Tennessee, USA

Published volumes in this Series

The Interphalangeal Joints
William H. Bowers

The Paralysed Hand
Douglas W. Lamb

Dupuytren's Disease
Robert M. McFarlane, D. A. McGrouther and M. H. Flint

Fractures of the Hand and Wrist
Nicholas Barton

Unsatisfactory Results in Hand Surgery
Robert M. McFarlane

Volumes in preparation

Microsurgical Procedures
Viktor Meyer and Michael Black

Fingertip and Nailbed Injuries
Guy Foucher

The Thumb
James W. Strickland

Joint Replacement in the Upper Limb
William A. Souter

Congenital Malformations of the Hand and Forearm
Dieter Buck-Gramcko

Skin Cover in the Injured Hand
David M. Evans

Tumours of the Hand and Upper Limb
G. Bogurnill and E. Fleegler

THE HAND AND UPPER LIMB   VOLUME 6

Management of Pain in the Hand and Wrist

EDITED BY

C. B. Wynn Parry MBE MA DM DPhysMed FRCS FRCP

Formerly Director of Rehabilitation, Royal National Orthopaedic Hospital,
Stanmore, Middlesex; currently Director of Rehabilitation, King Edward VII Hospital, Midhurst, West Sussex, UK

FOREWORD BY

Douglas W. Lamb FRCS
Consultant Orthopaedic Surgeon, Princess Margaret Rose Orthopaedic Hospital, Edinburgh, UK

CHURCHILL LIVINGSTONE
EDINBURGH LONDON MELBOURNE NEW YORK AND TOKYO 1991

CHURCHILL LIVINGSTONE
Medical Division of Longman Group UK Limited

Distributed in the United States of America by Churchill Livingstone Inc., 1560 Broadway, New York, N.Y. 10036, and by associated companies, branches and representatives throughout the world.

© Longman Group UK Limited 1991

All rights reserved. No part of this publication may be reproduced, stored in a retrieval system, or transmitted in any form or by any means, electronic, mechanical, photocopying, recording or otherwise, without either the prior written permission of the publishers (Churchill Livingstone, Robert Stevenson House, 1–3 Baxter's Place, Leith Walk, Edinburgh EH1 3AF), or a licence permitting restricted copying in the United Kingdom issued by the Copyright Licensing Agency Ltd, 90 Tottenham Court Road, London W1P 9HE.

First published 1991

ISBN 0-443-04109-1

British Library Cataloguing in Publication Data
Management of pain in the hand and wrist.
  1. Man. Arms & shoulders. Pain
  I. Wynn Parry, C. B. (Christopher Berkeley) II. Series
  617.570472

Library of Congress Cataloging in Publication Data
Management of pain in the hand and wrist/edited by C. B. Wynn Parry.
    p. cm. — (The Hand and upper limb)
  Includes index.
  ISBN 0-443-04109-1
  1. Hand — Diseases — Treatment. 2. Wrist — Diseases — Treatment. 3. Intractable pain — Treatment.
  I. Wynn Parry, C. B. II. Series.
  [DNLM: 1. Hand. 2. Pain — physiopathology.
  3. Pain — therapy. 4. Wrist.]
  RC951.M318 1991
  DLC
  for Library of Congress   90-2341
                                                    CIP

Printed in Great Britain by The Bath Press, Avon

Foreword

The hand and upper limb series is planned to cover about a dozen common and important topics. A theme which is common to most of these is the presence of pain of varying type and severity. This often makes the management of the underlying condition so very much more difficult.

The Editorial Board felt that it would be very appropriate for an up-to-date review of the whole subject of pain. In particular, a volume covering the factors which predispose to disabling pain and the mechanisms by which this is interpreted by the human body would be valuable for surgeons at all levels of experience.

It is only when armed with this knowledge that the surgeon can interpret and understand the painful symptoms presented by the patient and initiate the most appropriate treatment.

There is nobody better equipped by his training, background and vast experience to be the Editor of such a volume than Dr C. B. Wynn Parry. He is an international authority on rehabilitation and his experience in restoring function of the upper limb and hand has been gained over many years in the management of those who have sustained injuries through industrial accident, the wounds of war and the accidents that lead to traction injuries of the brachial plexus, often associated with disabling intractable pain.

The editor has invited and obtained contributions from those who are recognised throughout the world as leaders in the interpretation of the mechanisms by which pain is relayed and controlled and the pathological processes which are involved.

New techniques are described which may be utilised to control pain, which may be such an important factor in limiting the recovery of function to the hand after injury, disease or operation. The information collected together here would not be obtainable elsewhere in any one source and should make this volume indispensable to the practising surgeon involved in the management of conditions affecting the upper limb.

1991 D.W.L.

Preface

Pain is a prominent and disabling feature of many disorders of the upper limb. Obviously successful treatment of pain depends on an accurate diagnosis and appropriate specific therapy. Painful rheumatic hands may need synovectomy of tendons and joints, replacement arthroplasty and second and third line drug treatment. A glomus tumour needs excision, painful entrapment neuropathies need decompression, but some painful states do not respond to specific therapy – causalgia may be worsened by repeated surgery, phantom pain and the pain of avulsion lesions of the brachial plexus may resist all drug therapy and may require radical measures such as the DREZ operation. Even these may not succeed in an appreciable proportion of patients. The challenge of what to do for the patient in whom every modality has been tried but yet suffers severe pain faces us all. The last 20 years has seen a quite remarkable explosion of treatment in chronic pain. Fundamental research in animals, particularly by Wall and his associates has revealed many of the pathophysiological mechanisms underlying damage to peripheral nerves.

The work of Loeser, Albe Fessard and Lombard has revealed the nature of the spinal and central nervous response to deafferentation and goes some way to explain the nature of phantom pain. This has led to the introduction of stimulation techniques, both peripheral such as TENS and central such as dorsal column stimulation. At the same time the new work revealing the major changes following nerve damage has made us wary of destructive lesions such as cordotomy and rhizotomy. The vast amount of work on the inflammatory process has led to a much greater understanding of the peripheral mechanisms in inflammatory arthritis.

We thus have more powerful drugs at our disposal and more refined surgical techniques. An appreciation of the importance of intensive rehabilitation has restored many more people to active life and work with subsequent relief of symptoms. However our new understanding of the nature of painful disorders has taught us the limitations of some of our approaches – Wall's exegesis of the peripheral and central effects of nerve damage has made us realise that surgery may well be contraindicated causing as it does further damage, more spontaneous discharges and more central effects of deafferentation.

The addition of clinical psychologists to the rehabilitation team has added a vital new dimension to the management of chronic pain. With their help it is now possible for patients to learn to cope with chronic pain by the use of behavioural therapy and operant conditioning techniques.

It is clear therefore that modern methods of treatment of pain embrace a whole range of options, and surgeons and physicians in this field need a sound understanding of the experimental work on nerve damage and a knowledge of the new modalities available including stimulation techniques and drug therapy and an appreciation of the role of clinical psychology.

It is impossible for surgeons to keep abreast of this field as the relevant work appears in a variety of journals not normally seen by clinicians and interdisciplinary fora combining basic science with clinical research are all too rare.

The Editorial Board therefore felt that we would

take this opportunity to review the present state of the art in relation to pain mechanisms as well as recent advances in management of chronic pain.

The reader will thus find this a rather unusual text. We hope though that it will serve to bring into focus the important fundamental work that has led us to a clearer understanding of why patients develop pain after nerve damage and loss of part or the whole of a limb, and the wide variety of approaches that are now available to help these unfortunate patients.

We have enlisted an outstanding panel of international experts: Professor Wall is the doyen of experimental physiologists in the field of peripheral nerve damage. His painstaking and brilliant experimental work with his many colleagues – Scadding, Devor, Gutnik, Fitzgerald, among many others, has totally changed our approach to the management of painful nerve disorders. In a characteristically provocative introductory chapter he reviews our present state of knowledge and relates it to the clinical situation.

For many years he and Dr Peter Nathan attended our Painful Nerve Clinic and made invaluable contributions to our thinking in this field – the co-operation of basic scientists and clinicians has proved exciting to us all, not least the patient who realises how much effort is being devoted by many different disciplines to this problem (Chapter 6).

It has long been known that the sympathetic nervous system must play a fundamental role in painful disorders of nerve. Barnes demonstrated in 1948 that sympathectomy could cure causalgia; Hannington Kiff showed us in 1971 that sympathetic blockade by guanethedine was more reliable than stellate blocks or surgical division of sympathetic nerves (all too likely to regenerate) and this has become a standard clinic tool in the treatment of painful limb states.

But how and why does it work and what is the role of the sympathetic nervous system?

Roberts has thought about this long and hard and has given us a convincing hypothesis which he explains in Chapter 2. This will inevitably lead to more experimental work and will for certain be of prime importance in developing new techniques of therapy. He takes us through a difficult field with exemplary clarity – surgeons will find it revealing – it answers for a start the question that has puzzled us all since Weir Mitchell's work of 1868 – why does pain commence in many cases immediately after a gunshot wound, long before there is time for the peripheral changes described by Wall to develop?

Ochoa is both an experimental scientist and a clinical neurologist. He has provided a series of case studies, whose problems are all too familiar to us in the clinic, in which he has tried to relate the clinical symptoms and signs to the possible underlying mechanisms and serves as an apotheosis as it were of Wall's and Robert's contributions.

It is well recognised that peripheral disorders can cause profound central changes at all levels of the nervous system – less well known but equally important is the fact that central disorders of the nervous system can cause pain in the limbs – the shoulder/hand syndrome as a symptom of brain tumour is one example – the thalamic syndrome, another. Schott is a neurologist with special interest in pain and describes the remarkable number of CNS disorders that can give pain in the upper limb and reminds us that we overlook this at our peril. In a text pitched at the high level of this whole series it would be inappropriate to review the diagnosis and treatment of all the painful disorders of the upper limb. There is therefore no section on the common conditions that are seen in the clinic. Painful fractures, De Quervain's syndrome, tenosynovitis for example will not be discussed. However certain disorders do present problems either because diagnosis is difficult or treatment controversial.

We thus asked Fisk to discuss osteoarthritis of the wrist. In this field he is prominent and his contribution is a distillation of a lifetime's experience in this complex problem.

There remain the sad cases of patients in whom everything has been tried – drugs, surgery, TENS, rehabilitation, with no relief of pain. A small but significant number of people can benefit from spinal and thalamic electrical stimulation. Siegfried is universally acknowledged as the most level headed exponent of these techniques in the world today. He steers us carefully between the heady optimism of certain units who report 95% cure but whose work is unconfirmed elsewhere and the gloom of those pioneers who showed initially brilliant results but declined to a tiny percentage of successes on long-term follow-up.

Finally we are all indebted to Nashold whose DREZ operation has revolutionised the lives of many patients with intractable phantom or avulsion pain.

Here is one destructive surgical procedure that is logical, for it seeks to destroy those cells that are firing spontaneously due to deafferentation and presumably causing pain.

Although the vast majority of patients with such disorders can and should be relieved by the various modalities described in this book, a few will need this procedure. Not to be overlooked is the appreciation by both patient and doctor that there is still one procedure to be considered – psychologically comforting, even though many patients will reject the offer. No doubt there are omissions. This is a text coloured by a personal view of a physician who has worked all his life with surgeons and hopefully sees both sides of the problem. It is hoped that the broad range of knowledge here displayed, both from basic science and from clinical experience will help to enlighten those practitioners whose pressure of work cannot allow them to sift through all the literature present and past to achieve an insight into this fascinating but difficult field.

London, 1991   C.B.W.P.

Contributors

Martha Cline MD
Department of Neurology, Neuromuscular Research Unit, Good Samaritan Hospital & Medical Center, Portland, Oregon, USA

W. Bruce Conolly FRCS FRACS FACS
Hand Unit, Sydney Hospital, Sydney, New South Wales, Australia

Geoffrey R. Fisk MB BS FRCS(Eng) FRCS(Ed)
Honorary Consultant Orthopaedic Surgeon, Harlow Group of Hospitals, Middlesex; Hunterian Professor, Royal College of Surgeons of England, UK

Ronald C. Kramis PhD
Neurological Sciences Institute, Good Samaritan Hospital & Medical Center, Portland, Oregon, USA

Paolo Marchettini MD
Director of EMG Laboratory and Associate Professor, Department of Neurology and Neuroorthopaedic Service, Istituto Scientifico San Raffaele and University of Milan, Italy

Blaine S. Nashold, Jr MD
Professor of Neurosurgery, Duke University Medical Center, Durham, North Carolina, USA

Jose L. Ochoa MD PhD DSc
Department of Neurology, Neuromuscular Research Unit, Good Samaritan Hospital, Oregon Health Sciences University, Portland, Oregon, USA

Michael Powell FRCS
Consultant Neurosurgeon, National Hospitals for Nervous Diseases, London, UK

William J. Roberts PhD
Senior Scientist & Chairman, Neurological Sciences Institute, Good Samaritan Hospital & Medical Center, Portland, Oregon, USA

Colin Shieff FRCS
Consultant Neurosurgeon, Royal Free Hospital, Hampstead, London, UK

G. D. Schott MD FRCP
Consultant Neurologist, National Hospitals for Nervous Diseases, London; Royal National Orthopaedic Hospital, London; Watford General Hospital, Watford, UK

Jean Siegfried MD
Professor of Neurosurgery, Klinik im Park, Seestrasse, Zurich, Switzerland

Patrick Wall FRS DM FRCP
Cerebral Functions Research Group, Department of Anatomy & Developmental Biology, University College, London, UK

C. B. Wynn Parry MBE DM DPhysMed, FRCS, FRCP
Formerly Director of Rehabilitation, Royal National Orthopaedic Hospital, Stanmore, Middlesex; currently Director of Rehabilitation King Edward VII Hospital, Midhurst, West Sussex, UK

Eduardo A. Zancolli MD
Chief of Surgery, National Rehabilitation Center, Buenos Aires; Professor of Orthopedics, Buenos Aires Medical University, Buenos Aires, Argentina

Contents

1. Mechanisms of pain in relation to the hand 1
   Patrick D. Wall

2. Sympathetically dependent pain: physiology and clinical expression 14
   William J. Roberts and Ronald C. Kramis

3. Lessons from human research on the pathophysiology of neuropathic pains in limbs 28
   Jose L. Ochoa, Paolo Marchettini and Martha Cline

4. Management of pain in the hand and wrist: central causes of peripheral pain 34
   G. D. Schott

5. The painful wrist: problems and solutions 48
   Geoffrey R. Fisk

6. Painful peripheral nerves and the painful stiff hand 69
   Christopher B. Wynn Parry

7. The management of traumatic neuroma in the hand 100
   W. Bruce Conolly

8. The painful hand: problems and solutions 114
   E. A. Zancolli

9. Neurostimulation techniques for intractable pain in the hand and wrist 139
   J. Siegfried

10. Phantom and avulsion pain 145
    B. S. Nashold Jr. and Colin Shieff

11. The management of malignant hand pain 162
    Michael Powell

Index 169

P. D. Wall

1 Mechanisms of pain in relation to the hand

THE PERSISTENCE OF A PERNICIOUS CLASSICAL APPROACH TO MECHANISMS

We are by nature classifiers, subdividers and atomisers. This has led to 50 years of 'scientific progress', at the end of which pain mechanisms could be expounded in a 15 minute medical school lecture, which could be summarised as follows. Pain is the sensation provoked by tissue damage. Tissue damage is detected by small myelinated A delta sensory afferents and by unmyelinated C afferents. These fibres end in the dorsal part of the dorsal horn, where they relay onto cells which project to the thalamus by way of the ventrolateral white matter of the spinal cord. End of lecture.

The lecture is so clear and precise and is delivered with such authority that it can be parroted by the dullest student; and usually is, for the duration of his professional life. The fact that he never sees a patient who fulfils the prediction that tissue damage and pain are exactly correlated does not shake his abiding faith in that great enlightening lecture. The fact that he can explain few pains and can treat even fewer leads him to classify patients as an infinity of exceptions to the proper patient in pain who exemplifies the simple purity of the mechanism he knows must exist.

Fortunately not all clinicians and scientists are dull and they have doubted the hard wired fixed atomic pain mechanism from the time of its conception. Just as it is rarely useful to consider the hand as five fingers stuck on the arm by way of the wrist, it is rarely useful to consider the nervous system as a collection of separate bits stuck together by glia and connective tissue. The triviality and inconsequential nature of the proposed pain mechanism led many clinicians and scientists to neglect the whole subject and to turn instead to consider only the nature of tissue damage. Now we need a new, mature approach to the way in which the normal or painful hand is integrated into the subtlest of our behaviours by way of the nervous system.

INNER AND OUTER SENSORY WORLDS OF THE HAND

If a hypodermic needle is pressed against a finger tip, it is perceived as a sharp object pitting the skin but existing in the outer world. If it penetrates the skin, a quite different perception predominates over the previous perception, even though the object persists. The rules of these two types of sensation differ greatly. Painful disorders may be a mixture of the two types.

The hand usually collects information about objects in contact with it by active exploration and manipulation. Passive reception of a stimulus is a rare event in real life although favoured in neurological examination. The improvement of sensation produced by movement goes beyond the advantage of overcoming the rapid adaptation of pressure detectors whose discharge fades if the object is stationary. Two point discrimination improves if the points are applied sequentially in imitation of movement rather than simultaneously, as happens with the passive application of a stationary stimulus. Even the simplest of textures is hardly discernible if passively applied. There is an improvement if the examiner moves the stimulus over the hand in imitation of the exploratory movements which would normally be made. However, it is active movement by the subject which reveals the full discriminating ability. This is shown dramatically in braille reading, where active scanning is superior to imitated identical movement applied by machine. Needless to say the presence of pain of whatever cause or nature interferes with the ability to move and therefore the ability to feel. This special role of active touch was discussed by Sherrington but really explored by Gibson (1968) and in a remarkable work by Revesz (1950). An active grasp is needed to give the impression of hardness whereas the same stimulus passively applied results in a feeling of pressure. As William James noted, two contacts are felt if an object is placed between the fingers but a single object is experienced if the fingers are squeezed together on the same object by active movement. In other words, active movement is necessary for haptic appreciation of the world in contact with the fingers. Without active movement, another world is apparent which not only lacks the details of the actively perceived world but is a disintegrated world in which the various independent bits of information cannot be formed into a connected whole. With all our senses we achieve a final analysis after the abrupt appearance of a novel event in a sequence of stages: attention, orientation and exploration. One of the defining characteristics of pain is that it takes precedence in seizing attention. Therefore when pain is provoked by finger movement, the normal sequence of analysis, i.e. attention, orientation and exploration, is instantly diverted from the outside world to the inside world. This 'blinds' the hand even though careful sensory examination, that is the detection of individual, passively applied stimuli, shows the hand to possess normal sensitivity.

In normal circumstances the hand acts in concert with the eye and the perceived haptic sensation is dominated by the visual. The hand has been called 'the tool of the eye'. A baby confirms its first visual experiences by reaching out and touching. An adult in the dark or blindfolded or blinded as an adult continues to use the hand according to the rules on the nature of the world out there which were first perceived by visual experience backed up by touch. The person blind from birth perceives with the hand in two quite different ways from those who have learned about the nature of the world out there with their hands serving and subserving the eyes. Dominant features of our visual world are the axes, vertical and horizontal. These are of little consequence in the pure haptic world (Millar 1978).

A much more important extension of this relates to the ability to integrate in the two sensory systems. The eye is capable of simultaneously detecting spatially separated events. Since the hand can only be in one place at a time, it has to construct the existence of wholes by detecting first one part and then another and remembering each part and then putting them all together to make the whole. The eye 'sees' a square as such and furthermore the square has a background. A finger tracing or drawing a square has to run sequentially along the sides and round the corners and finally has the immensely difficult task of deciding if the finger has returned to the start point. A circle and a spiral are visually obviously different but difficult to detect by touch because vision operates by simultaneous integration and touch by sequential construction. The differences between the two sensory worlds is shown with touching drama in the work by Revesz (1950) on the art of the blind, which differs strikingly depending on the time at which the person became blind and whether they are living in a world still dominated by memories of vision or one constructed ab initio from haptic experience. My reason for this apparent diversion from the topic of pain is to stress the artificiality of considering sensory modalities in isolation, let alone single nerve fibres or cells one by one.

Sensation and movement interact. Intentional exploratory movement, as we have said, does more than raise sensitivity; it reveals a quite special perceived world. Intentional executive movements have a quite separate effect on sensation. The effect is obvious and large and can easily be demonstrated by self experiment. Try wrenching a stopper from a jammed bottle. Examine the indentation on the fingers left by your painless effort. Get someone else to press your finger to produce a similar indentation. You are unlikely to stand a fraction of the stimulus you applied to yourself when it is applied by someone else. In other words, intentional movement can be associated with a marked increase of threshold. Sensation obviously affects movement as well as the other way round. This occurs both when the source of pain is in the region of the movement and in distant parts of the same segment. The shoulder–hand syndrome is an extreme example. I experienced a minor educational occurrence: I frequently dissect fibres from nerves using two sharpened jewellers' forceps, viewed through a high power dissecting microscope. For some time, I had a trivial shoulder pain which was of no marked intensity and easily ignored. When the pain was just detectable there was an obvious clumsiness in my ability to dissect with the hand on the side of the minimally and distant painful site. This is a threshold observation of what becomes a lame hand under more serious conditions.

There are good reasons to start with an examination of the hand's sensory world before launching into the technical details of pain mechanisms. First, it is evident that we should not expect to discover pain mechanisms in isolation as though they were the equivalent of a fire alarm system screwed onto a structure which had quite separate functions. Second, the presence of tissue damage or pain will interact with many other activities both by way of local neural circuitry as well as more distant complex cognitive processes. Lastly, pain and its consequences and intereactions are not the consequence of a fixed hard wired independent system but of a plastic interactive system likely to respond to subtle restorative therapies of the type introduced to the hand by Moberg (1964), Dellon (1981) and Wynn Parry (1966).

WHY DOES TISSUE DAMAGE GENERATE AN AFFERENT BARRAGE?

The typical example of tissue damage classically associated with pain is inflammation, with the other three cardinal signs of swelling, redness and heat. We can immediately dismiss the other three signs as the cause of the pain. Massive oedematous swelling is not necessarily painful. Maximal vasodilatation produced by heat or drugs is also not painful by itself. We must therefore seek a cause of the pain which may be coupled with the other changes but not necessarily dependent on them. We must reach into the inflamed tissue itself to discover which of the cellular and chemical changes cause the pain and which are independent correlates. One crucial clue comes from the simplest of clinical observations: pain is rarely continuous and then only in specific conditions. The commonest painful condition, as in arthritis, is that pain only occurs on movement and that a pain free position can be discovered. The significance of this common report is that there cannot be a continuous source of pain in operation rather that sensitisation has occurred so that normally innocuous movement now provokes pain. We should equally attend to the opposite report by patients in continuous pain, as in cases of causalgia, and be prepared to seek a different source of the afferent barrage.

The best known sources of sensitisation in inflamed tissue are E type prostaglandins and prostacyclin. They are the products of one arm of the breakdown in damaged tissue of arachidonic acid. This arm, the cyclooxygenase pathway, is the one blocked by aspirin and the many aspirin like non-steroidal anti-inflammatory agents. They are clearly useful and equally clearly inadequate for all forms and intensities of inflammatory pain.

The clue which led to the revelation of other inflammatory pain mechanisms came from the observation of the superior effectiveness of steroids as analgesic anti-inflammatory agents. Corticosteroids block both the cyclooxygenase breakdown pathway which produces prostaglandins and the lipoxygenase pathway which results in the release of leukotrienes into the tissue. The leukotrienes attract polymorphonuclear leukocytes into the tissue and are pain producing. The pain production of the leukotrienes seems to be dependent on the presence of the polymorphonuclear leukocytes which themselves breakdown and release pain producing agents. One of these is suspected to be a particular product of the lipoxygenase pathway of arachidonic acid breakdown, (8R,15S) – diHETE.

We have thus far considered only the pain producing consequences of tissue breakdown itself but the nerves themselves play a crucial part in three quite different ways. There is a neurogenic component to inflammation which was first described by Lewis as the triple response to tissue damage by way of the axon reflex. When unmyelinated afferents are excited, they release substances which are suspected to be peptides and include substance P. These substances have three separable effects, vasodilatation, neurogenic oedema and hyperalgesia. When tissue is not innervated, this component of inflammation is absent, which partially explains the poor inflammatory response in conditions such as diabetes and other examples of the fragile state of denervated tissue. The next neural effect on inflammation relates to the sympathetic efferents which have a role beyond their vascular control. The most striking action occurs when nerve is damaged and will be discussed in the next section. However, there is an algesic action of the sympathetic system where no gross nerve damage is apparent. For example, one of the best known pain producing substances released by damaged tissue, particularly from mast cells, is bradykinin. The hyperalgesia produced by bradykinin is blocked both by prostaglandin synthesis inhibitors and by sympathectomy. Thirdly, and most surprisingly, very recent work has identified a large group of unmyelinated afferents which are completely inexcitable in normal tissue. These amount to at least 40% of skin C-afferents and over 80% of such fibres from bladder or colon. They only become excitable in the presence of inflammation. They then respond to pressure and temperature. One might label such fibres as a special type of chemoreceptor. Nothing is known yet of which of the many components of inflammation switch on these normally silent fibres. Once activated these fibres are already known to take on quite new properties which include a local peripheral sensitivity to narcotics. We can therefore summarise the painful consequences of inflammation as being signalled from the periphery by the following seven independent but interacting factors:

1. Arachidonic acid breakdown
    a. Cyclooxygenase pathway – prostaglandins and prostacyclin
    b. Lipoxygenase pathway – leukotrienes
2. Polymorphonuclear leukocyte invasion and breakdown
3. Pain producing substances such as bradykinin
4. Neural components
    a. Axon reflex triple response of C-afferents
    b. Sympathetic efferents
    c. Activation of silent C-afferents.

WHY DOES NERVE DAMAGE GENERATE AN AFFERENT BARRAGE?

Immediate effects

When an axon is cut across there is an immediate violent and repetitive discharge in all types of axons (Wall & Gutnik 1974). However, this discharge dies down within seconds and the cut end becomes relatively insensitive for some time as the ends seal over. This period is unfortunately the calm before the storm.

Secondary effects

Within a day of an axon having been cut, the end seals over and sprouts begin to grow out. During the first week each axon sends out multiple sprouts, up to 50 from a single axon. These search out and probe surrounding tissue. Many curl back and run along intact axons towards the central nervous system. If an axon sprout suceeds in entering a Schwann cell tube, it continues to grow toward the periphery and the unsuccessful sprouts from that axon disappear. If axon sprouts fail to locate a distal Schwann cell, they probe for short distances into surrounding tissue. During the second week some of the multiple sprouts disappear but others remain to form a neuroma. If axons have been severed in a simple crush injury, many non-neural structures such as the basement membranes remain intact. In this situation, 100% of the severed fibres succeed in growing a sprout into a distal Schwann cell tube and will eventually reinnervate approximately the area of tissue which they previously innervated (Devor & Govrin-Lippmann 1979).

The extreme opposite injury, as in amputation, involves the section and ligation of nerves. Here the sprouts are trapped within the nerve sheath and form a terminal neuroma with only a few sprouts eventually escaping to make inappropriate connections with nearby tissue. An intermediate case is where a nerve has been cut across and then resutured. In experimental studies on rat sciatic nerve with very precise sectioning and immediate careful resuturing, it has been found that over 25% of axons fail to cross into the peripheral nerve. Therefore even under ideal conditions one must assume that such repairs will be only partially successful and will leave in the area of injury or surgery a substantial number of fibres forming a partial neuroma.

The properties of the outgrowing sprouts differ in three crucial ways from the normal nerve (Wall & Gutnick 1974).

1. Ongoing activity. As sprouts grow out, all types of sensory fibres begin to generate spontaneous nerve impulses. In the case of crushed nerves, where the sprouts are successfully penetrating into distal Schwann cells, this activity rises for about 7 days and then declines to zero. In the case of a cut-ligated nerve where all fibres form a neuroma, the activity of the sprouts reaches a peak at about 2 weeks and then declines to a low level over the next 2 weeks. These active sprouts then continue to produce nerve impulses indefinitely.

2. Mechanical sensitivity. Normal axons are relatively insensitive to mechanical distortion, although they can be activated by high-intensity stimuli, as everyone who has hit the ulnar nerve at the elbow knows. As nerve sprouts grow out and become spontaneously active they become extremely sensitive to slight mechanical distortion. This is the origin of the local tenderness associated with nerve injury and of the Tinel sign, where slight taps over a regrowing nerve elicit a sensation referred to the skin normally innervated by the cut nerve.

3. Sensitivity to adrenalin. Outgrowing sprouts become extremely sensitive to the alpha receptor action of adrenalin. Stimulation of the sympathetic system releases sufficient noradrenalin in the area of a neuroma to generate a powerful barrage of nerve impulses in sensory afferents. Since such afferent impulses will induce reflex sympathetic discharges, a situation of positive feedback exists. We have here an explanation of the various sympathetic dystrophies such as causalgia and Sudeck's atrophy. It also provides a rationale for sympathectomy and especially for the local application of guanethidine, introduced by Hannington-Kiff (1974). The exact action of the sympathetic system remains a mystery for two reasons. One is that there is a latency of seconds between the arrival of noradrenalin and the generation of the impulses. This delay cannot be explained by diffusion and suggests some intermediate processes. The second is that beta blockers have some effect on the chronic discharge of animal neuromas and some human conditions which is not expected, since the acute action of adrenalin or of sympathetic discharge is completely abolished by alpha blockers (Wall & Gutnick 1974).

Tertiary effects

As time goes by a small number of outgrowing axons may establish close contact with other sprouts. This may allow impulses to jump ephaptically from one axon to another and opens the possibility of some of the afferent barrage from a region of damage being formed by the direct transfer of efferent impulses into afferent nerve fibres (Seltzer & Devor 1979). In a second slow process, neighbouring intact nerves sense the degeneration of the cut axons. They send out sprouts which occupy at least part of the denervated zone (Devor & Govrin Lippmann 1979). This phenomenon explains the rapid phase of filling in of anaesthetic areas and may contribute to the abnormal sensations associated with the edge of such areas.

THE EFFECT OF AXONAL INJURY ON AXONS CENTRAL TO THE INJURY

There are practical as well as basic reasons for considering the central spread of the effects of injury other than the obviously important transmission of the nerve impulses from the injured area to the central nervous system. Noordenbos and Wall (1981) examined 7 patients who had developed pain and abnormal sensitivity in the area supplied by a single nerve which had been injured. They were treated unsuccessfully for periods ranging from 3–108 months by conservative methods. All then had the damaged nerve resected and in five cases a sural nerve graft was inserted. The patients were examined 20–72 months after the operation. In all 7 cases, pain had recurred in the same area as experienced before the operation. This unfortunate result suggests very strongly that peripheral nerve damage induces changes central to the lesion which are not reversed by treatment directed at the area of the original injury. We will now examine this central migration of changes related to pain which moves from the area of injury.

Immediate effects

The injury discharge which results from the section of axons and the discharge from intact terminals in damaged tissue will be conducted centrally over the afferent fibres.

Secondary changes

The distal axon separated from the cell body degenerates and the cut axon sprouts. The central part of the cut axon was classically presumed to remain essentially intact although chromatolysis occurs in the cell bodies. Some cells die if regeneration fails. However it now seems that there are at least three types of central changes of practical importance.

1. Activity in dorsal root ganglia (DRG). Some days after peripheral nerve section, generation of nerve impulses begins in the region of the DRG (Wall & Devor 1983). In the rat, after sciatic section, this rises to a maximum after about 3 weeks and declines slowly over subsequent months but never ceases as long as the neuroma exists. At the same time these ganglia become very sensitive to mechanical distortion and to circulating adrenalin. Lesions in the dorsal roots do not cause changes in the DRG cells (Czeh et al 1977). In other words, there is evidence that some signal, presumably a transported chemical, moves from the periphery to the ganglion cell but does not move from the spinal cord to these cells. There are two different sources of abnormal peripheral afferent nerve impulses in chronic pain, one from the region of injury and one from the DRG.

2. Loss of peptides and chemicals. The DRG cells synthesise proteins and peptides which are then transported to the peripheral terminals and to the spinal cord terminals. Each peptide has its proponent as playing some part in neurotransmission. Peptides are certainly released from nerve terminals and have powerful actions on nerve cells. When a peripheral nerve has been cut, the presence of these chemicals in the spinal cord afferent terminals in the substantia gelatinosa drops very substantially (Barbut et al 1981). Much to the surprise of many who believed that these chemicals represented neurotransmitters, stimulation of the central end of the cut nerve produces the same excitation of spinal cord cells as is produced by a volley in an intact nerve (Wall & Devor 1981; Wall et al 1981; Woolf & Wall 1982). The fact is one of a number which raises severe doubts about the function of these substances as normal transmitters (Wall & Fitzgerald 1982). However the substances have some function. Alternative possibilities for that function are that these substances control overall excitabilities with long-term courses of action rather than producing the brief and dramatic inhibitions or excitations which are characteristic of classical neurotransmitters. Whatever may be their function, it is clear that their concentrations change after peripheral injury and these changes could be a link in the slow changes of postsynaptic function which we will discuss in the next section.

3. Changes of conduction velocity. All axons central to a nerve lesion decrease their conduction velocity. In rat sciatic nerve this change begins by 3 days after nerve section and continues for long periods of time (Wall & Devor 1981). If the nerve fibre eventually successfully regenerates and again establishes a contact with peripheral tissue these changes slowly reverse. We do not know if this change has any functional consequence but it is certainly a sign of the widespread central changes induced by peripheral lesions and it provides a useful clinical sign.

Tertiary changes

Atrophy of the central terminals of sensory afferents

Some investigators reported that the terminals of fine afferent fibres show electron microscope changes within 6 days of sciatic nerve section in rats. Others have not been able to detect these changes. 'Reactive cells' which are not nerve cells and whose nature remains a matter of speculation accumulate around the afferents in the dorsal horn and are a further example of the cord responding to peripheral damage.

Degeneration of some dorsal root ganglion cells

We have shown a number of changes sweeping centrally from nerve damage. It is perhaps not surprising that for some cells these changes are lethal. Cell death and consequent degeneration of central axons is particularly apparent in trigeminal lesions. Even after tooth extraction, some obvious degeneration is apparent in the trigeminal nuclei. In limb nerves, the changes are slower and more scattered but eventually produce a substantial loss of afferent fibres. This means that in chronic nerve lesions such as in amputation, some spinal cord cells are anatomically deafferented following this transganglionic degeneration. It is well known that root lesions can produce severe deafferentation syndromes, and we can expect that one of the factors in pain following chronic peripheral nerve lesions will be due to irreversible but scattered degeneration of spinal cord afferents.

Partial reversals

By 2 weeks after peripheral nerve section, there is severe depletion of chemicals in the spinal cord terminals of some afferent fibres. However, after 6 months some of these chemicals begin to reappear, particularly the fluoride-resistant acid phosphatase and substance P. It was first thought that this might represent collateral sprouting from intact neighbouring afferents which moved in to occupy the area evacuated by the affected afferents. This is evidently not the case, since resectioning of the originally damaged nerve is again followed by a disappearance of the chemicals. These very slow changes indicate that the central nervous system shows signs of change which continue for many months after a peripheral nerve lesion.

THE EFFECT OF PERIPHERAL INJURY ON CELLS IN THE SPINAL CORD

Immediate effects

It is now useful to restrict the term 'gate control' to the rapidly acting mechanisms which receive and control the transfer of impulses from the input afferent fibres to cells which in turn trigger the various effector systems and which evoke sensation (Melzack & Wall 1965; Wall 1978). There are four components of the gate control.

The afferents

Nociceptive afferents terminate in precisely localised regions. The C-afferent terminals are limited to the two outer laminae. A deltas also end in this area and some extend to a zone in the mid-dorsal horn, lamina 5. We must also consider low-threshold afferents in relation to pain mechanisms for two reasons.

1. Tenderness is partly explained by a sensitisation of nociceptors, but in some pathological states, such as referred pain, innocuous stimuli to normal tissue produce pain. Impulses from low-threshold afferents may summate with those from nociceptors.

2. Inhibition of the central effect of nociceptors is produced by low threshold afferents, the basis of transcutaneous electrical nerve stimulation and dorsal column stimulation.

Segmental interactions within the dorsal horn

The cells which receive incoming afferents are arranged in 6 laminae. These cells are not simply collecting information from particular types of afferents and transmitting them to their destination: the role of these cells, like all central nervous system cells, is to select and compute combinations of the signals which impinge on them. Some combinations sum and aid each other. Other combinations evoke inhibitions so that one input excludes the effect of the other. These inhibitory and excitatory interactions require the presence of interneurons. Laminae 1 and 2, in particular, contain cells which are well suited to be such interneurons.

Descending controls

Many structures in the brain project into the dorsal horn and have mainly inhibitory effects on the firing of dorsal cells. The inhibition of nociceptive responses in cord produced by electrical stimulation of some of these structures appears to correlate well with behavioural analgesias. Emphasis has been placed on the raphe nuclei and the reticular formation as the origin of descending control, but there are other sources: spinal segments, dorsal column nuclei, vestibular nuclei, the olive, trigeminal nuclei, locus coerulus, tectum, red nucleus, hypothalamus, pyramidal tract etc. All of these could play a role in inducing analgesias or hyperpathias, but unfortunately we know little of their relative importance and nothing of the actual circumstances in which they come into action.

The transmission cells

The outcome of the synaptic decisions made in the dorsal horn and trigeminal nuclei are collected by several different types of cell, which send their axons to distant structures. Many of these systems contain information about the presence of injury. We must remain extremely cautious in assigning to any one system the responsibility for triggering pain. The easiest fact to forget is the discovery of Schiff, confirmed by Basbaum (1973), that bilateral hemisections of the cord separated by two segments do not abolish painful reactions. Short-chain polysynaptic systems (Noordenbos 1959) may play a crucial role.

Of the long-running pathways it has been traditional to emphasise the spinothalamic tract. However, that emphasis comes first from the success of anterolateral cordotomy, which was taken to be the equivalent of cutting the spinothalamic tract, neglecting the many other projection systems which are cut in that operation. Second, the emphasis comes from the classical but completely unproven assumption that pain is the product of thalamo-cortical systems. Positive evidence suggests that, if the thalamus is involved, then systems feeding to medial thalamus are more important and that the most powerful correlation between the firing of cells and of painful behaviour has been found in caudal brain stem in reticular formation (Casey 1971).

Secondary changes in spinal cord after injury: connectivity control

It is not enough to consider only an abrupt stimulus of the type used in experimental laboratories. Pain as felt by our patients is unfortunately a continuing process. Furthermore, as we shall see, it is not enough to propose that ongoing pain is simply a repetition of a series of responses to a series of abrupt stimuli. We have already seen how the periphery changes the nature of the afferent barrage with time. Now we must ask if the receiving mechanism within brain and spinal cord also changes under conditions of ongoing injury detection.

Prolonged central changes triggered by nerve impulses

It is a common clinical and personal experience that minor deep injuries such as a twisted ankle result in prolonged pain and tenderness which spread far from the site of injury while apparently equivalent cutaneous injuries result in more spatially and temporally restricted sensory disorders. Similar differences have been noted by comparing the effects of experimental noxious stimuli to skin and to deep tissue in man (Lewis & Kellgren 1939; Lewis 1942; Hockaday & Whitty 1967). Skin lesions are associated with pain and tenderness in the immediate region of the damage while deep lesions are in addition associated with distant referred areas of pain and tenderness. With an acute experimental lesion such as the injection of 0.2ml of 6% saline the cutaneous effect is a rapidly rising pain peaking in less than a minute and then dying down although a triple response spreads some centimetres from the punctate lesion. In deep tissue, as described in detail by Hockaday & Whitty (1967), there is a three-stage time course: immediate local pain followed by distant pain followed by distant tenderness which may persist for a day.

It is evident that there are central changes as well as peripheral changes of the primary and secondary inflammatory type which must be invoked to explain the widespread effects of peripheral damage. Woolf (1983) showed that peripheral thermal injury in decerebrate rats results in a prolonged increase in the excitability of the flexor reflex. Part of this increase has to be attributed to changes within the spinal cord since a delayed peripheral sensory blockade of the area of injury does not abolish the increased excitability. We decided to examine this phenomenon with cutaneous and muscle afferent barrages (Wall & Woolf 1984). Twenty conditioning stimuli at C fibre strength in the sural cutaneous nerve at 1Hz produced a marked increase in the flexor reflex lasting about 5 min. However, if the same type of conditioning stimulus originates from muscle nerve, the flexor reflex is enhanced for up to 90 min. Brief tetanic contraction of muscle fibres or nerve section is sufficient to trigger similar prolonged changes. A related phenomenon has been observed in lamina 1 cells when punctate deep skin burns were placed outside the cells' receptive field (McMahon & Wall 1984). After 10–15 min the excitability of the cells increased and the receptive field of the cells moved to incorporate the area of injury.

C fibre activity is required to trigger these central changes, since they only occur if the conditioning stimuli activate C fibres. Furthermore, they do not occur if the conditioning nerve has been treated with capsaicin, a selective C fibre neurotoxin. It is important to stress that although triggered by C fibres, the change is not sustained by the continuation of the triggering barrage because local anaesthesia of the conditioning nerve fails to abolish the central change once established. These changes may represent a model for the central component of tenderness. There is a particularly evocative clue: if a peripheral nerve is cut, there are prolonged central changes which we will discuss below. However, there are 3 changes relevant to the present phase:

1. Short-latency, short-duration excitation of central cells by C-afferents, which are cut in the periphery, is either normal or increased
2. The peptide content of the C afferents is decreased
3. The prolonged increased excitability of the flexor reflex induced by C afferents is abolished.

A possible way to link these 3 facts together is to propose that peptides are not rapid neurotransmitters but are responsible for the long latency, long-duration increased excitability. Narcotics are particularly effective in abolishing these prolonged central increases of excitability.

Changes in the spinal cord inevitably change the impulses transmitted to the brain, which in turn will alter the descending feedbacks from brain back to the spinal cord. The most dorsal of dorsal horn cells, the marginal cells in lamina 1, are particularly well placed to receive the unmyelinated fibre input since they lie in exactly the region of termination of the C afferents. These cells project in a recently discovered pathway to the midbrain (McMahon & Wall 1985) and their axons run in the contralateral dorsolateral spinal cord white matter. Cutting this pathway has no effect on acute pain. However, cutting the pathway greatly exaggerates and accelerates chronic painful reactions. This exaggeration occurs whether in the ascending or the descending loop of the control circuit. We have therefore discovered a control circuit which was expected to be involved in triggering pain, but in fact normally reduces prolonged painful responses while having no effect on acute pain.

In summary, when tissue is damaged in the periphery, the central nervous system receives an afferent barrage from nociceptors which produce rapid central inhibitions and excitations as determined by a gate control mechanism. Subsequent to this rapid phase, slow-onset long-duration changes are triggered by impulses in unmyelinated afferents, particularly those originating from deep tissue. These central changes consist of widespread increases of excitability of nerve cells projecting to the brain and to reflex circuits. The increases of excitability are so great that previously ineffective inputs become effective. The practical effect of this is that some cells which were previously excited only by nociceptors now respond to low-threshold inputs. It is highly likely that this provides a basis for the widespread secondary tenderness or allodynia which characterises so many pains. In this pathological state, the nervous system has been reorganised with less specificity, less somatotopy and less precise timing. Furthermore, there are slowly acting brain to spinal cord circuits which control the extent of this spinal cord plasticity.

Tertiary changes in spinal cord following nerve or root damage

If a peripheral nerve is cut, changes sweep centrally to produce changes in the central terminals, particularly of C fibres. As these changes take place there is a progressive decrease in the ability of these cut fibres to evoke primary afferent depolarisation, particularly in the terminals of the axons which have been cut (Wall & Devor 1981). While the ability of both A and C fibres to excite spinal cord cells remains, there is a failure of their ability to inhibit. Nerve section is followed by a severe decline of various interactive inhibitions, i.e. A on A, A on C and to a lesser extent C on C inhibitions (Woolf & Wall 1982). This decline of inhibition is sensitive to the type of damage which the nerve has sustained. While section of the nerve produces the described loss of inhibitions, crush of the nerve sufficient to induce complete peripheral degeneration does not produce the decrease of inhibition. It will be seen that these changes are a form of homeostatic mechanism. After a decreased input as a result of deafferentation, the cord reacts to increase the remaining input by diminishing inhibitions.

Spinal cord cells changes after peripheral nerve damage

Cells responding to peripheral stimuli are quite precisely arranged within the spinal cord (Brown 1981). Medial cells respond to distal stimuli and lateral cells to proximal areas. In other words, the dermatome is represented transversely in the cord. The presence of this map implies that if the foot is made anaesthetic by cutting the sciatic and saphenous nerves, a large area in the medial part of the dorsal horn in the lumbar enlargement, the foot area, loses its input. Cells which formerly responded to stimulation of the foot now fail to respond to any natural stimuli. They are deafferented in a functional sense, even though the anatomical structures of the proximal afferent nerves remain intact. This situation continues in the rat for 3–4 days, but then large numbers of these formerly deafferented cells begin to respond to stimuli applied to proximal innervated tissue. In other words, some change has occurred by which intact afferents which were formerly ineffective now excite cells which have expanded their receptive fields to incorporate innervated peripheral structures (Devor & Wall 1981a,b). It is believed that this process is caused by the slow unmasking of existing anatomical structures rather than by the sprouting of anatomically new afferent connections. This process has considerable clinical significance in explaining some of the irradiations of sensation and increased effectiveness of stimuli, so characteristic of the edge of denervated areas and of amputation stumps.

The role of unmyelinated afferents in these changes

We have said that the anatomical and chemical changes we have observed central to a nerve lesion in the cut axons themselves are particularly apparent in the unmyelinated fibres. We therefore wondered what would be the effect of lesions limited almost entirely to unmyelinated fibres; and have done this using capsaicin. If given as a single dose to neonatal rats or mice this compound permanently destroys some 95% of the C fibres. For a more subtle and controlled effect we have applied capsaicin for 15 minutes to a single nerve in adult rats (Ainsworth et al 1981; Wall & Fitzgerald 1981, 1982). There are marked chemical changes in the chemistry of the central terminals of the C fibres which mimic the effects of nerve section. There is a marked expansion of the receptive field of the cells supplied by the treated nerve in spite of the fact that the A fibres remain intact and able to drive the cell (Wall et al 1981). We have repeated these experiments on the mouse infraorbital nerve in order to be able to take advantage of the most precise somatotopic map known (Wall et al 1982a). In normal mouse somatosensory cortex there are cylinders of cells, the barrels, clearly visible with light microscopy. Developmental and physiological studies show that each barrel is related to a single whisker. If mice are treated with capsaicin the barrels are present anatomically but now the receptive fields of cells have expanded to incorporate many whiskers.

These results taken together suggest a new role for the unmyelinated fibres and the following hypothesis. C fibres could be continually transporting from the periphery chemicals which constitute messages about the nature and state of the tissue in which the fibres terminate. If the tissue is damaged or if the nerve is cut across, a new chemical message will be transmitted since the fibre ends will now lie in a novel chemical environment. We know that the chronic changes we have described do not take place if the nerve impulses alone are blocked with chronic tetrodotoxin (Wall et al 1982b). We also know that nerve crush which leaves the sprouting nerve surrounded by some intact membrane does not induce such changes. Therefore it seems likely that chemical transport mechanisms are involved. Since capsaicin treatment imitates many of the central effects of whole nerve section it is reasonable to propose that C fibres are responsible for transporting a chemical message.

The proposal that there is a continuous slow chemical signalling system connecting tissue to the central nervous system by way of C afferents has received recent strong support. If a continuous supply of nerve growth factor is provided to the cut end of a nerve, there is a considerable decrease of the central consequences of the nerve damage (Fitzgerald et al 1985). The chemistry of C fibres depends on the tissue they innervate (McMahon et al 1984). Furthermore, if cutaneous and muscle nerve are cross-anastomosed in the adult both the chemistry of the fibres and their central effects change (McMahon & Gibson 1987; McMahon & Wall 1987). There is therefore the probability that C fibres detect chemically the nature of the tissue in which they terminate not only in the extreme conditions of nerve damage but also when pathology takes over their normal target tissue.

Within the central nervous system, it is now clear that a considerable plasticity of connection is retained in the adult nervous system. These pathological changes of connection do not necessarily involve any morphological sprouting of new connections. It becomes more and more apparent that fast, slow and chronic changes of the routing of nerve impulses can be achieved by at least three mechanisms which alter the effectiveness of existing anatomical connections.

WHAT THEN IS THE RELATIONSHIP BETWEEN TISSUE DAMAGE AND PAIN?

From what has been said above, it is obvious that there will be no fixed simple relationship. Every observant clinician knows that to be true from the first few patients he sees. He does not need scientists to tell him such an obvious and difficult fact. The role of the clinical and basic scientist is to define, explain and hopefully manipulate the factors which cause the variation. The problem with the classical mechanism which I mocked in the first section is that it is a rigidly fixed system in which response automatically follows stimulus unless there is a gross section of the pain pathway or some mental disturbance. Following this model, doctors with closed minds have examined peripheral tissue for signs of damage, checked the transmission pathways and asked the patient what he felt. If there was a mismatch in the three answers, these doctors diagnosed a mental abnormality. These are the doctors who have dismissed an army of amputees with phantom pains by telling them, 'it is all in the head'. They were wrong. They were also wrong about some pains which seemed to match the existing and obvious peripheral injury. For example, part of postoperative pain now appears to be the long-term central consequence of the afferent barrage during the operation as well as the consequence of the healing injury at the time the pain is felt. Finally they were wrong in neglecting the distant tenderness which is such an obvious and troublesome component of pain even when damaged tissue can be identified. For example if ischaemic heart muscle can produce pain and tenderness in the arm, an arthritic finger is surely likely to produce pain and tenderness in other parts of the hand?

Faced with a reactive nervous system and with multiple components, the tactic for clinician and for scientist is to start in the periphery and to work centrally, step by step, seeking an origin of the painful pathology. The crucial locations evolve with time.

The periphery in the immediate vicinity of damage

We have described 7 components in the reaction of tissue to damage, each of which affects the afferent barrage from the region of injury. They appear in a timed spatial sequence. We know little of the factors which make them disappear. There could be the neural equivalent of the fibrous tissue scar in which nerve ends remain sensitised long after other signs of damage have gone.

The peripheral nerve

The massive injury discharge which follows acute section dies down within seconds. However, the sprouts which grow from cut nerve develop new properties of mechanical sensitivity, spontaneous activity and response to the sympathetic system. These changes mature over weeks. They also sweep centrally and change the chemistry and physiology of the dorsal root ganglia and central terminals of the afferent fibres.

The spinal cord

At least 3 mechanisms control the consequences of arrival of signals from damaged tissue.

The gate control

Rapidly acting mechanisms dependant on the input from nearby afferents and from distant afferents and from descending controls from the brain determine subsequent transmission.

Connectivity control by impulses

The arrival of injury signals, particularly by way of unmyelinated afferents from deep tissue, triggers widespread hyperexcitability of central neurons which is sustained by central mechanisms (Wall & Woolf 1984). This mechanism relates to the narcotic sensitive pains and widespread secondary hyperalgesia.

Connectivity control by transport

When nerves or roots have been cut, the change of chemicals, such as nerve growth factor, which arrive on central cells changes the physiology of central cells so that they show the hyperexcitable deafferentation states. These are associated with narcotic resistant pains and tenderness.

Subsequent central stages

The first 3 stages contain a cascade of changes which sweep centrally from the point of damage. Each stage adds more information which may increase or decrease the pain provoking message. Distraction, placebos, anxiety, muscle tension and such factors will all converge and influence the final outcome. At no stage is there a sudden transition from an organic to a mental explanation. All stages will play their part simultaneously and sequentially. All stages are therefore targets for combined diagnosis and therapy.

REFERENCES

Ainsworth A, Hall P, Wall P D et al 1981 Effects of capsaicin applied locally to adult peripheral nerve. II Anatomy and enzyme and peptide chemistry of peripheral nerve and spinal cord. Pain 11: 379–388

Barbut D, Polak J M, Wall P D 1981 Substance P in spinal cord dorsal horn decreases following peripheral nerve injury. Brain Research 205: 289–298

Basbaum A I 1973 Conduction of the effects of noxious stimulation by short-fibre systems in the spinal cord of the rat. Experimental Neurology 40: 699–716

Brown A G 1981 Organization in the rat spinal cord. Springer-Verlag, Berlin

Casey K L 1971 Responses of bulboreticular units to somatic stimuli eliciting escape behaviour in the cat. International Journal of Neuroscience 2: 15–28

Czeh G, Kudo N, Kuno M 1977 Membrane properties and conduction velocity in sensory neurones following central or peripheral axotomy. Journal of Physiology 270: 165–180

Dellon A L 1981 Evaluation of sensibility and re-education of sensation in the hand. Williams & Wilkins, Baltimore

Devor M, Govrin-Lippmann R 1979 Selective regeneration of sensory fibres following nerve crush injury. Experimental Neurology 65: 300–315

Devor M, Wall P D 1981a The effect of peripheral nerve

injury on receptive fields in the cat spinal cord. Journal of Comparative Neurology 199: 277–291.

Devor M, Wall P D 1981b Plasticity in the spinal cord sensory map following peripheral nerve injury in rats. Journal of Neuroscience 1(7): 679–684

Fitzgerald M, Wall P D, Goedert M, Empson P C 1985 Nerve growth factor counteracts the neurophysiological and neurochemical effects of chronic sciatic nerve injury. Brain Research 332: 131–141

Gibson J J 1968 The senses considered as perceptual systems. Allen & Unwin, London

Hannington-Kiff J G 1974 Pain relief. Heinemann, London

Hockaday J M, Whitty C W M 1967 Patterns of referred pain in the normal subject. Brain 90: 481–496

Lewis T 1942 Pain. Macmillan, London

Lewis T, Kellgren J H 1939 Observations relating to referred pain, visceromotor reflexes and other associated phenomena. Clinical Science 4: 47–71

McMahon S B, Gibson S 1987 Peptide expression is altered when afferent nerves reinnervate inappropriate tissue. Neuroscience Letters 73: 3–8

McMahon S B, Wall P D 1984 Receptive fields of rat lamina 1 projection cells move to incorporate a nearby region of injury. Pain 19: 235–247

McMahon S B, Wall P D 1985 Electrophysiological mapping of brainstem projections of spinal cord lamina I cells in the rat. Brain Research 333: 19–26

McMahon S B, Wall P D 1989 Changes in spinal reflexes after cross anastomosis of cutaneous and muscle nerves in the adult rat. Nature 342: 272–274

McMahon S B, Sykova E, Wall P D, Woolf C J, Sibson S J 1984 Neurogenic extravasation and substance P levels are low in muscle as compared to skin in the rat hindlimb. Neuroscience Letters 52: 235–240

Melzack R, Wall P D 1965 Pain mechanisms: a new theory. Science 150: 971–979

Millar S 1978 Aspects of memory for information from touch and movement. In: Gordon G (ed) Active touch. Pergamon, Oxford

Moberg E 1964 Aspects of sensation in reconstructive surgery of the upper extremity. Journal of Bone and Joint Surgery 46: 817–825

Noordenbos W 1959 Pain. Elsevier/North Holland, Amsterdam

Noordenbos W, Wall P D 1981 Implications of the failure of nerve resection and graft to cure chronic pain produced by nerve lesions. Journal of Neurology, Neurosurgery and Psychiatry 44: 1068–1073

Revesz G 1950 Psychology and art of the blind. Longman, Green, London

Seltzer Z, Devor M 1979 Ephaptic transmission in chronically damaged peripheral nerves. Neurology 29: 1061–1064

Wall P D 1978 The gate control theory of pain mechanisms. A re-examination and re-statement. Brain 191: 1–18

Wall P D, Devor M 1981 The effect of peripheral nerve injury on dorsal root potentials and on transmission of afferent signals into the spinal cord. Brain Research 209: 95–111

Wall P D, Devor M 1983 Sensory afferent impulses from dorsal root ganglia as well as from the periphery in normal and nerve injured rats. Pain 17: 321–339

Wall P D, Fitzgerald M 1981 Effects of capsaicin applied locally to adult peripheral nerve. I. Physiology of peripheral nerve and spinal cord. Pain 11: 363–377

Wall P D, Fitzgerald M 1982 If substance P fails to fulfil the criteria as a neurotransmitter in somatosensory afferents, what might be its function? CIBA Foundation Symposium 91. Pitman, London, pp 249–266

Wall P D, Gutnick M 1974 Ongoing activity in peripheral nerves: 2. The physiology and pharmacology of impulses originating in a neuroma. Experimental Neurology 43: 580–593

Wall P D, Woolf C J 1984 Muscle but not cutaneous C-afferent input produces increases in the excitability of the flexion reflex in the rat. Journal of Physiology 356: 443–458

Wall P D, Waxman S, Basbaum A I 1974 Ongoing activity in peripheral nerve. III. Injury discharge. Experimental Neurology 45: 576–589

Wall P D, Fitzgerald M, Gibson S J 1981 The response of rat spinal cord cells to unmyelinated afferents after peripheral nerve section and after changes in substance P levels. Neuroscience 6: 2205–2215

Wall P D, Fitzgerald M, Nussbaumer J C, Van der Loos H, Devor M 1982a Somatotopic maps are disorganised in adult rodents treated with capsaicin as neonates. Nature 295: 691–693

Wall P D, Mills R, Fitzgerald M, Gibson S J 1982b Chronic blockade of sciatic nerve transmission by tetrodotoxin does not produce central changes in the dorsal horn of the spinal cord of the rat. Neuroscience Letters 30: 315–320

Woolf C J 1983 Evidence for a central component of post injury pain hypersensitivity. Nature 306: 686–688

Woolf C J, Wall P D 1982 Chronic peripheral nerve section diminishes the primary afferent A-fibre mediated inhibition of rat dorsal horn neurones. Brain Research 242: 77–85

Wynn Parry C B 1966 Rehabilitation of the hand, 2nd edn. Butterworth, London

W. J. Roberts and R. C. Kramis

2 Sympathetically dependent pain: physiology and clinical expression

INTRODUCTION

Clinical studies indicate that sympathetic nervous system activity is causally related to pain in disorders as diverse as reflex sympathetic dystrophy, rheumatoid arthritis, Raynaud's disease, and acute herpes zoster. The first 3 of these disorders commonly involve the hand, and the latter does so occasionally.

Potential mechanisms of sympathetic involvement in pain have been the subject of speculation since Leriche (1916) first demonstrated alleviation of causalgic pain by periarterial sympathectomy. No single, simple mechanism appears able to explain all clinically observed characteristics of sympathetically dependent pain. However, recent experiments have provided information about specific sympathetic and central neural mechanisms involved in the painfulness of differing conditions.

In this chapter, we first review clinical evidence of sympathetic involvement in several painful syndromes, all of which can involve the hand. Then, after discussing several hypotheses about potential underlying mechanisms, we re-examine the syndromes to determine which mechanisms are most likely to subserve the pain in each condition.

CLINICAL SYNDROMES WITH SYMPATHETICALLY DEPENDENT PAIN

RSDS and causalgia

In reflex sympathetic dystrophy syndrome (RSDS) and causalgia, both of which commonly involve the hand, a causal relationship exists between sympathetic efferent activity and pain (Janig & Kollmann 1984; Wiesenfeld-Hallin & Hallin 1984; Schott 1986). The causal nature of the relationship is clearly demonstrated when sympathetic innervation of the painful region is blocked. This abolishes or greatly reduces the spontaneous pain and mechanical allodynia (touch-evoked pain) which characterise these disorders. Sympathetic innervation of painful peripheral regions can be selectively blocked by: local anaesthetic block of the relevant sympathetic ganglia (Loh & Nathan 1978; Wang et al 1985); sympathectomy (Shumacker 1948; Barnes 1953); guanethidine-induced depletion of transmitter from peripheral sympathetic terminals (Hannington-Kiff 1974; Loh et al 1980; Bonelli et al 1983); and administration of alpha-adrenergic blocking agents (Ghostine et al 1984).

Reflex sympathetic dystrophy syndrome (RSDS) is commonly precipitated by accidental trauma; however, it can also be precipitated by surgical procedures (Bonica 1979). For example, RSDS develops in about 5% of patients who undergo surgery for carpal tunnel release (Lankford 1982). The mechanisms through which surgery and/or accidental trauma precipitate RSDS are described in the sections describing the vicious circle and SMP hypotheses (pp. 16–17).

RSDS can also develop in the distal limbs following lesions of the central nervous system, even in the absence of peripheral trauma (Loh et al 1981; Schott 1986; Gellman et al 1988). This pain is sympathetically dependent in that it can be effectively treated by sympathetic ganglion block or by regional infusion of guanethidine, which depletes sympathetic transmitter in the painful region.

The appearance of sympathetically dependent pain referred to the periphery following central lesions suggests that sensitisation or disinhibition of central neurons is important in the development of sympathetically dependent pain. Even when the precipitating event for RSDS is peripheral trauma, the essential dysfunction giving rise to the persistent pain may be the persistent sensitisation of central neurons rather than some peripheral dysfunction. This concept is developed fully in subsequent presentations of the vicious circle and SMP hypotheses.

Inflammatory rheumatoid arthritis

This is another painful condition in which pain has been alleviated by sympathetic intervention. Reports state that rheumatic pain is reduced by sympathectomy (Herfort 1956) and by regional depletion of sympathetic efferent transmitters (Levine et al 1986a). These reports of reduced arthritic pain in humans following sympathetic intervention have been substantiated by animal studies. For example, rats sympathectomised prior to the production of adjuvant-induced arthritis showed delayed development of tenderness and swelling and less severe joint degeneration than did rats with intact sympathetic systems. Mechanisms by which sympathetic efferent activity can exacerbate painful effects of arthritis are discussed more fully later.

Raynaud's disease

This is a disorder characterised by aching pain and vasospasm in the hands and/or feet (Raynaud 1862; Carter et al 1988). Sympathetic involvement in Raynaud's disease is indicated by symptomatic improvement in many individuals following treatments that interfere with peripheral sympathetic function. Improvement has been demonstrated with each of the following procedures: systemic administration of alpha–adrenoreceptor antagonists (Nielsen et al 1983); regional depletion of noradrenaline with guanethidine (Hannington-Kiff 1974; Loh et al 1980); and sympathectomy or local anaesthetic blockade of sympathetic ganglia (Blunt & Porter 1981).

The physiological mechanisms underlying *Raynaud's phenomenon* may be different from those responsible for Raynaud's disease. In Raynaud's phenomenon, tissue pathology is present with aching pain and vasospasm. Sympathetic block provides symptomatic relief in some individuals but is completely ineffective in others. Microneurographic recordings have failed to reveal sympathetic hyperactivity in patients with Raynaud's phenomenon, suggesting that the pain may be due to factors unrelated to sympathetic tonus (Fagius & Blumberg 1985; Cotton & Khan 1986: Wollersheim et al 1987). Thus, the physiological basis for pain in Raynaud's phenomenon appears to be quite complex. The efficacy of sympathetic intervention in many individuals (Blunt & Porter 1981) suggests, however, that a sympathetic component exists.

Herpes zoster

The infection is expressed most commonly in the face or thorax; however, it may also develop in the C6–7 dermatomes, which include part of the hand (Juel-Jensen et al 1970). During the acute phase, herpetic pain is rapidly and markedly reduced by sympathetic block (Colding 1969; Olsen & Ivy 1981; Toyama 1982; Milligan & Nash 1985). Recent reviews of the clinical literature on herpes zoster and post-herpetic neuralgia have emphasised that few studies of sympathetic involvement have been well controlled (Loeser 1986; Higa et al 1988). However, the many reports of symptomatic improvement with sympathetic block strongly suggest a sympathetic role in the exacerbation of zoster pain. Sympathetic blocks are reportedly much less effective for treatment of post-herpetic pain than acute herpetic pain; however, use of sympathetic blocks during the acute phase of the disease may reduce the incidence of post-herpetic neuralgia (Toyama 1982).

Postsympathectomy neuralgia

PSN paradoxically is a frequent complication of sympathectomy performed to alleviate chronically painful conditions. It is characterised by spontaneous deep, aching, or sometimes burning pain which usually begins 1–2 weeks following surgical sympathectomy. Muscle tenderness in response to deep pressure and hyperaesthesia in response to touch may also be present. Clinical reports indicate that the PSN typically is perceived to be proximal to the sympathectomised region (Tracy & Cockett 1957; Raskin et al 1974). This proximal, non-sympathectomised region sometimes shows signs of sympathetic hyperactivity, e.g. excessive sweating (Tracy & Cocket 1957). As indicated in a later analysis, we think that PSN is a deafferentation syndrome induced by sympathectomy and exacerbated by sympathetic efferent activity in the painful area.

SYMPATHETIC MECHANISMS AND PAIN

Several plausible hypotheses have been advanced to explain the physiological basis for sympathetic involvement in pain. No single hypothesis offers an adequate explanation for all of the painful syndromes known to have sympathetic involvement, and more than one mechanism may pertain to single syndromes. Four hypotheses are presented in this section; each is accompanied by experimental evidence for and against the hypothesis. In the subsequent section, these hypotheses are discussed in relation to specific clinical syndromes.

Vicious circle hypothesis

Livingston (1943), writing about causalgia and reflex sympathetic dystrophy, proposed that trauma in the periphery creates '. . . afferent impulses that eventually create an abnormal state of activity in the internuncial neuron centers of the spinal cord . . .'. The internuncial disturbance, he suggested, results in abnormal motor neuron responses in both the lateral horn (sympathetic pre-ganglionic neurons) and the anterior horn (skeletal motor neurons). These responses, in turn, produce vasomotor changes, muscle spasm, and other effects that '. . . may furnish new sources for pain and new reflexes . . .', thus creating a vicious circle of painful neural activity. He speculated that the 'underlying factor of prime importance is the central disturbance'. Livingston also suggested that the disturbed internuncial pool of spinal neurons would not only change motor function but would also 'change the routing of sensory impulses . . . .'.

Livingston's suggestion that the central disturbance is of prime importance has been endorsed by experienced clinical observers who report that sensations evoked by normally non-noxious stimuli are *consistently abnormal* (painful) whereas peripheral signs of sympathetic function, such as skin temperature and colour, are not consistently abnormal (Shumacker 1948; Sunderland 1976; Loh & Nathan 1978; Bonica 1979; Tahmoush et al 1983). Although signs of sympathetic hyper- or hypofunction often occur in association with sympathetically dependent pain, it is not clear from clinical findings that *abnormal* sympathetic function is necessary for the pain. It is possible that *normal* sympathetic efferent activity may produce sufficient afferent activity to elicit pain in the presence of *abnormal* central excitability (see SMP hypothesis).

Although Livingston speculated that the '. . . routing of sensory impulses in spinal centers . . .' is changed to produce central hyperexcitability, he did not identify the particular types or classes of spinal neurons affected. Later, Tahmoush (1981) and Roberts (1986) proposed that the most likely candidate is the spinal wide–dynamic–range (WDR) neuron, which receives input from both nociceptive and non-nociceptive primary afferents. These neurons are more dramatically sensitised by nociceptor activity than are nociceptor-specific neurons, which receive input only from primary afferent nociceptors (Mendell & Wall 1965; Kenshalo et al 1982; Cook et al 1987). However, Price et al (1989) have suggested that the central hyperexcitability occurs in neurons other than WDR neurons. This suggestion resulted from their observation that their patients with sympathetically dependent pain showed mechanical but not thermal allodynia and from the knowledge that WDR neurons mediate responses to both thermal and mechanical stimuli. Additional discussion of WDR involvement in sympathetically dependent pain is included in the next section.

In summary, there is agreement among many clinical investigators that Livingston's concept of an altered central state applies to patients with causalgia/RSDS. However, there is no consensus that *abnormal* sympathetic efferent activity is consistently related to or necessary for the occurrence of pain in these syndromes; *normal* sympathetic efferent activity, in conjunction with abnormal central conditions, may be sufficient. Some features of Livingston's vicious circle hypothesis are encompassed in the SMP hypothesis below, which proposes that development of sympathetically maintained pain involves changes in specific types of spinal neurons.

SMP hypothesis

Sympathetically maintained pain (SMP) is defined as *spontaneous* burning or aching pain that can be abolished by blocking sympathetic efferent activity in the painful region (Roberts 1986). The fact that a precipitating event commonly precedes the development of SMP suggests that it is not initiated by sympathetic actions. Once present, however, the pain is maintained by sympathetic actions. This maintenance is clearly demonstrated by clinical findings (cited earlier) that the pain disappears when sympathetic function in the painful region is blocked. SMP occurs in disorders such as RSDS and causalgia, and it may be one component of a complex painful condition in disorders such as acute herpes zoster. In advanced cases, SMP is commonly associated with tissue dystrophy; however, dystrophy is not always present, and it is therefore not necessary for the occurrence of SMP (Sunderland 1976; Loh & Nathan 1978; Bonica 1979).

The SMP hypothesis proposes that:

1. trauma, which most commonly precipitates SMP, does so by activating primary afferent nociceptors
2. trauma-induced nociceptor activity excites and sensitises spinal wide–dynamic–range (WDR) neurons
3. sensitised WDR neurons respond at painfully high rates to input from either nociceptive or non-nociceptive afferents
4. the 'spontaneous pain' that is SMP results from sympathetic activation of low-threshold touch receptors (see below) which causes sensitised WDR neurons to discharge at high rates
5. the mechanical allodynia (sometimes called hyperalgesia) that accompanies SMP results from mechanical activation of the same or similar non-nociceptive afferents which cause sensitised WDR neurons to discharge at abnormally high rates (Roberts 1986).

According to the SMP hypothesis, the essential dysfunction leading to pain is a persistent hyperexcitability of spinal WDR neurons. WDR neurons are part of a central pain 'pathway' and receive excitatory input from both nociceptors and non-nociceptors. Sympathetic efferent activity directly or indirectly excites *non-nociceptive mechanoreceptors* (touch receptors), and the resulting afferent activity drives the hyperexcitable WDR neurons to painfully high rates of activity. It is important to note that once the syndrome is established, activity in *nociceptive afferents* is not necessary in order that pain occur. Instead, painful levels of activity are produced in spinal WDR neurons by *non-nociceptive afferents*.

The SMP hypothesis provides an explanation for the alleviation of spontaneous and allodynic pain by sympathetic block. The block presumably abolishes spontaneous pain by reducing tonic excitatory input to WDR neurons from *sympathetically-activated* low-threshold touch receptors. Similarly, sympathetic block abolishes or reduces allodynia by reducing sympathetically-induced input from touch receptors onto WDR neurons, making these neurons less excitable and therefore less responsive to *mechanically-activated* touch receptors. During a sympathetic block, noxious stimuli are still perceived as painful because primary afferent nociceptors innervating the extremities are not affected by the sympathetic block.

Results from electrophysiological studies in experimental animals led to and provide consistent support for the SMP hypothesis. The essential findings are the following:

1. Many non-nociceptive, low-threshold mechanoreceptors can be activated by sympathetic efferent activity, whereas most nociceptors cannot (reviewed in Roberts 1986). Note: these findings suggest that sympathetic efferent activity will activate only non-nociceptive afferents in patients with SMP. Supporting evidence from human studies will be presented later.

2. Many spinal WDR neurons are responsive to *sympathetically-evoked* afferent activity, whereas

nociceptor-specific spinal neurons are not (Roberts & Foglesong 1986; Roberts & Foglesong 1988a). Note: these findings suggest that WDR neurons are capable of mediating sympathetically-maintained pain and that nociceptor specific neurons are not.

3. Trauma in the periphery activates spinal WDR neurons and sensitises them to mechanically- and sympathetically-evoked afferent activity (Roberts & Kramis 1988; see also Mendell & Wall 1965; Kenshalo et al 1982; Cook et al 1987). Note: trauma induces the sensitisation of WDR neurons, thereby allowing them to respond at 'painful' rates to afferent input from non-nociceptive afferents.

The concept that sensitised WDR neurons can produce pain has been supported by Mayer et al (1975), who reported that, in humans, stimulation of the axons of WDR neurons at low rates produced non-painful sensations, whereas stimulation of the same population of axons at higher rates (e.g. 25 Hz) produced pain.

In summary, there is remarkably good evidence from physiological studies to support the SMP hypothesis. This hypothesis suggests that the essential dysfunction resulting in SMP is hyperexcitability of spinal WDR neurons. The spontaneous pain is mediated in the periphery by sympathetically-activated, low-threshold touch receptors (mechanoreceptors). It is not clear why SMP develops in some, but not in most, individuals after trauma.

Neuroma hypothesis

The neuroma hypothesis presented here incorporates mechanisms proposed by several investigators to explain the physiological basis for sympathetically dependent pain that occurs after injury to a major nerve. It is derived primarily from results of studies with experimental neuromata in animals (Korenman, Devor & Janig 1981; Devor 1983; Habler et al 1987). The hypothesis is that sympathetic efferent activity produces pain by exciting damaged or regenerating nociceptive afferents in neuromata formed after nerve damage. Excitation is proposed to occur either by noradrenergic depolarisation of regenerating terminals of nociceptive afferent fibres or by ephaptic (electrical) transmission between adjacent sympathetic efferent and damaged nociceptive afferent axons.

The neuroma hypothesis is supported by experimental studies showing that some injured nerve fibres associated with neuromata become responsive to sympathetic efferent activity or to application of noradrenaline (Wall & Gutnick 1974; Devor & Janig 1981; Korenman & Devor 1981; Scadding 1981). However, the validity of the hypothesis in relation to clinical syndromes is difficult to reconcile with the following findings:

1. Afferent fibres ending in experimentally-induced neuromata take days to become sensitive to sympathetic actions (Scadding 1981). In contrast, causalgic pain develops almost immediately or within hours in most cases (Shumacker 1948; Scadding 1981; Devor 1983). Thus, the time course of the disorder in humans is not similar to the time course of changes in afferent sensitivity in animal studies.

2. Anaesthetic nerve blocks *distal* to a neuroma–in–continuity can block causalgic pain in some individuals (Livingston 1943; Doupe et al 1944; Barnes 1953). Similarly, causalgic pain is reduced or abolished in some individuals by guanethidine infusion *distal* to a site of nerve injury (Loh & Nathan 1978). These procedures would not affect sympathetic/somatic interactions in the more proximal neuroma, suggesting that neural activity originating distal to the neuroma causes or is necessary for causalgic pain.

3. The incidence of causalgia is reported to be less after complete nerve transection than after partial nerve injury (Sunderland 1976). This finding suggests that the coexistence of many regenerating sympathetic efferent and primary afferent fibres is not a sufficient condition for causalgia.

4. The sympathetically-activated afferent fibres recorded from experimental neuromata probably have not been nociceptive afferents, as they had conduction velocities indicative of myelinated afferent fibers (Wall & Gutnick 1974; Scadding 1981; Korenman & Devor 1981), and most myelinated afferents are not nociceptors. Some of the activated fibres had conduction velocities typical of small myelinated fibres, which can be nociceptors. However, activity in myelinated nociceptive afferents evokes sensations of pricking pain, not the burning pain of causalgia.

Burning pain is evoked by activation of nonmyelinated afferents, but sympathetic activation of this type of afferent has been demonstrated in only one study (Habler et al 1987). In this study, non-myelinated (C) afferents associated with neuromata–in–continuity in cats could be sympathetically activated. However, it is not clear that the sympathetically activated C-fibres were nociceptors. Many C-fibres in cats are non-nociceptive mechanoreceptors, and many of these are known to respond to sympathetic efferent activity (Roberts & Elardo 1985).

Thus, physiological studies have not provided convincing evidence that primary afferent nociceptors ending in neuromata are sympathetically activated. It should also be noted that the use of paralytic drugs in neuroma experiments may have led to exaggeration of the afferent activity associated with neuromata (Burchiel & Russell 1987).

In summary, experiments in humans and other animals have shown that nerve injury produces changes in the properties of damaged afferent fibres, making some more responsive to sympathetic efferent actions and more spontaneously active. However, the physiological studies have been primarily studies of myelinated afferent fibres, most of which probably have been non-nociceptive. Sympathetically-evoked activity in non-nociceptive afferents could contribute to the pain of causalgia by increasing the excitatory input to spinal WDR neurons (see SMP hypothesis); however, that mechanism has not been described as part of a neuroma hypothesis. Sympathetic effects that occur within a neuroma seem not to explain either the rapid onset of causalgic pain or the relief produced by procedures applied distal to the neuroma. Thus, the neuroma hypothesis described at the beginning of this section seems inadequate to explain many aspects of clinical, sympathetically-dependent pain associated with nerve injury.

Nociceptor sensitisation hypothesis

The mechanism of sympathetically dependent pain proposed here is derived primarily from studies of sympathetic involvement in arthritic conditions (Levine et al 1987; Levine et al 1988). The hypothesis is that primary afferent *nociceptors* are sensitised by *pro-inflammatory substances* released into peripheral tissues either directly from *sympathetic efferent terminals* or indirectly from *non-neuronal cells* in response to sympathetic efferent activity. This sympathetic mechanism presumably contributes to pain only in the presence of undetermined cofactors or under unusual conditions, because, in normal tissue, sympathetic efferent activity does not result in pain. Sympathetically released substances likely to be involved in the sensitisation of nociceptors include prostaglandins and perhaps purines and peptides, as discussed below.

Some prostaglandins strongly sensitise nociceptors (Ferreira et al 1973; Mense 1981; Hepplemann et al 1985; Martin et al 1987), and sympathetic activity causes prostaglandins to be released from cells located near sympathetic neuroeffector junctions (Hedqvist 1977; Moore 1985). It has also been proposed that prostaglandins may serve as sympathetic co-transmitters in sympathetic postganglionic neurons and thus may be released directly from sympathetic terminals (Stjarne 1972; Levine et al 1986b). In either case, sympathetic efferent activity would increase the level of nociceptive afferent activity by sensitising nociceptors, and thus would exacerbate the pain.

Other substances, well-demonstrated to be sympathetic co-transmitters, are sometimes released from sympathetic efferent terminals and may affect nociception. These are non-adrenergic, non-cholinergic substances such as peptides and purines (Burnstock 1976; Lundberg & Hokfelt 1983; Pernow et al 1988). Their release from sympathetic terminals is most prominent when high rates of sympathetic activity occur (Lundberg et al 1981; Lundberg et al 1986; Bartfai et al 1988), as after trauma. The relevant effects exerted by these substances include: potentiation of the effects of noradrenaline; vasoconstriction, and direct effects on primary afferent nociceptors (Juan & Lembeck 1974; Hakanson et al 1986; Burnstock 1986). Each of these effects, directly or indirectly, could increase activity in primary afferent nociceptors, thus contributing to pain.

The extent to which non-adrenergic, non-cholinergic sympathetic transmitters contribute to sympathetically dependent pain remains largely to be explored. For a review of sympathetic co-transmission, the reader is referred to Burnstock (1986) and Hokfelt et al (1986).

SYMPATHETIC MECHANISMS IN SPECIFIC CLINICAL SYNDROMES

Reflex sympathetic dystrophy syndrome and causalgia

Definitions

No consensus has been reached in the clinical or scientific literatures on a definition for the reflex sympathetic dystrophy syndrome (RSDS). As a result, patient populations and therapeutic outcomes are not directly comparable across studies, and physiological mechanisms subserving RSDS are difficult to establish. For the purposes of this chapter, we will consider RSDS as a syndrome characterised primarily by, firstly, *spontaneous* burning or aching pain, and secondly, by mechanical allodynia (painful response to touch), both of which are disproportionate to the severity of the injury and are alleviated by sympathetic block. Causalgia will be considered here to be a special case of RSDS – involving injury to a major peripheral nerve.

The inclusion of the criterion that the pain and allodynia be alleviated by sympathetic block follows the proposal by Shumacker (1948) that an essential diagnostic criterion for RSDS or causalgia is '. . . temporary, complete, or nearly complete alleviation [of pain] during sympathetic procaine anaesthesia'. This proposal has been adopted by some (e.g. Sweet & Poleti 1985) but not all clinical investigators (e.g. Schwartzman & McLellan 1987). Failure to include this criterion may result in failure to distinguish between individuals with sympathetically maintained pain and others with very similar symptoms but very different pathophysiology. For example, the spontaneous burning pain and allodynia in patients with a swollen extremity can be mediated either by nociceptive or non-nociceptive primary afferents, and only one type is alleviated by sympathetic block (Ochoa 1986; Campbell et al 1988a; Cline et al 1989).

Pain resulting from dystrophic changes is not discussed here because dystrophy and pain are not consistently related in the early stages of RSDS (Sunderland 1976; Bonica 1979). We discuss only those physiological mechanisms of RSDS that are associated with *sympathetically maintained pain* (SMP), defined as spontaneous pain that is alleviated by sympathetic block.

Mechanisms

The remainder of this section is a review of evidence from both clinical and animal studies relating to sympathetically maintained pain (SMP) in RSDS. The evidence indicates that the essential dysfunction is a persistent hyperexcitability of spinal wide–dynamic–range neurons and that the sympathetically-evoked afferent activity responsible for chronic SMP is carried by afferent fibres that normally subserve sensations of touch/pressure, not pain. These mechanisms are described in the SMP hypothesis (Roberts 1986) presented earlier in the chapter.

Evidence

Sympathetically maintained pain in RSDS can be abolished by selective block of large diameter myelinated afferents as described below (Wallin et al 1976; Ochoa et al 1988; Campbell et al 1988b). These afferents normally subserve the non-nociceptive sensations of touch and pressure. The disappearance of sympathetically-maintained pain when these afferents alone are blocked is strong evidence that the pain is mediated by non-nociceptive rather than nociceptive afferents.

The selective block of large diameter afferents is accomplished by placing a blood pressure cuff on the limb proximal to a region of SMP and inflating it above systolic pressure. Nerve conduction block occurs gradually over time, beginning with the largest fibres and progressing to the smaller fibres. When this type of pressure block is done in patients with SMP, the first sensory changes that occur are the simultaneous loss of SMP, allodynia and tactile sensibility. These sensory changes occur early during the compression block, at a time when the pains induced by pinprick, noxious heat and noxious cold are still perceived correctly. The persistence of these noxious sensations indicates that small myelinated and nonmyelinated nociceptive afferents remain capable of conducting action potentials. Thus, the disappearance of SMP cannot be due to nociceptor blockade. This finding clearly indicates that activity in large-diameter touch/pressure afferents is responsible for the spontaneous pain.

In order for activity in touch/pressure afferents to produce pain, central pain pathways must be hyperexcitable – as suggested by findings from clinical studies (Sunderland 1976; Loh & Nathan 1978; Tahmoush 1981). Hyperexcitability of spinal wide–dynamic–range (WDR) neurons has, in fact, been demonstrated in numerous physiological studies (Mendell & Wall 1965; Kenshalo et al 1982; Cook et al 1987), and these neurons are thought to participate in the conscious assessment of painful stimuli (Maixner et al 1986). WDR hyperexcitability can be induced by peripheral trauma, resulting in increased WDR responding to sympathetically-evoked afferent activity (Roberts et al 1987). The increased responding to sympathetically-evoked afferent activity persists long after the trauma-induced primary afferent activity ceases (Roberts & Kramis 1988).

Direct evidence that non-nociceptive, touch/pressure afferents are capable of eliciting pain in patients with SMP has been provided by Price et al (1989). They showed that selective electrical stimulation of only large diameter afferents innervating an area with SMP evokes a painful sensation in patients, but does not do so in normal human subjects. These results are consistent with the hypothesis that the central neurons involved in pain are hyperexcitable, as proposed by the SMP hypothesis (Roberts 1986).

The fact that chronic SMP occurs in the absence of any apparent physical stimulus, coupled with the knowledge that this pain is mediated by activity in touch/pressure fibres, requires the touch/pressure afferents to be active in the absence of mechanical stimulation. This requirement conflicts with findings from humans and other animals, which have shown that most touch/pressure afferents are not spontaneously active (Burgess & Perl 1973). This apparent conflict can be resolved by data from recent studies of sympathetic effects on primary afferent fibres in animals. These have shown that some types of non-nociceptive afferents innervating mammalian skin are activated by sympathetic efferent activity (Roberts et al 1985; Roberts & Foglesong 1988b). There is also evidence from microneurographic studies indicating that mechanoreceptors can be sympathetically activated in humans (Hallin & Wiesenfeld-Hallin 1983; Soininen et al 1983). Thus, sympathetic efferent activity may provide the stimulus necessary for spontaneous SMP to occur (Roberts 1986).

Although there is good evidence that the physiological mechanisms described above are responsible for SMP, other mechanisms may also contribute to pain in SMP patients. In fact, many patients appear to suffer from a combination of painful conditions involving both touch/pressure and nociceptive afferents (Ochoa 1986).

In summary, the evidence reviewed above indicates that chronic SMP results from sympathetic activation of non-nociceptive afferent fibres, as described in the SMP hypothesis (Roberts 1986). These afferents most likely excite hyperexcitable WDR neurons, which, according to animal experiments, are the only nociceptive spinal neurons responsive to sympathetically-evoked afferent activity (Roberts & Foglesong 1988a). *Initiation* of spinal neuron hyperexcitability may result from activation of primary afferent nociceptors or from central lesions that change the excitability of WDR neurons. Tonic sympathetic activation of afferents projecting to these spinal neurons seems important to the *maintenance* of hyperexcitability. Other mechanisms involved in the initiation and maintenance of hyperexcitability probably exist, but remain to be determined.

Inflammatory rheumatoid arthritis

The findings that the pain associated with rheumatoid arthritis is significantly reduced by sympathetic blocks suggest a causal relationship between sympathetic efferent activity and rheumatoid pain (Herfort 1956; Levine et al 1986a). Animal studies also suggest that sympathetic efferent fibres contribute to the inflammation of joints in adjuvant-induced arthritis, as beta-adrenergic antagonists reduce the severity of joint injury (Levine et al 1988). It remains to be determined whether sympathetic efferents affect inflammation independently, or, more likely, by acting in concert with other compounds such as substance–P, released by primary afferent nociceptors (Levine et al 1987).

The identity of the afferent fibres that mediate pain from arthritic joints has not been determined in clinical studies; however, recordings from primary afferent fibres innervating joints in experimental animals have shown that nociceptive afferents are sensitised in inflamed joints and respond strongly to gentle movements (Guilbaud et al 1985; Grigg et al 1986). Sympathetic efferent activity has been reported to sensitise nociceptive afferents, either directly or indirectly (Nakamura & Ferreira 1987), and thus nociceptor sensitisation seems to be a likely mechanism of sympathetic involvement in arthritic pain.

It should be noted that the nociceptor activity associated with inflammation is likely to produce hyperexcitability in spinal WDR neurons. This hyperexcitability would then contribute to an SMP-like condition if the hyperexcitable neurons with joint input also receive input from mechanoreceptors that can be sympathetically driven. However, tests of sympathetic effects on non-nociceptive afferents innervating arthritic joints have not been reported.

Raynaud's disease

Raynaud (1862) proposed that exaggerated sympathetic activity caused the aching pain and vasospasm that characterise this disease, and this view is supported by some clinical findings, which show that many patients with Raynaud's disease are improved by sympathetic block (reviewed earlier).

Alternatively, vasospasm may result from other mechanisms, including: abnormal direct vascular sensitivity to cold; hyperreactive receptor mechanisms in vascular smooth muscle; and non-neural, locally released or circulating vasoactive substances (Vanhoutte & Janssens 1980; Olsen 1987; Wollersheim et al 1987; Seibold & Terregino 1986). These alternative mechanisms must be given serious consideration, as microneurographic studies in humans with Raynaud's disease have not provided clear evidence of sympathetic hyperactivity (Fagius & Blumberg 1985).

Any mechanism, including sympathetic efferent activity, that produces excessive vasoconstriction may cause or exacerbate pain by producing accumulations of metabolic products or, if prolonged, ulcers (Cousins & Bridenbaugh 1988; Spittell 1983). It is also possible that a reduction in tissue temperature consequent to vasoconstriction may contribute directly to pain in the absence of metabolic products or ulcers.

Physiological studies of the effects of cooling on primary afferent fibres have shown that some high-threshold cold receptors and some C–polymodal nociceptors are activated by temperatures as high as 20°C. Such temperatures can be attained in vasoconstricted digits when vasoconstricted tissue is exposed to cold weather conditions or even at cool room temperatures (Chery-Croze 1983; LaMotte & Thalhammer 1982). Sympathetic efferent activity can also activate cold-specific afferent fibres at normal skin temperatures via undetermined mechanisms (Davies 1985).

Sympathetic efferent activity in Raynaud's phenomenon may also contribute to pain through the release of nociceptor sensitising substances, via mechanisms discussed earlier in the section on rheumatoid arthritis.

The extent to which these various mechanisms contribute to Raynaud's disease or Raynaud's phenomenon remains undetermined. In the absence of an animal model for Raynaud's disease, carefully designed clinical studies are needed to determine which mechanisms are involved in specific cases.

Herpes zoster

Many clinical studies have indicated a causal relationship between sympathetic efferent activity and the pain of acute herpes zoster, as reviewed earlier. The inflammation and tissue damage associated with the vesicular eruptions in herpes zoster is undoubtedly sufficient to sensitise and activate primary afferent nociceptors. However, sympathetic efferent actions appear to exacerbate the pain associated with the disease. At least two physiological mechanisms may subserve this sympathetic action in herpes zoster.

First, substances released from sympathetic efferent terminals or released from non-neural cells in response to sympathetic activity are likely to contribute to the activation and sensitisation of nociceptors in inflamed skin (Coderre et al 1984;

Levine et al 1986b; Nakamura & Ferreira 1987). Second, sympathetically-evoked activity in low-threshold afferents would likely summate with nociceptor activity to excite spinal WDR neurons, as proposed in the SMP hypothesis. The latter mechanism is consistent with the clinical finding that very gentle mechanical stimulation, such as hair movement which activates only low-threshold mechanoreceptors, is very painful in severe cases of herpes zoster.

Thus, it is likely but unproven that the sympathetic system contributes to the pain in herpes zoster both by contributing to the sensitisation and activation of primary afferent nociceptors and by activation of low-threshold mechanoreceptors, whose spinal terminals converge with those of nociceptors onto WDR neurons.

Postsympathectomy neuralgia

The neuralgia that develops in many patients after a sympathectomy is performed to treat a painful condition in the periphery has a delayed onset and is localised *proximal* to the region that is sympathetically denervated (Tracy & Cockett 1957; Raskin et al 1974). Roberts and Kramis (1989) integrated these clinical findings with anatomical and physiological findings from animal studies and proposed that: firstly, postsympathectomy neuralgia (PSN) results from deafferentation-induced hyperactivity of spinal neurons having convergent input from both visceral and somatic tissues; and secondly, sympathetic efferent activity to the newly painful region contributes to the 'neuralgia' by activating non-nociceptive primary afferents. The hypothesis is derived from the following data and concepts:

1. Visceral and/or vascular afferents projecting through the sympathetic trunk are transected during sympathectomy. For example, cardiac afferents are transected by cervicothoracic sympathectomy (White & Sweet 1969; Foreman 1986; Hobbs et al 1989), and some afferents from pelvic viscera and blood vessels in the proximal limb regions are probably transected by lumbar sympathectomy (Janig & McLachlan 1986; Meyers & Katz 1988). The anatomical pathways followed by afferents from the pelvic and lower abdominal viscera are particularly variable. This variability in the number of afferent fibres in the sympathetic trunk may partially determine the severity of PSN following trunk transection.

2. The retrograde changes or cell death that follows transection of primary afferent fibres, specifically visceral/vascular afferents, produces partial denervation (deafferentation) of spinal neurons and subsequent development of denervation hyperactivity in these neurons. Denervation hyperactivity (Loeser & Ward 1967) is a well demonstrated phenomenon which has been invoked to explain pain associated with other syndromes, e.g. brachial plexus avulsion pain and phantom limb pain. The extent to which peripheral axotomy (vs plexus avulsion or dorsal root section) can produce central hyperactivity is undetermined (for related reviews see Mendell 1984 and Pubols & Sessle 1987).

3. Visceral afferents project almost exclusively to 'viscerosomatic' spinal neurons, i.e. neurons which receive input from both visceral and primarily *proximal* somatic afferents (Milne et al 1981; Foreman et al 1988; Chandler et al 1988). It is these proximal somatic areas that become painful in PSN.

4. Most viscerosomatic neurons are wide-dynamic-range neurons (Hancock et al 1975; Cervero 1983; Cervero & Tattersall 1986). Thus, the spinal neurons partially deafferented and made hyperactive by sympathectomy would be the same type of neuron that, when sensitised, provides a basis for sympathetically maintained pain in RSDS and causalgia.

5. Sympathetic efferents that terminate proximal to the sympathectomised area would, according to animal studies, activate WDR neurons by exciting non-nociceptive afferents in the proximal region. Data supporting activation of primary afferents by sympathetic efferents have been cited above in the discussions of the SMP hypothesis. When sympathetic tonus in the proximal area is excessive, as in some patients (Tracy & Cockett 1957), PSN would likely be particularly intense.

The natural history of PSN is consistent with the hypothesis that this pain involves deafferentation hyperactivity of spinal neurons, and the proximal location of PSN is consistent with known patterns of convergence of visceral and somatic afferent fibres onto spinal WDR neurons. These consistencies provide strong support for the hypothesis described above.

SUMMARY

The clinical findings reviewed in this chapter indicate that the sympathetic nervous system contributes to spontaneous pain in a variety of different syndromes, including RSDS, acute herpes zoster, rheumatoid arthritis, and Raynaud's disease. Some of these disorders are not commonly known to have sympathetic involvement; however, responses to diagnostic blocks of sympathetic function have indicated a causal relationship between sympathetic efferent activity and pain in many patients suffering from these syndromes.

Two very different mechanisms for sympathetic exacerbation of pain emerge from this analysis. One is sympathetic activation of non-nociceptive primary afferent mechanoreceptors (touch/pressure receptors), which produces painful levels of activity in hyperexcitable spinal WDR neurons. The second mechanism involves sympathetically-enhanced sensitisation and/or activation of primary afferent nociceptors through substances released by sympathetic efferent terminals. The essential dysfunction in the first mechanism is hyperexcitability of spinal neurons involved in pain. The essential dysfunction in the second is hyperexcitability of primary afferent nociceptors.

The first of these mechanisms, involving non-nociceptive afferents, appears to be precipitated by events such as trauma or acute herpes zoster that activate primary afferent nociceptors, or by disorders of the central nervous system that result in hyperexcitability of spinal pain pathways.

The second of these mechanisms, involving sensitised primary afferent nociceptors, commonly involves an inflammatory process. In this process, sympathetic efferent activity contributes to inflammation and to the sensitisation of nociceptors.

One of the most common events that precipitates the development of SMP is surgery. In view of the physiological mechanisms discussed here, the incidence of post-surgical sympathetically-maintained pain could be minimized by intraoperative and postoperative block of primary afferent nociceptors.

REFERENCES

Barnes R 1953 The role of sympathectomy in the treatment of causalgia. Journal of Bone and Joint Surgery 35B: 172–180

Bartfai T, Iverfeldt K, Fisone G, Serfozo P 1988 Regulation of the release of coexisting neurotransmitters. Annual Review of Pharmacology and Toxicology 28: 285–310

Blunt J R, Porter J M 1981 Raynaud syndrome. Seminars in Arthritis and Rheumatism 10: 282–302

Bonelli S, Conoscente F, Movilia P G, Restelli L, Francucci B, Grossi E 1983 Regional intravenous guanethidine vs stellate ganglion block in reflex sympathetic dystrophies: a randomized trial. Pain 16: 297–307

Bonica J J 1979 Causalgia and other reflex sympathetic dystrophies. In: Bonica J J, Liebeskind J C, Albe-Fessard D G (eds) Advances in pain research and therapy. Raven, New York, pp 141–166

Burchiel K J, Russell L C 1987 Has the amount of spontaneous electrical activity in experimental neuromas been overestimated? Somatosensory Research 5: 63–75

Burgess P R, Perl E R 1973 Cutaneous mechanoreceptors and nociceptors. In: Iggo A (ed) Handbook of sensory physiology. Springer-Verlag, Berlin, pp 29–78

Burnstock G 1976 Do some nerve cells release more than one transmitter? Neuroscience 1: 239–248

Burnstock G 1986 The changing face of autonomic neurotransmission. Acta Physiologica Scandinavica 126: 67–91

Campbell J N, Raja S N, Meyer R A 1988a Painful sequelae of nerve injury. In: Dubner R, Gebhart G F, Bond M R (eds) Proceedings of the Vth world congress on pain. Elsevier, Amsterdam, pp 135–143

Campbell J N, Raja S N, Meyer R A, MacKinnon S E 1988b Myelinated afferents signal the hyperalgesia associated with nerve injury. Pain 32: 89–94

Carter S A, Dean E, Kroeger E A 1988 Apparent finger systolic pressures during cooling in patients with Raynaud's syndrome. Circulation 77: 988–996

Cervero F 1983 Somatic and visceral inputs to the thoracic spinal cord of the cat: effects of noxious stimulation of the biliary system. Journal of Physiology (London) 337: 51–67

Cervero F, Tattersall J E H 1986 Somatic and visceral sensory integration in the thoracic spinal cord. In: Cervero F, Morrison J F B (eds) Visceral sensation. Progress in brain research. Elsevier, Amsterdam

Chandler M J, Hobbs S F, Bolser D C, Foreman R D 1988 Could spinothalamic tract (STT) transmit muscle afferent input to primary motor cortex (MI) in monkeys? Society for Neuroscience Abstracts 14(Pt 1): 181

Chery-Croze S 1983 Painful sensation induced by a thermal cutaneous stimulus. Pain 17: 109–137

Cline M A, Ochoa J, Torebjork H E 1989 Chronic hyperalgesia and skin warming caused by sensitized C-nociceptors and antidromic vasodilatation. Brain (in press)

Coderre T J, Abbott F V, Melzack R 1984 Behavioral evidence in rats for a peptidergic-noradrenergic interaction in cutaneous sensory and vascular function. Neuroscience Letters 47: 113–118

Colding A 1969 The effect of regional sympathetic blocks in the treatment of herpes zoster. Acta Anaesthesiologica Scandinavica 13: 133–141

Cook A J, Woolf C J, Wall P D, McMahon S B 1987 Dynamic receptive field plasticity in rat spinal cord dorsal horn following C-primary afferent input. Nature 325: 151–153

Cotton L T, Khan O 1986 Raynaud's phenomenon: a review. International Angiology 5: 215–36

Cousins M J, Bridenbaugh P O 1988 Neural blockade in clinical anaesthesia and management of pain. Lippincott, Philadelphia

Davies S N 1985 Sympathetic modulation of cold-receptive neurones in the trigeminal system of the rat. Journal of Physiology 366: 315–329

Devor M 1983 Nerve pathophysiology and mechanisms of pain in causalgia. Journal of the Autonomic Nervous System 7: 371–384

Devor M, Janig W 1981 Activation of myelinated afferents ending in a neuroma by stimulation of the sympathetic supply in the rat. Neuroscience Letters 24: 43–47

Doupe J, Cullen C, Chance G 1944 Post-traumatic pain and the causalgic syndrome. Journal of Neurology, Neurosurgery and Psychiatry 7: 33–48

Fagius J, Blumberg H 1985 Sympathetic outflow to the hand in patients with Raynaud's phenomenon. Cardiovascular Research 19: 249–53

Ferreira S H, Moncada S, Vance J R 1973 Prostaglandins and the mechanism of analgesia produced by aspirin-like drugs. British Journal of Pharmacology 49: 86–97

Foreman R D 1986 Spinal substrates of visceral pain. In: Yaksh T L (ed) Spinal afferent processing. Plenum, New York, pp 217–242

Foreman R D, Hobbs S F, Chandler J J, Bolser D C 1988 Differences in viscerosomatic input to spinothalamic (STT) cells projecting to VPLc and VPLo thalamus in monkeys. Society for Neurosciences Abstracts 14(Pt 1): 121

Gellman H, Eckert R R, Bott M J, Sakiomura I, Waters R L 1988 Reflex sympathetic dystrophy in cervical spinal cord injury patients. Clinical Orthopaedics and Related Research 233: 126–131

Ghostine S Y, Comair Y G, Turner D M, Kassell N F, Azar C G 1984 Phenoxybenzamine in the treatment of causalgia. Report of 40 cases. Journal of Neurosurgery 60: 1263–1268

Grigg P, Schaible H G, Schmidt R F 1986 Mechanical sensitivity of group III and IV afferents from posterior articular nerve in normal and inflamed cat knee. Journal of Neurophysiology 55: 635–643

Guilbaud G, Iggo A, Tegner R 1985 Sensory receptors in ankle joint capsules of normal and arthritic rats. Experimental Brain Research 58: 29–40

Habler H J, Janig W, Koltzenburg M 1987 Activation of unmyelinated afferents in chronically lesioned nerves by adrenaline and excitation of sympathetic efferents in the cat. Neuroscience Letters 82: 35–40

Hakanson R, Wahlestedt C, Ekblad E, Edvinsson L, Sundler F 1986 Neuropeptide Y: coexistence with noradrenaline. Functional implications. In: Hokfelt T, Fuxe K, Pernow B (eds) Progress in brain research, vol 68. Elsevier, Amsterdam, pp 279–287

Hallin R G, Wiesenfeld-Hallin Z 1983 Does sympathetic activity modify afferent inflow at the receptor level in man? Journal of the Autonomic Nervous System 7: 391–397

Hancock M B, Foreman R D, Willis W D 1975 Convergence of visceral and cutaneous input onto spinothalamic tract cells in the thoracic spinal cord of the cat. Experimental Neurology 47: 240–248

Hannington-Kiff J G 1974 Intravenous regional sympathetic block with guanethidine. Lancet I: 1019–1020

Hedqvist P 1977 Basic mechanisms of prostaglandin action on autonomic neurotransmission. Annual Review of Pharmacology and Toxicology 17: 259–279

Heppelmann B, Schaible H G, Schmidt R F 1985 Effects of prostaglandins E_1 and E_2 on the mechanosensitivity of group III afferents from normal and inflamed cat knee joints. In: Fields H L et al (eds) Advances in Pain research and therapy. Raven, New York, pp 91–101

Herfort R A 1956 Extended sympathectomy in the treatment of advanced rheumatoid arthritis. New York Journal of Medicine 56: 1292

Higa K, Dan K, Manabe H, Noda B 1988 Factors influencing the duration of treatment of acute herpetic pain with sympathetic nerve block: importance of severity of herpes zoster assessed by the maximum antibody titers to varicella-zoster virus in otherwise healthy patients. Pain 32: 147–158

Hobbs S F, Chandler M J, Bolser D C, Foreman R D 1989 Functional organization of visceral spinal afferent input to C_3 to T_6 spinothalamic tract (STT) cells in monkeys. The Faseb Journal Abstracts, Part I 3(3): A680

Hokfelt T, Holets V R, Staines W et al 1986 Coexistence of neuronal messengers – an overview. In: Hokfelt T, Fuxe K, Pernow B (eds) Coexistence of neuronal messengers – a new principle in chemical transmission. Progress in brain research. Elsevier, Amsterdam, pp 33–70

Janig W, Kollmann W 1984 The involvement of the sympathetic nervous system in pain. Arzneimittel-Forschung/Drug Research 34: 1066–1073

Janig W, McLachlan E M 1986 The sympathetic and sensory components of the caudal lumbar sympathetic trunk in the cat. Journal of Comparative Neurology 245: 62–73

Juan H, Lembeck F 1974 Action of peptides and other algesic agents on paravascular pain receptors of the isolated perfused rabbit ear. Naunyn-Schmiedeberg's Archives of Pharmacology 283: 151–164

Juel-Jensen B E, MacCallum F O, Mackenzie A M R, Pike M C 1970 Treatment of zoster with idoxuridine in dimethyl sulphoxide. Results of two double-blind controlled trials. British Medical Journal 4: 776–780

Kenshalo D R, Leonard R B, Chung J M, Willis W D 1982 Facilitation of the responses of primate spinothalamic cells to cold and to tactile stimuli by noxious heating of the skin. Pain 12: 141–152

Korenman E M D, Devor M 1981 Ectopic adrenergic sensitivity in damaged peripheral nerve axons in the rat. Experimental Neurology 72: 63–81

LaMotte R H, Thalhammer J G 1982 Response properties of high-threshold cutaneous cold receptors in the primate. Brain Research 244: 279–287

Lankford L L 1982 Reflex sympathetic dystrophy. In: Green D P (ed) Operative hand surgery. Churchill Livingstone, New York, p 563

Leriche R 1916 De la causalgie envisagée comme un nevrite

du sympathetique et de son traitement per la denudation et l'excision des pleuxus nerveux perarteriels. Presse Medicale 24: 178–180

Levine J D, Fye K, Heller P, Basbaum A I, Whiting-O'Keefe Q 1986a Clinical response to regional intravenous guanethidine in patients with rheumatoid arthritis. Journal of Rheumatology 13: 1040–1043

Levine J D, Taiwo Y O, Collins S D, Tam J K 1986b Noradrenaline hyperalgesia is mediated through interaction with sympathetic postganglionic neurone terminals rather than activation of primary afferent nociceptors. Nature 323: 158–160

Levine J D, Goetzl E J, Basbaum A I 1987 Contribution of the nervous system to the pathophysiology of rheumatoid arthritis and other polyarthitides. Rheumatic Diseases Clinics of North America 13: 369–383

Levine J D, Coderre T J, Helms C, Basbaum A I 1988 β_2-adrenergic mechanisms in experimental arthritis. Proceedings of the National Academy of Science 85: 4553–4556

Livingston W K 1943 Pain mechanisms, a physiologic interpretation of causalgia and its related states. MacMillan, New York, pp 83–127

Loeser J D 1986 Herpes zoster and postherpetic neuralgia. Pain 25: 149–164

Loeser J D, Ward A A 1967 Some effects of deafferentation on neurons of the cat spinal cord. Archives of Neurology 17: 629–636

Loh L, Nathan P W 1978 Painful peripheral states and sympathetic blocks. Journal of Neurology, Neurosurgery and Psychiatry 41: 664–671

Loh L, Nathan P W, Schott G D 1981 Pain due to lesions of central nervous system removed by sympathetic block. British Medical Journal 282: 1026–1028

Loh L, Nathan P W, Schott G D, Wilson P G 1980 Effects of regional guanethidine infusion in certain painful states. Journal of Neurology, Neurosurgery and Psychiatry 43: 446–451

Lundberg J M, Hokfelt T 1983 Co-existence of peptides and classical neurotransmitters. Trends in Neuroscience 6: 325–333

Lundberg J M, Anggard A, Fahrenkrug J 1981 Complementary role of vasoactive intestinal polypeptide (VIP) and acetylcholine for cat submandibular gland blood flow and salivary secretion. I. VIP release. Acta Physiologica Scandinavica 113: 317–327

Lundberg J M, Rudehill A, Sollevi A, Theodorsson-Norheim E, Hamberger B 1986 Frequency- and reserpine-dependent chemical coding of sympathetic transmission: differential release of noradrenaline and neuropeptide Y from pig spleen. Neuroscience Letters 63: 96–100

Maixner W, Dubner R, Bushnell M C, Kenshalo D R, Oliveras J L 1986 Wide-dynamic-range dorsal horn neurons participate in the encoding process by which monkeys perceive the intensity of noxious heat stimuli. Brain Research 374: 385–388

Martin H A, Basbaum A I, Kwiat G C, Goetzl E J, Levine J D 1987 Leukotriene and prostaglandin sensitization of cutaneous high-threshold C- and A-deltamechanonociceptors in the hairy skin of rat hindlimbs. Neuroscience 22: 651–659

Mayer D J, Price D D, Becker D P 1975 Neurophysiological characterization of the anterolateral spinal cord neurons contributing to pain perception in man. Pain 1: 51–58

Mendell L M 1984 Modifiability of spinal synapses. Physiological Reviews 64: 260–324

Mendell L M, Wall P D 1965 Responses of single dorsal cord cells to peripheral cutaneous unmyelinated fibres. Nature 206: 97–99

Mense S 1981 Sensitization of group IV muscle receptors to bradykinin by 5-hydroxytryptamine and prostaglandin E_2. Brain Research 225: 95–105

Meyers R R, Katz J 1988 Neuropathology of neurolytic and semidestructive agents. In: Cousins M J, Bridenbaugh P O (eds) Neural blockade in clinical anesthesia and management of pain. Lippincott, Philadelphia, pp 1031–1052

Milligan N S, Nash T P 1985 Treatment of post-herpetic neuralgia. A review of 77 consecutive cases. Pain 23: 381–386

Milne R J, Foreman R D, Giesler G J, Willis W D 1981 Convergence of cutaneous and pelvic visceral nociceptive inputs on to primate spinothalamic neurons. Pain 11: 163–183

Moore P K 1985 Prostanoids: pharmacological, physiological and clinical relevance. Cambridge University Press, Cambridge

Nakamura M, Ferreira S H 1987 A peripheral sympathetic component in inflammatory hyperalgesia. European Journal of Pharmacology 135: 145–153

Nielsen S L, Vitting K, Rasmussen K 1983 Prazosin treatment of primary Raynaud's phenomenon. European Journal of Clinical Pharmacology 24: 421–423

Ochoa J 1986 The newly recognized painful ABC syndrome: thermographic aspects. Thermography 2: 65–107

Ochoa J, Roberts W J, Cline M A, Dotson R 1988 Unpublished observations

Olsen E R, Ivy H B 1981 Stellate block for trigeminal zoster. Journal of Clinical NeuroOpthalmology 1: 53–55

Olsen N 1987 Centrally and locally mediated vasomotor activities in Raynaud's phenomenon. Scandinavian Journal of Work and Environmental Health 13: 309–312

Pernow J, Kahan T, Hjemdahl P, Lundberg J M 1988 Possible involvement of neuropeptide Y in sympathetic vascular control of canine skeletal muscle. Acta Physiologica Scandinavica 132: 43–50

Price D D, Bennett G J, Rafii A 1989 Psychophysical observations on patients with neuropathic pain relieved by a sympathetic block. Pain 36: 273–288

Pubols L M, Sessle B J 1987 Effects of injury on trigeminal and spinal somatosensory systems. Liss, New York

Raskin N H, Levinson S A, Hoffman P M, Pickett J B E, Fields H L 1974 Postsympathectomy neuralgia. American Journal of Surgery 128: 75–78

Raynaud A G M 1862 De l'asphyxic locale et de la gangrene symmetrique des extremetes. Ribnoux, Paris

Roberts W J 1986 A hypothesis on the physiological basis for causalgia and related pains. Pain 24: 297–311

Roberts W J, Elardo S M 1985 Sympathetic activation of unmyelinated mechanoreceptors in cat skin. Brain Research 339: 123–125

Roberts W J, Foglesong M E 1986 A neuronal basis for sympathetically maintained pain. Thermology 2: 2–6

Roberts W J, Foglesong M E 1988a I. Spinal recordings indicate that wide-dynamic-range neurons mediate sympathetically maintained pain. Pain 34: 289–304

Roberts W J, Foglesong M E 1988b II. Identification of afferents contributing to sympathetically evoked activity in wide-dynamic-range neurons. Pain 34: 305–314

Roberts W J, Kramis R C 1988 Sympathetic activation of hyperactive WDR neurons following receptive field trauma. Society for Neurosciences Abstracts 14: 563

Roberts W J, Kramis R C 1989 Sympathetic nervous system influence on acute and chronic pain. In: Fields H L (ed) Pain syndromes in neurology. Butterworth, London (in press)

Roberts W J, Elardo S M, King K A 1985 Sympathetically-induced changes in the responses of slowly-adapting type I receptors in cat skin. Somatosensory Research 2: 223–236

Roberts W J, Foglesong M E, Kramis R C 1987 Enhancement of sympathetically evoked activity in sensitized WDR neurons is dependent on conditioning stimulus modality. Society for Neurosciences Abstracts 13: 991

Scadding J W 1981 Development of ongoing activity, mechanosensitivity and adrenaline sensitivity in severed peripheral nerve axons. Experimental Neurology 73: 345–364

Schott G D 1986 Mechanisms of causalgia and related clinical conditions: the role of the central and of the sympathetic nervous systems. Brain 109: 717–738

Schwartzman R, McLellan T L 1987 Reflex sympathetic dystrophy. Archives of Neurology 44: 555–561

Seibold J R, Terregino C A 1986 Selective antagonism of S_2-serotonergic receptors relieves but does not prevent induced vasoconstriction in primary Raynaud's phenomenon. Journal of Rheumatology 13: 337–340

Shumacker H B 1948 Causalgia. III. A general discussion. Surgery 24: 485–504

Soininen K, Jarvilehto T, Aleksandrov T I, Shvyrkow V B 1983 Task dependence of activity in human peripheral mechanoreceptive units. Proceedings 7th International Congress, Electromyography, Munich S12

Spittell J A 1983 Vasospastic disorders. In: Clinical vascular disease. Davis, Philadelphia

Stjarne L 1972 Prostaglandin E restricting noradrenaline secretion – neural in origin. Acta Physiologica Scandinavica 86: 574–576

Sunderland S 1976 Pain mechanisms in causalgia. Journal of Neurology, Neurosurgery and Psychiatry 39: 471–480

Sweet W H, Poletti C E 1985 Causalgia and sympathetic dystrophy (Sudeck's atrophy). In: Aronoff G M (ed) Evaluation and treatment of chronic pain. Urban and Schwarzenberg, Baltimore, pp 149–165

Tahmoush A J 1981 Causalgia: redefinition as a clinical pain syndrome. Pain 10: 187–197

Tahmoush A J, Mallet J, Jennings J R 1983 Skin conductance, temperature, and blood flow in causalgia. Neurology 33: 1483–1486

Toyama N 1982 Sympathetic ganglion block therapy for herpes zoster. Journal of Dermatology 9: 59–62

Tracy G D, Cockett F B 1957 Pain in the lower limb after sympathectomy. Lancet I: 12–14

Vanhoutte P M, Janssens W J 1980 Thermosensitivity of cutaneous vessels and Raynaud's disease. American Heart Journal 100: 263–265

Wall P D, Gutnick M 1974 Ongoing activity in peripheral nerves: the physiology and pharmacology of impulses originating from a neuroma. Experimental Neurology 43: 580–593

Wallin G, Torebjork E, Hallin R 1976 Preliminary observation on the pathophysiology of hyperalgesia in the causalgic pain syndrome. In: Zotterman Y (ed) Sensory functions of the skin in primates with special reference to man. Pergamon, Oxford, pp 489–502

Wang J K, Johnson K A, Ilstrup D M 1985 Sympathetic blocks for reflex sympathetic dystrophy. Pain 23: 13–17

White J C, Sweet W H 1969 Pain and the neurosurgeon. Thomas, Springfield, pp 528–534

Wiesenfeld-Hallin Z, Hallin R G 1984 The influence of the sympathetic system on mechanoreception and nociception. A review. Human Neurobiology 3: 41–46

Wollersheim H, Cleophas T, Thien T 1987 The role of the sympathetic nervous system in the pathophysiology and therapy of Raynaud's phenomenon. VASA (Supplementum 18): 54–63

J. L. Ochoa, P. Marchettini and M. Cline

3   Lessons from human research on the pathophysiology of neuropathic pains in limbs

INTRODUCTION

In the realm of sensory dysfunction, the application of basic research methods and of scientific thinking to the investigation of patients supplements basic animal research. It may also provide unique lessons on the subject researched, and on research itself. The following case histories of a handful of selected patients with neuropathic pain exposes conceptual points which are either currently confused, debated or accepted uncritically. Some of those concepts clarify when the clinical case is approached scientifically.

NEURAL SOURCE RELATIVE TO SYMPTOMATIC LOCALISATION OF NEUROPATHIC PAIN

Pain localised to the source contrasting with projected neuropathic pain

When the finger points at the moon, the fool looks at the finger.

ANCIENT PROVERB

Case history 1

Miss Susan S. was in her late fifties when she was referred for a second neurological consultation to the National Hospital, London, in May 1970. Her chief complaint was pain in the left ring finger, started some 30 years earlier 'while bathing in the Black Sea'. Thereafter, cold immersion would fairly consistently trigger or exaggerate her pain. Mechanical stimulation of the tip of the symptomatic digit, even by gentle touch, would also evoke pain which forced her to readapt her technique as a typist. Five years earlier, when first referred to the National Hospital, a postgraduate neurologist in training from Australia became impressed by some impairment of sensation on the ulnar side of the symptomatic hand and, accordingly, launched electrophysiological and radiological testing for possible ulnar nerve or brachial plexus lesion. Results were normal. By that time, the patient had long discovered that warming the finger helped relieve pain and had developed the habit of putting the finger inside her mouth whenever possible. In view of that, the patient was discharged on antidepressants.

On a second referral, a more naive neurologist-in-training failed 'to look at the moon'; but looked at the finger itself. The report reads: 'There is a swelling in the medial aspect of the distal phalanx of the left ring finger: it is soft, the overlying skin is normal, it is partly subungual and exquisitely painful. It has been there since 1940. I have little doubt that this is a glomus tumor and with her enthusiastic approval, I put her name on our waiting list to be admitted for treatment'.

X-rays showed a soft tissue swelling which, upon surgical removal by Mr Wilson at the Royal National Orthopaedic Hospital, was confirmed histologically to be a glomus tumour. The majority of such tumours, when situated in the fingers, occur in females, a large proportion being Jewish. When Miss S. was seen one month following surgery, she was very grateful and in no pain.

Comment. When people learn that what *feels* the pain is the finger of the brain (rather than the finger of the hand) and when neurologists learn that the pain will *project* to the finger of the hand regardless of the site of origin of the nerve impulses in the neural channels that connect finger to brain, it becomes natural to search for lesions in the nervous system in patients complaining of limb pains with neuropathic characteristics. This strategy is usually rewarded because, rather than indicating *local* pathology, the localised symptom reflects projection to the physical endings of the sensory line of an afferent event initiated further proximally. Of course, the 'finger of the brain' will also hurt if nerve endings themselves are actually irritated in the finger of the hand, and it does pay to include the latter in the examination.

Projected pain contrasting with referred neuropathic pain: Neurogenic pain from skin and neurogenic pain from deep tissues

Case history 2

Dr William S., a dentist, progressively developed a painful muscle spasm in the left hand in relation to voluntary activation during dental work. Symptoms had started several years earlier following what was thought to be an ulnar nerve injury at elbow level, sustained during surgery under general anaesthesia. Some time after the onset of the syndrome, the patient noticed additional pain in the chest, which would regularly associate with the pain in the hand. The localisation of the chest pain and its suggested relationship to voluntary effort led Dr S. to self-diagnose angina, for which he personally arranged for stress EKG, with negative results. Neurological examination and conventional nerve conduction studies revealed no deficit of motor, sensory or reflex functions. But the syndrome involved irritative symptoms and signs, rather than deficit phenomena. Therefore, to further investigate the pathophysiological basis of the complaints, the patient consented to microneurographic recordings and microstimulation in his ulnar nerve at wrist level, aimed at disclosing neural correlates underlying the pains.

On multiple occasions, intraneural electrical microstimulation in muscle nerve fascicles reproduced both his hand and chest pain, with or without associated muscle spasm. When present, muscle contraction was stereotyped in that it involved contraction of the abductor digiti minimi and volar interossei. Further, the hand posture produced by the electrically induced contraction mimicked that occurring spontaneously, as previously videotaped for comparison.

Comment. The case of Dr S., who was fully investigated at the Department of Neurology, University of Wisconsin, Madison, in 1985, illustrates a number of points of interest in the field of neuropathic pain, providing a dramatic example of pain originating in muscle afferents. It has been shown in volunteers that pain evoked by intraneural microstimulation of *muscle nerve fascicles* has a distinct muscle cramp quality. It is *projected* to the region of the pertinent muscle belly, and is often also *referred* remotely relative to the nerve endings in the receptive field of the nerve. Favourite areas of referral for median nerve (Torebjork et al 1984) and for ulnar nerve (Marchettini et al 1990) are shoulder, scapular region and lateral chest wall. These features of localisation, together with the subjective quality of the pain, carry differential meaning, since pain evoked by activation of nociceptor afferents in *skin nerve fascicles* does not have a cramp-like subjective quality; it is either sharp and pricking, or dull burning, and has no tendency towards remote proximal referral; it projects accurately to the receptive field of activated sensory units (Torebjork & Ochoa 1980; Ochoa & Torebjork 1989; Torebjork & Ochoa 1989).

The case also illustrates a fact often neglected or ignored, namely that normal sensory nerve action potentials and conduction velocity only attest ability of large calibre fibres to conduct impulses, but do not assess the status of small calibre fibres concerned with pain. Further, ectopic impulse generation also eludes conventional electrodiagnosis, even when it occurs in large calibre sensory fibres (Ochoa 1987). Abnormal impulse generation is known to underlie positive sensory phenomena such as neuropathic paraesthesiae and, perhaps, pains (Ochoa & Torebjork 1980; Nordin et al 1984; Ochoa et al 1987).

SOURCES OF ABNORMAL AFFERENT ACTIVITY AND SPONTANEOUS VS PROVOKED NEUROPATHIC PAIN

Recurrent pain from ectopic impulse generation provoked by mechanical irritation of sensory fibres in peripheral nerves or roots

Case history 3

Mr Emmet W., also evaluated at University of Wisconsin, complained of episodes of intense paraesthesiae and pains in the left upper limb, consistently provoked by certain movements of the neck and clinically reproduced as positive foraminal sign of Spurling. The abnormal sensations were stereotyped in their subjective quality and in their localisation. They spread distally from axilla to ulnar aspect of the hand. Diagnosis of entrapment of the 8th cervical root due to herniated disc was straightforward on clinical, radiological and electrophysiological grounds. The patient consented to sampling with intraneural microelectrodes (microneurography) in an attempt to document the time relationships associating mechanical provocation through the Spurling manoeuvre, the verbalised sensory experience and the ectopic impulse activity anticipated to underlie the paroxysmal sensory symptoms. Seconds following initiation of the provocative manoeuvre, the patient would start describing a sequence of tingling, pins-and-needles and pain, and their gradual distal *marche*. On two separate recording sessions, when the sensations reached the hand, it became possible to record abrupt onset of paroxysmal, unitary bursting discharge, obviously conducted antidromically from an ulnar sensory nerve fascicle supplying symptomatic skin of the hand. Upon discontinuation of the Spurling manoeuvre, the symptoms gradually faded, the bursting discharge waned and ended prior to disappearance of the paraesthesiae (Ochoa et al 1987).

Convincing criteria ruled out the possibility that the discharges were locally induced at ulnar nerve recording level due to electrode movement.

Comment. This case provides unsurprising evidence that abnormal sensation as a symptom of damage to the afferent system may be due to epileptiform discharge from sensory pathways. Such afferent activity may also travel *antidromically* in the peripheral nervous system, a phenomenon potentially involved in the pathogenesis of certain other forms of neuropathic pain (Ochoa 1986). While this case also endorses microneurography as a powerful technique in the investigation of sensory function and dysfunction in man (Nordin et al 1984), it is unrealistic to regard that method as a routine option in electrodiagnosis.

Chronic spontaneous ongoing pain from primary damage to the peripheral sensory nervous system: peripheral vs centralised mechanisms

Case history 4

Mrs Cleo M. has a severe, chronic, progressive sensory neuropathy. Its aetiology remains undefined despite invasive specialised investigation. Symptomatology is dominated by a familiar combination of symptoms which proves puzzling to patients: profound loss of sensory acuity, side by side with intolerable spontaneous ongoing burning pain in hands and feet (anaesthesia dolorosa). Quantitative sensory testing, for thermal-specific and thermal pain submodalities, performed at the Department of Neurology, Good Samaritan Hospital, Portland, Oregon, revealed severe, nearly selective impairment of afferent functions served by small calibre nerve fibres in glove distribution, with global hypoaesthesia to all submodalities, tactile, thermal-specific and pain, in stocking distribution. Cutaneous nerve biopsy in the leg showed practical devastation of sensory fibres of all calibres, obviously explaining the global loss of sensation.

In the context of dying-back type peripheral neuropathy, it is most likely that the spontaneous pain of Mrs M. is due to spontaneous ectopic discharge originating in peripheral axons of surviving sensory units, as shown in acute animal experiments (Wall & Gutnick 1974). The burning quality suggests that unmyelinated nociceptor units are engaged (Ochoa & Torebjork 1989). Since a significant proportion of nociceptor units are disconnected from skin (as revealed by nerve biopsy), there is little opportunity for development of hyperalgesia or for development of antidromic vasodilatation, since both these phenomena require functional connection of axon to receptor or effector organs. For the same reason, therapeutic desensitisation of nociceptor endings should not be expected to relieve pain. These points will be discussed further below.

Case history 5

Mr William D. developed acute weakness, loss of sensation and reflexes, with eventual wasting of his left upper limb, as a consequence of a motor bicycle accident. The clinical and electrodiagnostic profile indicated root avulsion as opposed to brachial plexus injury. Pain became a prominent symptom, expressed in plural forms, as described by Wynn Parry (1980). Diagnostic local anaesthetic brachial nerve blocks failed to relieve the ongoing pain, although blocks temporarily abolished residual sensation in the limb.

It is unavoidable to interpret the ongoing pains of Mr D. as originating within the central nervous system, since firstly, irritation of central sensory pathways may undoubtedly evoke pain; secondly, experimental primary injury to peripheral nerve roots may induce secondary foci of neural discharge in dorsal horns, thalamus and even cortex (Lombard et al 1979); and thirdly, since primary sensory units supplying symptomatic areas were disconnected from their central projections, they therefore could not serve as effective sources of abnormal afferent activity.

Comment. Therapeutic surgical initiatives directed at the peripheral nervous system should be anticipated to provide relief for the first 3 patients described above, but for the case of the last patient, in particular, these initiatives should be avoided, as doomed to failure.

HYPERALGESIA IN NEUROPATHY
Chronically sensitised primary nociceptors
Case history 6

Mr Dennis O'K. was referred to the Sensory Disorders Clinic, University of Wisconsin, Madison, in September 1985 with the diagnosis of reflex sympathetic dystrophy. He had a 14-month history of unremitting burning pain in response to even light touch on the dorsum of his right hand. This mechanical hyperalgesia was the chronic local sequel of sunburn that led to temporary inflammation: calor, rubor and some swelling.

In addition to crippling mechanical hyperalgesia, there was burning pain in response to non-noxious elevation of temperature (heat hyperalgesia) and the symptomatic skin was thermographically warm. Spontaneous pain, when present, and mechanical hyperalgesia were strikingly improved by passive cooling of the hand. This state of 'erythralgia' (Lewis 1936), or 'ABC' syndrome (Ochoa 1986), as might have been anticipated, was refractory to sympathetic blocks (Ochoa 1990).

Cline et al (1989) describe in detail how microneurography directly documented the presence of sensitised C–nociceptors, confined to symptomatic skin, thus further identifying this human clinical syndrome with the experimental syndrome of sensitisation by local capsaicin (see Culp et al 1989). This hyperalgesic state was shown to be resistant to selective block of myelinated A fibres. This feature, coupled with a burning quality of the pain, further incriminate C nociceptors at the pathophysiological basis (Ochoa et al 1989).

The possible associated existence of secondary CNS dysfunction was considered, investigated through psychophysical estimates of pain during nerve stimulation which bypassed skin receptors, and ruled out by equivalent results for symptomatic and contralateral limb.

Comment. This case establishes nociceptor sensitisation as a viable abnormal mechanism in the production of chronic painful syndromes in man and calls for revision of criteria for 'sympathetic dystrophy'. This case also introduces an *ultradistal source* of abnormal afferent activity initiated at receptor level as the cause of pain.

The prominence of *thermal hyperalgesia* calls for incorporation of quantitative thermotest to the clinical routine in neuropathic pain patients (see recommendations by Asbury et al 1988), while the subclinical presence of deviation in temperature of symptomatic skin calls for incorporation of thermography in the evaluation of those patients (Ochoa 1986). In turn, microneurography again emerges as a powerful tool reserved for basic research of sensory mechanisms in patients.

Finally, this archetype of nociceptor sensitisation speculatively presents the optimal target for therapeutic desensitising strategies through the chronic use of neurotoxins, such as capsaicin.

Secondary central hyperexcitability?
Case history 7

Ms Linda R. lacerated her right ulnar nerve when she accidentally crashed her arm through a glass door in 1987. As a consequence, she developed an intractable chronic painful syndrome in the hand which featured:

1. spontaneous ongoing burning pain
2. mechanical hyperalgesia
3. cold hyperalgesia
4. deviations of temperature in symptomatic skin with predominant cold state.

The spontaneous pain and the (mechanical) hyperalgesic pain expressed some clinical differences; for example, the former was often described as burning in quality, while the latter was 'weird, creepy' and sometimes 'an unpleasantness not necessarily painful'. This 'weird' mechanical hyperalgesia had a clear *dynamic*, repetitive, on-off stimulus requirement, and disappeared during dissociated myelinated A fibre block performed proximal to the site of nerve injury. Ms R. experienced temporary abolition of pain and mechanical (and thermal) hyperalgesia both during sympathetic ganglion and regional guanethidine blocks.

Comment. The hyperalgesic pain induced by weak mechanical stimuli, which disappears during A-fibre block, may stem from activation of hyperexcitable *central* neurons by normally non-painful tactile input. Whatever the abnormal mechanism might be through which those neurons become hyperexcitable (Roberts 1986), their abnormal physiology could sufficiently explain both spontaneous pain and mechanical hyperalgesia, if not also thermal hyperalgesia.

On the other hand, it should be kept in mind

that there exists another distinct form of hyperalgesic pain induced by non-noxious mechanical stimuli. In contrast with the *dynamic*, on-off stimulus requirement described above, this second form of *static* mechanical hyperalgesia is elicited during sustained mechanical pressure. Further, it has a burning quality and persists during A fibre block, while C fibres continue to conduct. It is seen in patients with apparent C-nociceptor dysfunction and is experienced after capsaicin sensitisation (Ochoa et al 1989). Some patients express concomitantly both dynamic and static mechanical hyperalgesia. Actually, Ms R. was an example of both.

Finally, the temporary relief experienced during sympathetic blocks is often taken to indicate that the sympathetic system is both abnormal and, in some way, responsible for the painful syndrome. The frequent failure of sympathectomy to cure these patients, and other reasons, invite revision of those concepts (Ochoa 1989).

HOT AND COLD PATIENTS

While some patients may express both cold and heat hyperalgesia, the majority express either one or the other form of painful sensitivity to non-noxious temperature change, as illustrated by the two distinct examples described on page 31. An observation which must entail pathophysiological significance is that when attention is paid to the physical temperature of symptomatic parts, neuropathic pain patients cluster into well-defined descriptive categories: *hot* or *cold* patients.

Cold patients often exhibit regionally cold skin and express cold hyperalgesia: non-noxious low temperature hurts. They tend to improve symptomatically with warming, which is achieved either by passive immersion or by vasodilatation from blocking of sympathetic vasoconstrictor outflow. Hot patients often exhibit regionally warm skin and express heat hyperalgesia. Their symptomatic pains and mechanical hyperalgesia may be abolished transiently by cooling. Sympathetic blocks may exaggerate the temperature-determined pains in hot patients due to vasodilatation.

Since both types of patients often complain of burning pain and express hyperalgesia and vasomotor phenomena, they are conventionally confused into artificial unity, labelled as having 'causalgia-reflex sympathetic dystrophy' and are often condemned indiscriminately to sympathectomy, frequently with disappointing results. As mentioned above, hot patients may have sensitised peripheral C-nociceptors associated with antidromic vasodilatation, and their clinical profile is replicated by acute cutaneous application of capsaicin (Ochoa 1986; Cline et al 1989; Culp et al 1989). Since cold patients are the opposite of hot patients, the two profiles can be logically envisioned as closely related at an essential pathophysiological level. For hot patients, warm sensitive transducers may be leaky in excitable C-nociceptor membrane, thus facilitating depolarisation in response to weak thermal stimuli. C-nociceptor orthodromic activity would evoke pain sensation, while antidromic activity would evoke vasodilatation (Lewis 1936; Ochoa 1986; Cline et al 1989). For cold patients, perhaps cold-specific transducers are leaky, thus facilitating depolarisation at normally non-noxious low temperatures. Again, C-nociceptor orthodromic activity would evoke dull burning pain sensation but antidromic activity should cause skin warming from vasodilatation. The observed cooling could be reconciled firstly by interjection of sympathetic vasoconstrictor activity, excited reflexly by afferent activity (somatosympathetic reflex response; Sato & Schmidt 1973); and secondly, if sympathetic mediated vasoconstriction overrides warming from antidromic vasodilatation. The latter has been observed in humans (Ochoa et al 1989, 1990), whereas the former is easily triggered in humans by administration of afferent stimuli (Delius et al 1972; Hallin & Torebjork 1974). It is conceivable that if cold-specific transducers are leaky, not only in polymodal C-nociceptors but also in cold-specific afferents, which discharge ectopically, this input could naturally trigger somatosympathetic reflex vasoconstriction.

In support of this modified unifying hypothesis is the observation that patients may strikingly shift between cold and hot thermographic states (Ochoa 1989), and rats with the Bennett model of neuropathic pain may do the same (Bennett & Ochoa 1990). Nevertheless, the possibility that cold patients may be hot patients, originally expressing antidromic vasodilatation now under cover due to superimposed reflex sympathetic vasoconstriction, is unattractive: this would explain reversal of skin temperature from hot to cold, but not reversal of thermal hyperalgesia.

REFERENCES

Asbury A K, Porte D, Genuth S M, Griffin J, Halter J B, Kimura J, Kuller L H, McLeod J G, Ochoa J L, Ward J D 1988 Report and recommendations of the San Antonio conference on diabetic neuropathy. Diabetes Care 11: 592–597

Bennett G J, Ochoa J L 1990 Thermographic observations on rats with experimental neuropathic pain. In preparation

Cline M, Ochoa J, Torebjork H E 1989 Chronic hyperalgesia and skin warming caused by sensitized C nociceptors. Brain 112: 621–647

Culp W J, Ochoa J, Cline M, Dotson 1989 Heat and mechanical hyperalgesia induced by Capsaicin. Cross modality threshold modulation in human C nociceptors. Brain 112: 1317–1331

Delius W, Hagbarth K-E, Hongell A, Wallin B G 1972 Manouevers affecting sympathetic outflow in human skin nerves. Acta Physiologica Scandinavica 84: 177–186

Hallin R G, Torebjork H E 1974 Single unit sympathetic activity in human skin nerves during rest and various manoeuvers. Acta Physiologica Scandinavica 92: 303–317

Lewis T 1936 Vascular disorders of the limbs, described for practitioners and students. MacMillan, London

Lombard M C, Nashold B S, Pelissier T 1979 Thalamic recordings in rats with hyperalgesia. In: Bonica J J, Liebeskind J C, Albe-Fessard D G (eds) Advances in pain research and therapy, vol 3. Raven, New York, pp 767–772

Marchettini P, Cline M, Ochoa J L 1990 Innervation territories for touch and pain afferents of single fascicles of the human ulnar nerve. Mapping through intraneural microrecording and microstimulation. Brain. In press

Nordin M, Nystrom B, Wallin U, Hagbarth K-E 1984 Ectopic sensory discharges and paresthesiae in patients with disorders of peripheral nerves, dorsal roots and dorsal columns. Pain 20: 231–245

Ochoa J L 1986 The newly recognized painful ABC syndrome: thermographic aspects. Thermographic 2: 65–107

Ochoa J L 1987 Mechanisms of symptoms in neuropathy. In: Ellingson, R J, Murray N M F, Halliday A M (eds) The London symposia (EEG suppl 39). Elsevier, Amsterdam

Ochoa J L 1990 Neuropathic pains from within: personal experiences, experiments, and reflections on mythology. In: Dimitrijevic M R (ed) Recent achievements in restorative neurology: Altered sensation and pain. Karger, Basel, 100–111

Ochoa J L, Torebjork H E 1980 Paresthesiae from ectopic impulse generation in human sensory nerves. Brain 103: 835-853

Ochoa J L, Torebjork E 1989 Sensations evoked by intraneural microstimulation of C nociceptor fibres in human skin nerves. Journal of Physiology 415: 583–599

Ochoa J L, Cline M, Dotson R, Marchettini P 1987 Pain and paresthesias provoked mechanically in human cervical root entrapment (sign of spurling). Single sensory unit antidromic recording of ectopic, bursting, propagated nerve impulse activity. In: Pubols L M, Sessle B J (eds) Effects of injury on trigeminal and spinal somatosensory systems. Liss, New York, pp 389–397

Ochoa J L, Dotson R, Cline M A, Yarnitsky D, Marchettini P 1990 Antidromic vasodilatation overridden by somatosympathetic reflex vasoconstriction in man. Intraneural stimulation and thermography. Society for Neuroscience Abstracts. In press

Ochoa J L, Roberts W J, Cline M A, Dotson R, Yarnitsky D 1989 Two mechanical hyperalgesias in human neuropathy. Society for Neuroscience Abstracts 15: 472

Roberts W J 1986 A hypothesis on the physiological basis for causalgia and related pains. Pain 24: 297–311

Sato A, Schmidt R F 1973 Somatosympathetic reflexes: afferent fibers, central pathways, discharge characteristics. Physiological Reviews 53: 916–947

Torebjork H E, Ochoa J L 1980 Specific sensations evoked by activity in single identified sensory units in man. Acta Physiologica Scandinavica 110: 445–447

Torebjork H E, Ochoa J L 1990 Receptor characteristics and sensory attributes of nociceptors with myelinated (A) fibres innervating the glabrous skin of the human hand. Brain research. In press

Torebjork H E, Ochoa J L, Schady W 1984 Referred pain from intraneural stimulation of muscle fascicles in the median nerve. Pain 18: 145–156

Wall P D, Gutnick M 1974 Properties of afferent nerve impulses originating from a neuroma. Nature 248: 740–743

Wynn Parry C B 1980 Pain in avulsion lesions of the brachial plexus. Pain 9: 41–53

G. D. Schott

4 Management of pain in the hand and wrist: central causes of peripheral pain

INTRODUCTION

It is often not obvious to patients, and not always obvious to doctors, that pain experienced in a particular area can be due to disease that is located far away. Whilst pain in the hand is far more commonly due to local causes, diseases of the central nervous system (brain and spinal cord) occasionally produce pain in the hand, presumably through mechanisms of reference or projection. Thus pain results from stimulation of pathways whose peripheral end projects to the extremity, and whose central projection gives rise to conscious appreciation of pain. In this chapter, it is proposed to deal with those centrally generated sensory disturbances of the hand which patients call painful. These include dysaesthesiae, paraesthesiae and hyperpathia, as well as strictly 'painful' conditions, since these disagreeable sensations often co-exist and may be difficult to distinguish, though different mechanisms may well underlie the different types of painful sensation.

The areas from which central pain may arise can be anywhere in the central nervous system; certain areas, however, more commonly give rise to pain, such as the thalamic region, the lower brainstem and the spinal cord, whereas lesions of the cortex and mid–brain infrequently cause pain. Rarely specific, the quality of pain may include aching, stinging, bruised or burning sensations, and the latter, especially if accompanied by extreme hypersensitivity to innocuous stimuli such as light touches, puffs of wind or contact with clothing, produce pain described as causalgic. Central pain is often poorly localised, and sometimes peculiar distributions of pain occur, such as involvement of just a few fingers of one hand or half the hand; this may be erroneously considered hysterical, because the pain does not obviously conform to a root or peripheral nerve distribution.

DIAGNOSIS AND INVESTIGATION

Diagnosing a central rather than peripheral cause for hand pain is not always easy. Consideration of a central cause should arise if the cause of the pain is uncertain, if the signs do not fit with the symptoms, if there are upper motor neuron signs, if there are neurological signs outside the hand, and if disease of the central nervous system is known to be present or to have occurred in the past. Examples of relevant past events include previous stroke, a whiplash injury or cerebral trauma, and relapsing and remitting neurological problems which might suggest multiple sclerosis.

The selection of investigations for a possible neurological cause depends on the clinical circumstances. When the cause is unknown, it may be better to err on the side of over-investigation, especially if this can be carried out non-invasively, and if surgery is being contemplated. In addition, failure of surgery to the periphery to resolve pain in the hand should lead to consideration of more extensive investigation and review of the underlying cause. Neurophysiological and radiological investigations are the main methods of diagnosing central lesions. Although neurophysiological investigations were initially employed in assessment of peripheral problems such as the carpal tunnel syndrome, these investigations may be very useful in assessment of diseases of the central nervous system and exclusion of peripheral problems. For example, pain in the hand attributed to the carpal tunnel syndrome should be reconsidered if the increasingly sophisticated neurophysiological techniques now available (Lancet 1985) show no evidence supporting the diagnosis. Similar considerations apply to studies of ulnar nerve function. Conventional neurophysiological investigations may be useful in determining whether pain in the hand is due to a post-ganglionic lesion indicating a peripheral cause, or a pre-ganglionic and perhaps central cause. Examples where this assessment is useful include investigation of brachial plexus injuries where the extent of spinal cord, root or plexus involvement after trauma is uncertain, and in assessing upper limb pain associated with malignancy or irradiation in the apical region when intraspinal damage may also occur. Somatosensory evoked potential studies may be valuable in assessing sensory aspects of plexus, root and posterior column function. Most studies, however, have employed techniques which assess large-diameter fibre function, although methods which involve stimulation of small-diameter, pain-subserving fibres are being developed (Bromm 1985).

The choice of radiological investigations in elucidating central causes of hand pain again depends on the clinical circumstances. For instance, plain radiographs of the cervical spine, sometimes with oblique and flexion and extension views, give valuable information on spinal canal dimensions, size of root exit foramina, spinal stability and a number of congenital and acquired diseases. For diseases of the cervical spinal cord itself, the method of choice is probably magnetic resonance imaging (MRI scanning), which can delineate structural and inflammatory lesions non-invasively, but with the limited availability of this technique at present, myelography, sometimes with computed tomography (CT scanning), is highly effective although invasive. It does, however, also enable the CSF to be examined, which is helpful in assessing infective, malignant and inflammatory diseases such as multiple sclerosis.

CONDITIONS CAUSING CENTRAL PAIN

Central causes of pain in the hand can be divided into cerebral and spinal disorders; there are in addition causes which may involve the peripheral and central nervous systems at the same time (such as some traumatic brachial plexus injuries, malignancy and post-herpetic neuralgia), and causes of hand pain where the precise site of damage is unclear (e.g. the shoulder–hand syndrome). Hand pain from central causes may be unilateral or bilateral, often giving a valuable clue to localisation of the lesion. Thus disorders localised to a cerebral hemisphere typically give rise to contralateral hand pain, but the further caudally the lesion lies, the more likely is bilateral pain to be present.

Cerebral disease

Cerebrovascular disease

Strokes are probably the commonest cause of cerebral disease resulting in pain affecting the upper limb and hand, although how often pain occurs is unknown. The classical disorder is the thalamic syndrome, described first by Dejerine and Roussy in 1906. Typically a small infarct is present in or near the thalamus, resulting, in its complete form, in contralateral hemiplegia, hemianaesthesia, ataxia and choreoathetosis, and pain. It is the pain which is the cardinal feature of the thalamic syndrome, the other features being variable, though it may be impairment of temperature and pain sensibility which is the commonest associated abnormality (Leijon et al 1989). Different somatosensory evoked potentials have been reported as differentiating between various sensory and pain features of the thalamic syndrome (Mauguière & Desmedt 1988). A particularly unfortunate phenomenon sometimes encountered in an initially hypoalgesic or analgesic area is the change over weeks or months to severe and persistent pain in that area. The hand is a part of the body not uncommonly involved in the thalamic syndrome, the pain often being deep, burning and accompanied by hyperpathia; pain is often spontaneous but can also be accompanied by induced pain. It may also be associated with other conditions such as pain from immobility and the shoulder–hand syndrome. Although Dejerine & Roussy (1906) termed the condition the thalamic syndrome, and their patients had vascular lesions in or around the thalamus, the same type of pain can arise from different lesions in the same area (e.g. tumour) and from lesions elsewhere in the central nervous system, such as from vascular lesions elsewhere in the nervous system, tumours, trauma and multiple sclerosis (Riddoch 1938; Cassinari & Pagni 1969). Thus pain in the hand from central causes within the brain does not indicate a specific site nor a specific cause. Perhaps the minimal form of this phenomenon is pain that just affects the corner of the mouth and ipsilateral hand, the cheiro–oral syndrome; it has recently been appreciated that this syndrome, too, does not have a specific underlying anatomical substrate, having been described in lesions of the thalamus, pons and mid-brain (Valzelli 1987).

Epilepsy

Epilepsy as a cause of pain is rare (Young & Blume 1983). Fine (1967) however has drawn attention to the elderly patient with post-hemiplegic pain. Some of these patients experience severe paroxysmal pain in the hemiplegic limbs accompanied by twitchings or other movements of those limbs. Although the EEG did not show changes typical of epilepsy, he concluded the pain was a manifestation of epilepsy and he reported relief of pain with anticonvulsants.

Migraine

Apart from these paroxysmal post-hemiplegic pains, pain in the extremities following cerebrovascular accidents is usually persistent, though it may slowly subside and disappear with time. Episodic pain can, however, also arise in association with migraine, and limb pain including involvement of the hand is rarely appreciated but probably occurs more frequently than is usually recognised (Guiloff & Fruns 1988). The pain may be associated with ipsilateral weakness and other sensory symptoms, and is often ipsilateral to the headache. The phenomenon is more of interest in considering theories of central pain than as a problem in orthopaedic management.

Parkinson's disease

Compared with cerebrovascular disease, extrapyramidal disease is not so commonly associated with pain in the hand; indeed, logically, a disease until recently thought to be confined to these motor pathways would be painless. However, patients with Parkinson's disease may develop a frozen shoulder (Riley et al 1989), the shoulder–hand syndrome (Charcot 1868; Sicard 1921) and contractures of the fingers (Kyriakides & Langton Hewer 1988), as well as rather more non-specific cramps and pains in the limbs (Schott 1985). Indeed, up to 10% of patients with Parkinson's disease may complain of pain as their first symptom and such pain may involve the hand with neuralgic pains and painful finger spasms (Lees 1981).

Dystonia

Dystonic conditions also produce hand pain and are notoriously difficult to diagnose. It is not uncommon for patients to present to the orthopaedic surgeon with pain in the hand that has been attributed to ulnar or median nerve compression, thoracic outlet syndrome or cervical radiculopathy (Schott 1983). It is only when a careful history is obtained, and in particular the precipitating activities noted, that it becomes clear that the cause is some form of dystonia. Asking the patient to carry out the activity which causes pain reveals the bizarre posture that is the hallmark of these disorders, of which writer's cramp is a typical example (Sheehy & Marsden 1982). There are numerous other examples of such occupational dystonias affecting the hand, ranging from telegraphists' and typists' cramps to cramps induced by playing specific musical instruments (Lockwood 1989) or other activities such as throwing darts (for references, see Lees 1985). Since the accounts patients give appear so bizarre and signs are absent except when the specific activity is being carried out, there naturally is a tendency to view the complaint as one of hysteria. There is no doubt, however, that these curious conditions are organic, though the mechanisms remain unknown (see Sheehy & Marsden 1982). Pain appears to be due largely to mechanical factors related to muscle spasms and abnormal finger and hand posture. Treatment is often very unsatisfactory. Drugs such as anticholinergic agents and benzodiazepines, numerous physical and psychiatric methods of therapy, and more recently local injections of botulinum toxin (Cohen et al 1989) have all been tried, with unpredictable response; orthopaedic and other surgical measures on the limb are virtually always ineffective. Indeed, peripheral trauma may itself induce long-lasting involuntary movements and pain, perhaps through central mechanisms (Schott 1986a).

Cervical cord disease

Although unilateral pain in the hand suggests a contralateral focal aetiology, bilateral hand pain can occur from central causes, although it is rare for the origin to be in the cerebral hemispheres. Bilateral upper limb pain, however, is not uncommonly seen in spinal cord disease, usually from involvement of the dorsal root entry zones or intraspinal sensory pathways. Causes of cervical cord disease giving rise to hand pain include spinal compressive and ischaemic lesions (such as spondylitic spine disease, trauma and spinal tumour), inflammatory disorders (in particular, multiple sclerosis), and cavitating lesions of the cord (especially syringomyelia).

Cervical spondylosis and other compressive lesions

Hand pain due to disease of the spinal cord is most commonly due to cervical spondylosis. This degenerative condition increases with advancing age and is almost universal by the fifth decade, though fortunately neurological damage occurs less often. Those patients who do develop symptoms and signs are more likely to have one or more predisposing factor such as a congenitally narrow spinal canal, a history of previous cervical trauma when acute symptoms may develop, and bony anomalies such as the Klippel-Feil syndrome and Paget's disease; systemic atherosclerosis does not seem to be particularly relevant (Nurick 1975). Pain in the hand commonly occurs in association with cervical nerve root damage in the dermatome of the nerve segment involved, usually C6, C7, C8 or T1, although the precise area of pain within the hand that results from root involvement at a particular level is variable (Benini 1987).

The symptoms of cervical spondylosis are heterogeneous. The reason is that compression may be at one or several levels, can produce unilateral or bilateral symptoms and signs, can involve the spinal cord or spinal nerve roots, or both, and with varying degrees. Thus 'cervical spondylosis may simulate a number of other disorders of the spinal cord as well as of the brachial plexus and peripheral nerves of the upper limbs' (Brain et al 1952).

It is not always easy to localise the level of the lesion causing pain and other sensory disturbances in the hands. This is well illustrated in a report of hand pain due to lesions much higher in the cervical spine. Thus Good et al (1984) reported 13 patients with cervical spondylosis and high compressive myelopathy between C3 and C5. These patients presented with 'numb, clumsy hands' with loss of postural sense in the fingers; 6 of these patients had tingling and dysaesthesiae of the hands which were severe in 5; the legs were comparatively unaffected and neck symptoms were mild. Noteworthy is that in only 4 patients was a high cervical myelopathy suspected, the initial diagnosis having included peripheral neuropathy and carpal tunnel syndrome. Thus a benign and potentially treatable condition of the upper cervical spine can give rise to painful sensory disturbances in the hands, which might easily and erroneously be attributed to radicular or peripheral nerve involvement. (Similar inconsistency of localisation affecting the motor system has been reported, with weakness and wasting from denervation of the hands due to lesions far higher than the lower cervical and upper thoracic roots (Stark et al 1981; Alani 1985.) The condition of painful and numb hands is not diagnostic of a high spondylitic lesion. Similar symptoms can be due to high cervical or foramen magnum tumours (Symonds & Meadows 1937). Indeed, numbness and tingling in the hands and fingers were reported in 54 of 57 patients with tumours at the foramen magnum (Yasuoka et al 1978).

Radiological and neurophysiological investigations are required to delineate the contribution of central and peripheral factors, though clinical signs such as the presence of lower motor and sensory neuron features and focal reflex abnormalities will often provide helpful information in elucidating the problem. It is clear, however, that the mechanisms of pain due to spinal disease, both at segmental level and when the disorder is higher than might be anticipated, remain confusing. Recent studies using CT myelography have only partially clarified the anatomical and clinical features in the case of cervical spondylosis (Yu et al 1986). Thus the shape of the spondylitic deformity bears some relationship to symptomatology (for instance, lateral deformity of the cord often correlates with root signs), but radiculopathy can occur without cord deformity if the lesion is close to or inside the intervertebral foramen (analogous to sciatica from the lateral recess syndrome in the lumbar spine). It is also unclear why some individuals with severe spondylosis who sustain neck trauma never develop symptoms, whereas others who do develop pain have scant evidence of spondylosis.

An important issue that has been considered extensively is the role of spinal cord ischaemia. Factors in favour of an ischaemic component include those patients who fail to improve as might be expected after decompressive surgery, and the effects of obstruction of thin walled veins which drain upwards from the lower to the higher cervical region. The latter may be of particular relevance, since venous obstruction from whatever cause might result in hypoxia at a lower level, accounting for symptoms in the hands when the lesion is several segments higher. Evidence from animal experiments tends to confirm this 'distant' hypoxia and might lend support for the concept of cord compression giving rise to impairment of the microcirculation of the cord at the same or lower levels (Taylor & Byrnes 1974). Detracting from the ischaemic component and favouring a mechanical compressive aetiology, however, are some of the factors referred to above: the increased incidence of spondylitic changes in individuals with a narrow spinal canal, the effects of movement of the cervical spine which may occur with trauma, and the benefit of decompressive surgery – although these features do not exclude an ischaemic component as well.

Treatment of pain in the hand due to cervical spondylitic myelopathy and cervical root irritation is controversial; in particular, the indications for surgical intervention are a source of continuing discussion. Much of the problem in assessing the place of any particular treatment (conservative or surgical) is due to the paucity of information on natural history, the mixture of radicular and myelopathic features, the often small surgical series describing numerous types of procedures, and sometimes inadequately described clinical features and limited follow-up studies. These problems and the contribution of surgical management of cervical spondylosis have been critically assessed by Monro (1984). She concludes that surgery has a limited role in the management of radiculopathy, the results of surgery for myelopathy are inconsistent and there is a lack of uniformity of opinion. Indeed, the same problems confront the assessment of simple measures such as the benefits of a variety of physiotherapy procedures (British Association of Physical Medicine 1966) and even the use of a collar (Huston 1988).

Spinal tumour

The features encountered in cervical spondylosis may closely resemble those due to spinal tumour. Indeed pain has been described as a constant symptom of spinal tumours, often exacerbated by coughing and sneezing and worse at night (Moersch et al 1951). Pain may be due to involvement of the neck and spine, of the cord, or of the spinal nerve roots, and thus pain in the hand may be mistakenly attributed to a cause such as cervical spondylosis, especially since the signs may be minimal (Moersch et al 1951). Mistaken diagnosis is well recognised, and conditions such as disc disease, 'fibrositis', syringomyelia and multiple sclerosis have been confused with a spinal tumour (Bloom et al 1955), and inappropriate surgery for conditions such as carpal tunnel compression has been undertaken. The presence of pain in particular, including pain in the upper limb and hand, requires appropriate investigation, and delineation of a suspected spinal tumour calls for the opinion of an appropriate specialist.

Spinal trauma

Trauma affecting the cervical spine, particularly with hyperextension and flexion injuries, may give rise to severe pain in the upper limbs, including the hand. The typical picture is associated with weakness greater in the upper than lower limbs, variable sensory loss and urinary retention, suggesting damage to the centre of the spinal cord. The symptoms usually occur very acutely, and the pain has been sufficiently severe in the early stages to raise the possibility of upper limb fractures. The pain may later change to hyperpathia, usually then subsiding over some weeks, although sometimes residual hypoalgesia and parasthesiae in the fingers may persist. The cause may be due to damage of the spinothalamic tracts and their decussation (Hopkins & Rudge 1973). In addition, persistent dysaesthesiae may develop, with an incidence estimated at from 11–94%; these sensory disturbances may affect the hands if the injury is sufficiently high, and result in severe incapacity (Davidoff et al 1987).

Syringomyelia

Of particular relevance to orthopaedic surgeons because of the various orthopaedic problems that may occur, syringomyelia is an important although rare condition and may produce severe pain. Although classically associated with analgesia in the hands from spinothalamic dysfunction, and hence problems such as painless burns, the reverse situation may obtain, and severe pain which often affects the neck, shoulders and upper limbs including the hands can occur. Indeed, pain is the commonest and sometimes much the earliest symptom, and various orthopaedic procedures such as carpal tunnel decompression and other operations at the wrist and thoracic outlet have been erroneously carried out for this condition (Williams 1979). Also noteworthy is that Charcot's joints, of which syringomyelia is a well-known cause, often involve the upper limbs and, at least before the advent of sophisticated methods of investigations led to early treatment, these joints were very often painful.

The mechanism of pain in syringomyelia is probably complex, and could arise from involvement of the spinal cord and nerve roots, associated joint disease, and anomalies such as cerebellar ectopia. In the past, the clinical features were thought to be dependent upon the anatomy and dimensions of the intraspinal cyst cavity, at least in respect of spinal cord dysfunction. However, MRI scanning has recently enabled localisation of the intramedullary cyst to be assessed more precisely (and non-invasively), and no significant relationship between the clinical features and dimensions of the syrinx has been found (Grant et al 1987). Thus the mechanism of the clinical features including the pain of syringomyelia, as well as the role of surgery, needs to be reconsidered. Treatment of syringomyelia falls within the province of the neurosurgeon. With regard to pain, syringoperitoneal shunting has been described as a useful therapeutic procedure; thus of 29 patients with syringomyelia reported in a recent series, 19 experienced pain in the neck, shoulder and upper limbs and 14 were improved with surgery (Suzuki et al 1985).

Multiple sclerosis

The final cause of cervical cord disease giving rise to hand pain to be discussed is that due to multiple sclerosis. This condition can obviously affect numerous areas of the central nervous system, and so it is rarely if ever possible to ascertain with certainty that a specific symptom is due to a single site of neural damage. Pain due to multiple sclerosis is usually apparent because of the clinical accompaniments, i.e. a history of relapsing and remitting neurological episodes and evidence of widespread cerebral and spinal involvement. The frequency of pain in multiple sclerosis is perhaps around 30% of patients, but it is impossible to ascertain both its true frequency and the frequency of involvement of a particular body part such as the hand (Clifford & Trotter 1984). Pain can occur through involvement of many different structures at many different sites, e.g. ascending sensory pathways in the spinal cord and brain, and dorsal root entry zones in the spinal cord. A variety of different types of pain may also be encountered, such as burning extremity pain, non-specific limb pain, painful extremity spasms, myalgia and cramps, and electric shock-like pains. Occasionally the pain may be radicular, and secondary changes due to abnormal posture, gait and joint abnormalities can all lead to pains that are additional to those due specifically to neural involvement from multiple sclerosis. Of the numerous methods of treatment that have been tried, antidepressant drugs have proven perhaps the most beneficial.

Peripheral disorders with a central component

There are at least 3 predominantly peripheral conditions in which a central component can co-exist and contribute to pain in the hand: brachial plexus injuries; malignant infiltration with and without sequelae of irradiation affecting the supraclavicular region; and herpes zoster affecting the lower cervical and upper thoracic roots. In each of these conditions, it may be difficult to delineate the degree of involvement of the nerve roots and trunk from spinal cord involvement.

Brachial plexus injuries

Pain in the hand due to brachial plexus injury is most often a result of damage to the preganglionic fibres (for review, see Wynn Parry 1980). Pain is usually severe, and is often permanent. This subject is dealt with elsewhere in this volume (see Ch. 6).

Malignancy and radiation damage of the brachial plexus

Pain in the hand due to malignant disease affecting the brachial plexus is often painful, and the most common underlying tumours are carcinoma of the breast and of the lung. When the lower trunk is involved, pain occurs along the inner aspect of the forearm and hand and this may be a very prominent feature; there are likely to be other features of C7, 8 and T1 root involvement. Sometimes, however, pain may be generated centrally when there is spread of malignancy through the intervertebral foramen, affecting not only the nerve roots but also causing spinal cord damage. There may be bony involvement as well, with destructive changes of the cervical spine evident even on plain radiographs. In some centres, myelography is carried out if metastatic plexopathy is suspected, but CT and MRI scanning may provide more detailed information non-invasively.

A common dilemma arises in the patient with pain in the hand and other features of root or plexus involvement or spinal cord involvement, who has had previous irradiation. Irradiation too can cause damage to the plexus, roots and spinal cord, and pain due to this cause would be a contraindication to further radiotherapy. Irradiation usually involves the upper trunk (C5, 6 and C7 roots), thus tending to cause hand pain less often. Features said to suggest malignant infiltration rather than irradiation are pain that is severe, hand weakness and a Horner's syndrome (Kori et al 1981). Other authors, however, report different experiences, and Thomas and Colby (1978) have stated, 'no single clinical symptom or sign permitted distinction between the two groups'. Unfortunately, a latency of well over 10 years can occur before pain from tumour recurrence appears, and so no time interval seems sufficiently long to preclude the onset of recurrence. Even if surgery is undertaken for intradural tumour extension or for biopsy of the plexus, it is unlikely to help pain.

The indications for surgery when irradiation damage is present remain controversial. Surgery can be considered at the earliest sign of neurological damage and should be viewed as a prophylactic measure to prevent further neurological damage; once pain has developed, however, the results of surgery are extremely disappointing (LeQuang 1989). At present few surgeons operate for post-irradiation brachial plexus lesions, and as with pain from malignant infiltration, conservative measures for pain relief are first required, such as transcutaneous electric nerve stimulation and sympathetic blockade; unfortunately, pain often continues unabated, and more radical forms of treatment such as root section, lesioning of the dorsal root entry zones, and cordotomy may be considered as part of the overall management of the patient with cancer (Foley 1985).

Post-herpetic neuralgia

Post-herpetic neuralgia is a painful condition that may be a sequel to localised herpes zoster infection (shingles) (for review, see Loeser 1986). The virus attacks the dorsal root ganglion, leading to nerve involvement at that segment, and there is involvement peripherally so that the whole length of the nerve and skin innervated by that nerve are affected, and there is central involvement so that the dorsal root and segment of spinal cord are involved as well. Following the acute infection, pain may continue, the development of prolonged pain (post-herpetic neuralgia) being largely a factor of age, with increasing incidence of persistent pain with advancing age. Although the dermatomes innervating the hand are comparatively infrequently involved, pain when it affects the hand may be due to the neuralgia itself, or to complicating factors such as the shoulder–hand or similar trophic sequelae, a phenomenon described over a century ago by Paget (1864).

The cause of the pain itself is uncertain. There is no doubt that haemorrhage and inflammatory changes occur in the dorsal root ganglion, following which nerve fibre damage occurs, but this is unselective, and there is no relationship between the histological appearance of the nerve and the presence of pain. It may well be, therefore, that the pain is due to central factors, including deafferentation. Studies of selected neurotransmittors in the segment of affected spinal cord have not been revealing (Watson et al 1988). Thus the contributions of the damaged spinal cord and the damaged peripheral nerve remain unclear, as does the precise mechanism of the pain. Also unsatisfactory is the poor response of post-herpetic neuralgia to treatment; of the numerous methods tried over several decades, only transcutaneous electric nerve stimulation, tricyclic antidepressant drugs and perhaps nerve blocks have stood the test of time.

The possibility that post-herpetic neuralgia can be prevented by treatment during the initial shingles infection remains unresolved: the use of steroids, sympathetic blockade and anti-viral agents such as acyclovir (with or without additional prednisolone) have been the most common methods tried, but extensive controlled trials are not available (for review see Jolleys 1989). For especially susceptible people, prophylactic vaccination against varicella infection may be a development of the future (Gershon 1987).

Miscellaneous conditions

Shoulder–hand syndrome

The shoulder–hand syndrome, a form of reflex sympathetic dystrophy (Doury et al 1981; Schwartzman & McLellan 1987), comprises pain and stiffness in the shoulder and pain in the ipsilateral hand. The pain is often burning, and may be accompanied by hyperpathia, thus merging with the more severe form of the condition, causalgia. This is further suggested by the trophic changes in the hand seen both in patients with the shoulder–hand syndrome and those with causalgia. The term shoulder–hand syndrome was first employed by Steinbrocker in 1947, in a paper with the title *The shoulder–hand syndrome. Associated painful homolateral disability of the shoulder and hand with swelling and atrophy of the hand*. By the following year he had recognised the condition as occurring also as a sequel to diseases of the central nervous system; of 42 cases described, 5 were associated with hemiplegia, 2 with post-herpetic neuralgia and 2 with cervical osteoarthritis (Steinbrocker et al 1948). In 1958 he summarised his experience (Steinbrocker & Argyros 1958), and identified 3 phases of the condition: initially a form of pseudo-inflammatory change lasting 3–6 months, then a similar period of partial or complete resolution, possibly with early trophic changes and beginning of contractures in the fingers, and finally atrophic or dystrophic changes with alteration of the soft tissues, contractures and 'frozen' fingers in partial flexion with demineralisation. These trophic changes in the hands, often with the radiological changes of osteoporosis of Sudeck (1900), are very similar to those seen in causalgia. The shoulder–hand syndrome may involve the elbow as well, as a tripartite disorder, and the syndrome may be bilateral. Even if clinically unilateral, investigation may reveal evidence of contralateral involvement, as indicated by isotope bone scanning and thermography (for references, see Schott 1986b). Moreover, bilateral involvement may be consecutive rather than simultaneous, and occasionally just both hands are involved.

The condition is poorly understood, not least because of the circumstances in which it can arise. Apart from occurring in association with peripheral damage to the limb, immobilisation and various systemic disorders such as after myocardial infarction, the shoulder–hand syndrome can occur in association with diseases of the central nervous system as mentioned above (e.g. Steinbrocker et al 1948; Rosen & Graham 1957; Steinbrocker & Argyros 1958; Thompson 1961). Such diseases include hemiplegia (Swan 1954; Moskowitz et al 1958; Eto et al 1980), in which the syndrome is said to occur in about 12% of cases (Davis et al 1977), also epilepsy, cerebral tumour (Vaernet 1952), spinal cord disease such as trauma (Wainapel 1984), following herpes zoster (Paget 1864; Richardson 1954; Graudal 1959), and use of anticonvulsant drugs, in particular phenobarbitone (Korst et al 1966). The frequency of the shoulder–hand syndrome in patients with cerebral tumours has been reported to be as high as 5%, and no less than 12% of the patients were receiving phenobarbitone (but not other anticonvulsants) (Taylor & Posner 1989). The condition may also occur with degenerative cervical spine disease, and whether it then occurs as a result of cord or root damage is uncertain; it was present in 20% of Steinbrocker's 146 cases reported in 1958.

The aetiology of this condition is not understood. The presence of pain which is often burning with hyperpathia, together with trophic features, the lack of significant motor, sensory or reflex changes or of any inflammatory disturbance indicates the likelihood that it is a form of causalgia. The evidence that such conditions are due to dysfunction of the central nervous system has been summarised elsewhere (Schott 1986b), and of course the fact that the shoulder–hand syndrome can occur in diseases strictly localised to the central nervous system lends support to central mechanisms being important. Indeed, the involvement of the central nervous system was suggested over a century ago (Brown-Séquard 1861). From a study of 7 cases of post-hemiplegic shoulder–hand syndrome for which autopsy evidence was available, there is evidence that involvement of the pre-motor cortex may be important in the generation of this syndrome when it follows strokes (Eto et al 1980). It may be that central sympathetic pathways are involved, a concept that would be supported by the best form of treatment, which is probably with sympathetic blockade. This can be carried out by stellate ganglion blockade performed in a number of ways, or by peripheral regional intravenous guanethidine infusion (for references, see Schott 1986b; Schwartzman & McLellan 1987). It should be noted that these techniques may be valuable, even when the lesion giving rise to the shoulder–hand syndrome is central, and proximal to the sympathectomised part (Loh et al 1981). If the hand can be made comfortable or pain free, vigorous physiotherapy then needs to be undertaken to the hand and if possible the shoulder, although the shoulder pain may not respond so readily as pain in the hand. It should be noted that steroids have also been used for decades, and Steinbrocker (Steinbrocker & Argyros 1958) has even questioned whether these are more effective than sympathetic blockade; good controlled studies are not available, and treatment inevitably tends to be given when dysfunction of the hand is already long standing. Prevention is therefore important, avoiding casts, splints and excessive manipulation, and encouragement of gentle graduated exercise and possibly injection of local anaesthetic into trigger points. Treatment with sympathetic blockade and steroids may lead to improvement in a third of cases, with moderate benefit in a half of cases, but it is not possible to give precise figures of response to treatment in this condition. Indeed, the large variety of treatments which have been tried with variable and unpredictable results indicates that treatment is often far from successful.

Phantom and referred pains

There can be few more curious causes of pain in medicine than that due to a phantom (Riddoch 1941; for review, see Sunderland 1978). Five to 10% of patients in whom a part of the body has been amputated, whether through trauma or through surgical intervention, experience pain in the non-existent part. It is commoner in the upper than the lower limb, and is mainly experienced in the periphery. Thus the hand is quite often affected, and pain is then referred particularly to the wrist, palm, knuckles and fingertips, and if a part has been removed for pain, continuing pain may be experienced where the initial pain was felt. Experience of a phantom of the missing part may not be painful, but often pain is a major feature, and it may be continuous, although with exacerbations; such exacerbations may occur spontaneously, or with percussion or other stimuli applied to the stump, or more generalised factors such as stress, fatigue, micturition and defaecation, or attempted movement of the phantom fingers. The phantom and phantom pain may be permanent, and the phantom phenomenon will not disappear unless the pain disappears. The phantom then tends slowly to shrink proximally (telescoping) until the hand or fingers are tucked up into the stump. Phantom phenomena in children, though described, are rare, and even more rare in congenital amputations (Weinstein & Sersen 1961).

The origin of the phantom phenomenon and phantom pain is unclear. Although an extensive mythology has grown up about this perplexing condition (Price & Twombly 1976), it is not a psychological disorder, and both central and peripheral factors have been considered important in its aetiology (British Medical Journal Editorial 1978). Though numerous methods of treatment have been employed, few treatment methods are even moderately successful (Sherman et al 1980).

Referred pain is a fascinating subject which has been studied for over a century. Pain, usually from a viscus, is felt in a more superficial and often remote site from its origin. With regard to pain in the hand, the most common referred pain is from the heart, and anginal pain referred down into the left (and less often right) arm and hand has been recognised frequently ever since the report by Sturge in 1883. Whilst the processes involved in referred pain have not been established, the phenomenon must involve central pathways probably in the spinal cord, perhaps through convergence mechanisms; it may be that long-standing focal abnormalities within the central nervous system can also be generated, which could be the basis for disorders such as the shoulder–hand syndrome following myocardial infarction referred to above (for review, see Procacci et al 1986).

Surely one of the most bizarre phenomena in clinical medicine must be the phantom arm and hand pain induced by angina (Cohen & Jones 1943)? Here a referred pain (angina felt in the upper limb) is appreciated in the non-existent limb that had been amputated many years previously. Transient recurrence of phantom left arm pain associated with herpes zoster affecting the left T2 dermatome has also been described (Wilson et al 1978).

MECHANISMS

Why and how disease of the central system can cause pain remain unknown, as has been pointed out repeatedly above. This is particularly tantalising because manipulation of the brain itself does not cause pain. It should also be emphasised that a rigid distinction between peripheral and central nervous disease is inappropriate, since diseases of the periphery also have major clinical, electrophysiological and chemical effects on the central nervous system. Moreover, the periphery influences central pain: for instance, local anaesthetic blocks of a limb or epidural anaesthesia may temporarily abolish central pain (Kibler & Nathan 1960), and a range of pain relieving measures including sympathetic blockade can be applied to the periphery, even when the cause of the pain lies centrally (Loh et al 1981). Furthermore, it may be that more than one disease occurring at the same time can cause summation of effects. This can certainly occur in the more peripheral nervous system; for instance, patients with carpal tunnel syndrome have a greater prevalence of lateral humeral epicondylitis, and a tendency to smaller cervical spine dimensions (Murray-Leslie & Wright 1976). The concept of double crush lesions in the peripheral nervous system has been considered by Upton & McComas (1973) but whether this could apply to the central nervous system is unknown.

Those parts of the central nervous system which are especially liable to cause pain when damaged have been mentioned above. It is damage to the grey matter which particularly tends to cause pain, for instance the posteroventrolateral nucleus of the thalamus in the thalamic syndrome, and the dorsal horn and central regions of the cord in spinal cord disease.

The pathophysiological mechanisms include a number of possible processes, any or all of which could be relevant (for review, see Cervero 1986). It is perhaps useful conceptually to consider that either excessive neural activity, or reduction of inhibition, could each give rise to pain.

1. Irritative or epileptic mechanisms: it could be postulated that an irritable focus, analogous to an epileptic focus, in damaged sensory pathways could give rise to pain. Recording from the midbrain, firing of neurons coinciding with paroxysms of pain in trigeminal neuralgia has been demonstrated in man (Nashold & Wilson 1966), and spontaneous activity on sampling single neurons in the human spinal cord just cranial to the damaged level in traumatic paraplegia has also been recorded (Loeser et al 1968). Anticonvulsant drugs have often been tried, unfortunately often with only limited benefit, but the fact that they sometimes work might support this hypothesis.

2. Inhibition: the realisation that inhibitory pathways are likely to be critical in modulating and preventing pain came late to the study of pain mechanisms. The two crucial observations were: first, the observation by Reynolds (1969) that (contrary to one's pre-conceptions) stimulation of the deep grey matter of a rat's brain allowed surgery on the abdomen and other painful procedures to be carried out apparently painlessly without anaesthesia; second, the demonstration that the central nervous system itself contained substances with potential analgesic properties (Hughes et al 1975). There is now considerable clinical evidence that stimulation of large fibres may inhibit the activity of pain-subserving fibres, as shown by methods such as rubbing, acupuncture and transcutaneous electric nerve stimulation. In the central nervous system, certain major descending pathways appear to inhibit the development of pain, pathways which can also be activated therapeutically, either chemically or physiologically (for review, see Basbaum & Fields 1984). The anatomical and physiological nature of these pathways has been studied extensively, though it is unclear whether damage to inhibitory pathways allows pain-subserving systems to act unopposed and hence result in the experience of pain.

TREATMENT

It should be realised that despite these major scientific developments, patients with central pain cannot easily be rendered pain free. Indeed, patients with central pain are still treated with relatively few, well tried substances and procedures. Throughout this chapter mention has been made of methods of treatment, but chronic pain due to lesions of the central nervous system often remains intractable and at best may only be improved. It is against this background that numerous destructive procedures on sensory pathways carried out from the periphery to cortex were tried in the past with generally poor long-term results. Such procedures have therefore now largely been abandoned (except for treatment for pain from malignant disease), and there has been a return to more conservative methods of treatment.

1. Drugs: these have included simple analgesics, phenothiazines, antidepressants (e.g. amitriptyline and L-tryptophan), anticonvulsants (e.g. carbamazepine, phenytoin and sodium valproate), antihistamines, anti-inflammatory drugs and numerous other drugs of a more speculative nature (e.g. naloxone, D-phenylalanine, anticholinesterases, steroids and calcitonin).

2. Procedures which block the sympathetic system: whilst these procedures are standard therapy for pain with a causalgic quality, including the shoulder–hand syndrome and other examples of reflex sympathetic dystrophy, they are often tried empirically in other conditions. For hand pain, block of the stellate ganglion may be carried out, as may peripheral chemical blockade with regional guanethidine using Bier's block, first described by Hannington-Kiff (1974). Occasionally dramatic relief of pain can occur, and generally a number of blocks are carried out. Few controlled trials, however, have been reported, and so most reports of benefit, whilst valid, remain anecdotal.

3. Stimulation procedures: these have generally replaced the former destructive procedures, and such stimulation techniques include intracerebral stimulation of the deep grey matter and dorsal column spinal stimulation, as well as stimulation of the periphery with transcutaneous electric nerve stimulation and acupuncture. The results in central pain are often far from satisfactory.

4. Peripheral destructive methods: these have become more refined, and dorsal root entry zone (DREZ) lesioning developed by Nashold has been employed particularly in deafferentation pain

(Nashold et al 1983). It is a neurosurgical technique not without hazard, but sometimes pain may be relieved even if central in origin.

5. Treatments using physical and psychological methods: these include various physiotherapy manoeuvres, attempts to return patients to useful work, psychological and psychiatric intervention and behavioural approaches. Such methods are often used in combination with drug and surgical treatments.

The therapy of pain is a very extensive and constantly developing subject. The reader is referred to textbooks (e.g. Swerdlow 1986) on the subject for details of techniques, discussion and references on this essential topic, which is the most important, if not the only, concern for the patient with pain.

REFERENCES

Alani S M 1985 Denervation in wasted hand muscles in a case of primary cerebellar ectopia without syringomyelia. Journal of Neurology, Neurosurgery and Psychiatry 48: 84–85

Basbaum A I, Fields H L 1984 Endogenous pain control systems: brainstem spinal pathways and endorphin circuitry. Annual Review of Neuroscience 7: 309–338

Benini A 1987 Clinical features of cervical root compression C5–C8 and their variations. Neuro-Orthopedics 4: 74–88

Bloom H J G, Ellis H, Jennett W B 1955 The early diagnosis of spinal tumours. British Medical Journal 1: 10–16

Brain W R, Northfield D, Wilkinson M 1952 The neurological manifestations of cervical spondylosis. Brain 75: 187–225

British Association of Physical Medicine 1966 Pain in the neck and arm: a multicentre trial of the effects of physiotherapy. British Medical Journal 1: 253–258

British Medical Journal Editorial 1978 Phantom limb pain. British Medical Journal 2: 1588–1589

Bromm B 1985 Evoked cerebral potential and pain. In: Fields H L, Dubner R, Cervero F (eds) Advances in pain research and therapy, vol. 9. Raven, New York, pp 305–329

Brown-Séquard C E 1861 Lectures on the diagnosis and treatment of the various forms of paralytic, convulsive, and mental affections, considered as effects of morbid alterations of the blood, or of the brain or other organs. Lancet 2: 29–30

Cassinari V, Pagni C A 1969 Central pain. Harvard University Press, Cambridge

Cervero F 1986 Neurophysiological aspects of pain and pain therapy. In: Swerdlow M (ed) The therapy of pain, 2nd edn. MTP, Lancaster, pp 1–29

Charcot J-M 1868 Sur quelques arthropathies qui paraissent dépendre d'une lésion du cerveau ou de la moelle épinière. Archives de Physiologie 1: 161–178; 379–400

Clifford D B, Trotter J L 1984 Pain in multiple sclerosis. Archives of Neurology 41: 1270–1272

Cohen H, Jones H W 1943 The reference of cardiac pain to a phantom left arm. British Heart Journal 5: 67–71

Cohen L G, Hallett M, Geller B D, Hochberg F 1989 Treatment of focal dystonias of the hand with botulinum toxin injections. Journal of Neurology, Neurosurgery and Psychiatry 52: 355–363

Davidoff G, Roth E, Guarracini M, Sliwa J, Yarkony G 1987 Function-limiting dysesthetic pain syndrome among traumatic spinal cord injury patients: a cross-sectional study. Pain 29: 39–48

Davis S W, Petrillo C R, Eichberg R D, Chu D S 1977 Shoulder-hand syndrome in a hemiplegic population: a 5-year retrospective study. Archives of Physical Medicine and Rehabilitation 58: 353–356

Dejerine J, Roussy G 1906 Le syndrome thalamique. Revue Neurologique 14: 521–532

Doury P, Dirheimer Y, Pattin S 1981 Algodystrophy. Springer, Berlin

Eto F, Yoshikawa M, Ueda S, Hirai S 1980 Posthemiplegic shoulder-hand syndrome, with special reference to related cerebral localization. Journal of the American Geriatrics Society 28: 13–17

Fine W 1967 Post-hemiplegic epilepsy in the elderly. British Medical Journal 1: 199–201

Foley K M 1985 The treatment of cancer pain. New England Journal of Medicine 313: 84–95

Gershon A A 1987 Live attenuated varicella vaccine. Annual Reviews of Medicine 38: 41–50

Good D C, Couch J R, Wacaser L 1984 'Numb, clumsy hands' and high cervical spondylosis. Surgical Neurology 22: 285–291

Grant R, Hadley D M, Macpherson P et al 1987 Syringomyelia: cyst measurement by magnetic resonance imaging and comparison with symptoms, signs and disability. Journal of Neurology, Neurosurgery and Psychiatry 50: 1008–1014

Graudal H 1959 Shoulder-hand syndrome and herpes zoster. Acta Rheumatologica Scandinavica 5: 157–163

Guiloff R J, Fruns M 1988 Limb pain in migraine and cluster headache. Journal of Neurology, Neurosurgery and Psychiatry 51: 1022–1031

Hannington-Kiff J G 1974 Intravenous regional sympathetic block with guanethidine. Lancet 1: 1019–1020

Hopkins A, Rudge P 1973 Hyperpathia in the central cervical cord syndrome. Journal of Neurology, Neurosurgery and Psychiatry 36: 637–642

Hughes J, Smith T W, Kosterlitz H W, Fothergill L A, Morgan B A, Morris H R 1975 Identification of two related pentapeptides from the brain with potent opiate agonist activity. Nature 258: 577–579

Huston G J 1988 Collars and corsets. British Medical Journal 296: 27

Jolleys J V 1989 Treatment of shingles and post-herpetic neuralgia. British Medical Journal 298: 1537–1538

Kibler R F, Nathan P W 1960 Relief of pain and

paraesthesiae by nerve block distal to a lesion. Journal of Neurology, Neurosurgery and Psychiatry 23: 91–98

Kori S H, Foley K M, Posner J B 1981 Brachial plexus lesions in patients with cancer: 100 cases. Neurology 31: 45–50

Korst J K van der, Colenbrander H, Cats A 1966 Phenobarbital and the shoulder-hand syndrome. Annals of the Rheumatic Diseases 25: 553–555

Kyriakides T, Langton Hewer R 1988 Hand contractures in Parkinson's disease. Journal of Neurology, Neurosurgery and Psychiatry 51: 1221–1223

Lancet Editorial 1985 Diagnosis of the carpal tunnel syndrome. Lancet 1: 854–855

Lees A J 1981 Early diagnosis of Parkinson's disease. British Journal of Hospital Medicine 26: 511–518

Lees A J 1985 Tics and Related Disorders. Churchill Livingstone, Edinburgh, pp 157–171

Leijon G, Boivie J, Johansson I 1989 Central post-stroke pain – neurological symptoms and pain characteristics. Pain 36: 13–25

LeQuang C 1989 Postirradiation lesions of the brachial plexus. Results of surgical treatment. Hand Clinics 5: 23–32

Lockwood A H 1989 Medical problems of musicians. New England Journal of Medicine 320: 221–227

Loeser J D 1986 Herpes zoster and postherpetic neuralgia. Pain 25: 149–1

Loeser J D, Ward A A, White L E 1968 Chronic deafferentation of human spinal cord neurons. Journal of Neurosurgery 29: 48–50

Loh L, Nathan P W, Schott G D 1981 Pain due to lesions of central nervous system removed by sympathetic block. British Medical Journal 282: 1026–1028

Mauguière F, Desmedt J E 1988 Thalamic pain syndrome of Dejerine-Roussy. Differentiation of four subtypes assisted by somatosensory evoked potentials data. Archives of Neurology 45: 1312–1320

Moersch F P, Craig W McK, Christoferson L A 1951 Spinal cord tumors with minimal neurologic findings. Neurology 1: 39–47

Monro P 1984 What has surgery to offer in cervical spondylosis? In: Warlow C, Garfield J (eds) Dilemmas in the management of the neurological patient. Churchill Livingstone, Edinburgh, pp 168–187

Moskowitz E, Bishop H F, Pe H, Shibutani K 1958 Posthemiplegic reflex sympathetic dystrophy. Journal of the American Medical Association 167: 836–838

Murray-Leslie C F, Wright V 1976 Carpal tunnel syndrome, humeral epicondylitis, and the cervical spine: a study of clinical and dimensional relations. British Medical Journal 1: 1439–1442

Nashold B S, Wilson W P 1966 Central pain. Observations in man with chronic implanted electrodes in the midbrain tegmentum. Confinia Neurologia 27: 30–44

Nashold B S, Ostdahl R H, Bullitt E, Friedman A, Brophy B 1983 Dorsal root entry zone lesions: a new neurosurgical therapy for deafferentation pain. Advances in Pain Research and Therapy 5: 739–750

Nurick S 1975 The cervical spine and paraplegia. In: Williams D (ed) Modern trends in neurology – 6. Butterworth, London, pp 167–182

Paget J 1864 Clinical lectures on some cases of local paralysis. Medical Times and Gazette 1: 331–332

Price D B, Twombly N J 1976 The phantom limb phenomenon. A medical, folkloric, and historical study. Georgetown University Press, Washington

Procacci P, Zoppi M, Maresca M 1986 Clinical approach to visceral sensation. Progress in Brain Research 67: 21–28

Reynolds D V (1969) Surgery in the rat during electrical analgesia induced by focal brain stimulation. Science 164: 444–445

Richardson A T 1954 Shoulder-hand syndrome following herpes zoster. Annals of Physical Medicine 2: 132–134

Riddoch G 1938 The clinical features of central pain. Lancet 1: 1093–1098; 1150–1156; 1205–1209

Riddoch G 1941 Phantom limbs and body shape. Brain 64: 197–222

Riley D, Lang A E, Blair R D G, Birnbaum A, Reid B 1989 Frozen shoulder and other shoulder disturbances in Parkinson's disease. Journal of Neurology, Neurosurgery and Psychiatry 52: 63–66

Rosen P S, Graham W 1957 The shoulder-hand syndrome: historical review with observations on seventy-three patients. Canadian Medical Association Journal 77: 86–91

Schott G D 1983 The idiopathic dystonias. A note on their orthopaedic presentation. Journal of Bone and Joint Surgery 65B: 51–54

Schott G D 1985 Pain in Parkinson's disease. Pain 22: 407–411

Schott G D 1986a Induction of involuntary movements by peripheral trauma: an analogy with causalgia. Lancet 2: 712–716

Schott G D 1986b Mechanisms of causalgia and related clinical conditions. Brain 109: 717–738

Schwartzman R J, McLellan T L 1987 Reflex sympathetic dystrophy. A review. Archives of Neurology 44: 555–561

Sheehy M P, Marsden C D 1982 Writers' cramp – a focal dystonia. Brain 105: 461–480

Sherman R A, Sherman C J, Gall N G 1980 A survey of current phantom limb pain treatment in the United States. Pain 8: 85–99

Sicard J-A 1921 Parkinsonisme et rhumatisme chronique. Revue Neurologique 28: 682–683

Stark R J, Kennard C, Swash M 1981 Hand wasting in spondylitic high cord compression: an electromyographic study. Annals of Neurology 9: 58–62

Steinbrocker O 1947 The shoulder-hand syndrome. Associated painful homolateral disability of the shoulder and hand with swelling and atrophy of the hand. American Journal of Medicine 3: 402–407

Steinbrocker O, Argyros T G 1958 The shoulder-hand syndrome: present status as a diagnostic and therapeutic entity. The Medical Clinics of North America 42: 1533–1553

Steinbrocker O, Spitzer N, Friedman H H 1948 The shoulder-hand syndrome in reflex sympathetic dystrophy of the upper extremity. Annals of Internal Medicine 29: 22–52

Sturge W A 1883 The phenomena of angina pectoris, and their bearing upon the theory of counter-irritation. Brain 5: 492–510

Sudeck P 1900 Uber die akute entzundliche Knochenatrophie. Archiv fur Klinische Chirurgie 62: 147–156

Sunderland S 1978 Nerve and nerve injuries, 2nd edn. Churchill Livingstone, Edinburgh, pp 424–458

Suzuki M, Davis C, Symon L, Gentili F 1985 Syringoperitoneal shunt for treatment of cord cavitation.

Journal of Neurology, Neurosurgery and Psychiatry 48: 620–627

Symonds C P, Meadows S P 1937 Compression of the spinal cord in the neighbourhood of the foramen magnum. Brain 60: 52–84

Swan D M 1954 Shoulder-hand syndrome following hemiplegia. Neurology 4: 480–482

Swerdlow M (ed) 1986 The therapy of pain, 2nd edn. MTP, Lancaster

Taylor A R, Byrnes D P 1974 Foramen magnum and high cervical cord compression. Brain 97: 473–480

Taylor L P, Posner J B 1989 Phenobarbital rheumatism in patients with brain tumor. Annals of Neurology 25: 92–94

Thomas J E, Colby M Y 1978 Radiation-induced or metastatic brachial plexopathy? Journal of the American Medical Association 222: 1392–1395

Thompson M 1961 Shoulder-hand syndrome. Proceedings of the Royal Society of Medicine 54: 679–681

Upton A R M, McComas A J 1973 The double crush in nerve-entrapment syndromes. Lancet 2: 359–362

Vaernet K 1952 2 cases of shoulder-hand syndrome in meningioma affecting the premotor region. Acta Psychiatrica et Neurologica Scandinavica 27: 201–209

Valzelli L 1987 About the cheiro-oral syndrome. Neurology 37: 1564–1565

Wainapel S F 1984 Reflex sympathetic dystrophy following traumatic myelopathy. Pain 18: 345–349

Watson C P N, Morshead C, Van der Kooy D, Deck J, Evans R J 1988 Post-herpetic neuralgia: post-mortem analysis of a case. Pain 34: 129–138

Weinstein S, Sersen E A 1961 Phantoms in cases of congenital absence of limbs. Neurology 11: 905–911

Williams B 1979 Orthopaedic features in the presentation of syringomyelia. Journal of Bone and Joint Surgery 61B: 314–323

Wilson P R, Person J R, Su D W, Wang J K 1978 Herpes zoster reactivation of phantom limb pain. Mayo Clinic Proceedings 53: 336–338

Wynn Parry C B 1980 Pain in avulsion lesions of the brachial plexus. Pain 9: 41–53

Yasuoka S, Okazaki H, Daube J R, MacCarty C S 1978 Foramen magnum tumors. Analysis of 57 cases of benign extramedullary tumors. Journal of Neurosurgery 49: 828–838

Young G B, Blume W T 1983 Painful epileptic seizures. Brain 106: 537–554

Yu Y L, Du Boulay G H, Stevens J M, Kendall B E 1986 Computer-assisted myelography in cervical spondylotic myelopathy and radiculopathy. Clinical correlations and pathogenetic mechanisms. Brain 109: 259–278

G. R. Fisk

5

The painful wrist: problems and solutions

INTRODUCTION

The painful wrist is one of the most crippling of disabilities, since there is almost no human activity in which the upper limb is not involved. Because of the large representation of the hand in the sensory cerebral cortex, pain has a serious effect on upper limb function. It not only brings about an inhibition of power in gripping, holding and manipulating objects but also hampers the versatility of movement on which many functions of the hand depend. Thus, pain will seriously affect skilled movement and may prejudice the sufferers' working capacity and put their employment at risk.

Many sports, hobbies and pastimes depend upon a fully functioning and painless wrist and hand, but the apprehension of inducing further pain in the wrist will often discourage pursuit of outside activities. Often, such sufferers find it difficult to place the hand and arm in a position of comfort and sleep is usually disturbed.

CLINICAL ASSESSMENT

Much information can be obtained from routine and careful assessment of the sufferer's disability and diagnosis may often be confidently made without recourse to complicated and time consuming investigations. It is important to record the age, occupation and sex of the patient and which is the dominant hand. It is of primary importance to enquire carefully into any history of injury or other factors which might have precipitated symptoms, such as unusual or excessive use of the upper limb.

The pattern of discomfort is usually revealing: the pain may be acute, intermittent or recurrent; it may be induced by movement or an attempt to use the hand; it may be generalised or localised; it may be lancinating, radiating or 'boring' in character and may be worse at night. An assessment of the range of movement should be carefully compared to the opposite side and this should include not only antero–posterior movement of the wrist but side-to-side deviation and rotation of the forearm, and should include a glance at the elbow and shoulder movements. Deformity should be noted, especially of the lower radius, when this is associated with some loss of movement. Swelling should be recorded and whether generalised, localised or associated with a specific anatomical structure. Active and passive movement may reveal clicks, crepitus or 'jumps' and the examiner must assess whether this arises from soft tissue structures, such as tendons and tendon sheaths, or bones and joints of the carpus.

Testing the power of grip is often an excellent method of assessing pain in the wrist. A dynamometer may be used for comparison of power in both hands (Leroy Young et al 1989) and this is usefully recorded on a scale. However, this method is open to many inaccuracies. Power grip can as easily be estimated by the patient grasping the examiner's index and middle fingers; while hypothenar power is assessed by hooking the little finger around the examiner's index finger and pinch grip by the attempt to pull apart the opposed thumb and index finger of the patient. Grasping the patient's forearm by the examiner's free hand will enable the examiner to judge the effort the patient is making in complying with these tests.

Sensory disturbance should be carefully investigated since in many cases there may be claims of widespread and ill-localised loss of sensation. Alteration in sweating of the hand is associated with a peripheral nerve lesion and this may be usefully tested by light stroking of the insensitive area by the examiner's finger tip. Resort to sophisticated tests, such as that devised by Moberg (1958), are thus rarely necessary. Motor power in the intrinsic and extrinsic muscles should be systematically examined and recorded on a motor chart (Seddon 1954). The colour of the hand may reveal circulatory problems, such as Raynaud's disease, as a source of pain.

INVESTIGATION

The diagnosis of the causes of pain in the wrist is usually evident following examination and clinical assessment, but confirmation may require special tests. It is essential to obtain high quality radiographs of the carpus and the standard views of posterior-anterior, including abduction and adduction views, an accurate lateral and two oblique views in semi-pronation and semi-supination. Tomographs may allow the examiner to visualise the

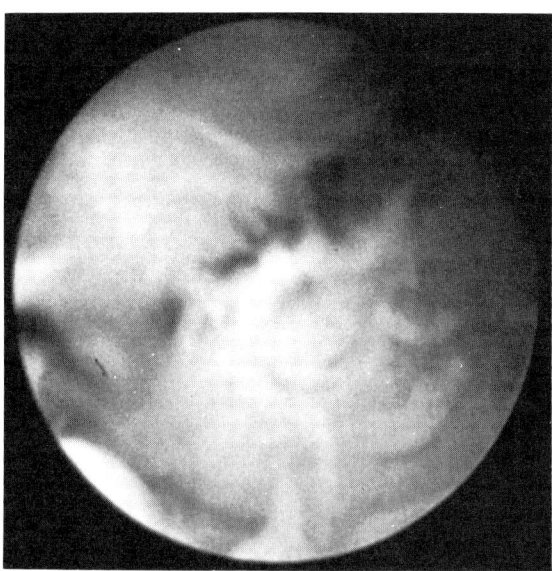

Fig. 5.1b Arthroscopy showing degenerative changes in the articular surfaces of the radius and lunate (courtesy of Mr J. K. Stanley).

carpus in 3 planes; contrast arthrography will reveal capsular and ligamentous rupture with the pattern of spread of the contrast medium. Scintigraphy will demonstrate 'hot spots', whereas the increasing use of the arthroscope may reveal unsuspected soft tissue lesions in the capsule, ligament and articular surfaces (Fig. 5.1a, b). Cine-radiography will reveal unusual or irregular movements of carpal bones. CAT scans and magnetic resonance imaging are occasionally helpful in the most difficult cases.

SOFT TISSUE INJURY

The 'sprained wrist' is perhaps the commonest cause of pain in the upper limb. Sprain is essentially a lay term used without specific connotation, but it may be defined as ligamentous or capsular injury without bony involvement. Much investigation and thought has been given to this type of injury over the last few years and there is now a much better understanding of the implication of ligamentous or capsular injury in the wrist which results in acute, intermittent or chronic pain; much more effective treatment is available than

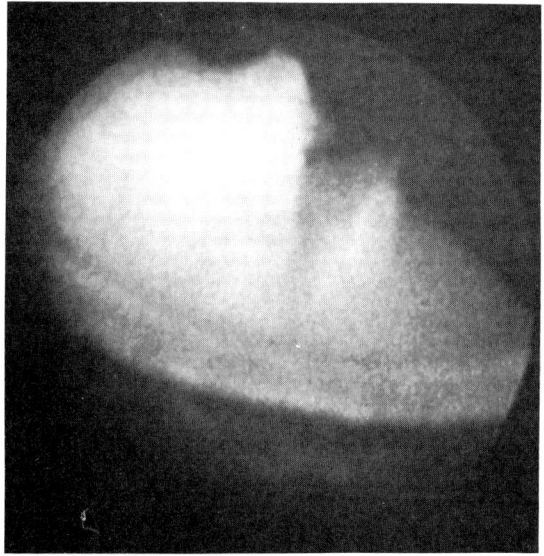

Fig. 5.1a Arthroscopy showing partial disruption of the scapho–lunate capsule.

the arbitrary symptomatic measures previously available.

Sprains of the wrist are almost always sustained by falls onto the outstretched hand or its forcible dorsiflexion by handlebar, crank or projectile. It is thus the soft tissue structures on the front of the wrist which are chiefly affected and the wrist is most vulnerable in a dorsiflexed position. There is nearly always a supination force exerted where the axis of rotation coincides with the shaft of the ulna. Much less commonly the dorsal ligaments are damaged when the hand is forced into palmar flexion. Experimental work by Mayfield (1956) and others has shown there is usually a sequential overloading and eventual rupture of wrist ligaments and capsules. This results in the severest forms in total disorganisation of the carpus, or less often in altered mechanics of the wrist with displacement of one bone from another. The effect of progressive increased stress forces the hand into dorsiflexion, supination and ulnar flexion with rupture of ligaments surrounding the lunate, so that there is first of all scapho–lunate rupture, then capito–lunate, triquetro–lunate and volar radio–carpal ligament failure.

Carpal instability

Any element of the ligamentous injury may produce carpal instability and much can be observed radiologically. It is important therefore to assess the degree of damage before treatment is offered and when major ligamentous rupture has been excluded the sprain may respond to immobilisation in a plaster cast or strapping for three weeks, followed by progressive use of the hand and physiotherapy. However, if such simple measures fail to relieve symptoms it is important to continue further X-ray studies to exclude bony lesions which may not have been evident in the original X-ray. X-ray examination may show that the scaphoid has become abnormally flexed within the carpus; this is commonly associated with rotation dorsalwards of the lunate and in about a quarter of cases the lunate rotates into volar flexion. These lesions have been termed by Linscheid et al (1972) 'dorsal intercalated carpal instability' and 'volar intercalated carpal instability' respectively (DICI and VICI).

A simple clinical test of carpal instability is an assessment of the ligamentous laxity in the two wrists by the 'drawer' sign (Fisk 1970). This test consists of assessing the antero-posterior excursion of the wrist. The examiner holds the forearm firmly and with the patient's hand in a neutral position moves it backwards and forwards on the forearm in a transverse plane comparing the laxity with the normal wrist. Early diagnosis of carpal instability is of the greatest importance since immobilisation often allows damaged ligaments to heal in anatomical alignment and without permanent lengthening. Where damage has been more severe or conservative treatment has failed, it is certainly possible to carry out open repair of the ligaments through an anterior approach on the front of the wrist using non-absorbable sutures. It necessarily follows that the damaged ligaments must be first identified, and 'cobbling up' of soft tissues on the front of the carpus is likely to be ineffective. It is sometimes necessary to repair the dorsal ligaments in the same way. Untreated carpal instability will give rise to persisting aching and weakness of the wrist, sometimes accompanied by episodes of clicking, 'jumping' and profound loss of grip. If left untreated carpal instability is almost invariably followed by osteoarthritic degeneration. If pain, weakness, instability and clicking persists, particularly in the presence of osteoarthritic degeneration, it is sometimes necessary to perform an arthrodesis. This may be limited to one or more joints of the carpus or in cases of persistent pain and weakness, panarthrodesis involving the whole of the carpus from the radius to the third metacarpal. The most obvious fusion and the easiest to perform is between the scaphoid and lunate bones and this will no doubt produce a much improved radiological picture. However, this joint is essential to antero–posterior and radial flexion so that stability may be achieved only with the loss of important function of the wrist and hand. Where there is gross deformity of the scaphoid and particularly when this is associated with intercarpal dislocation, 'tri–scaphi' fusion may bring about stability without significant loss of movement (Watson & Hempton 1980). This operation consists of fusion of the distal pole of the scaphoid with the trapezium and trapezoid bones. Panarthrodesis is a useful operation to salvage irremedial bone or joint damage in the carpus and the results are usually excellent.

The distal radio–ulnar joint

This is a potent and common source of pain. Localisation is not difficult to achieve but treatment is often arbitrary and ineffective. Fractures involving the inferior radio-ulnar joint (Fig. 5.2) are observed by X-ray examination and these should be carefully reduced and fixed as persisting deformity will lead to loss of rotation of the forearm. Fracture of the ulnar styloid is commonly seen in Colles' fracture and other injuries involving forced radial flexion. The avulsed fragment may give rise to tenderness and if it is large enough it may be successfully transfixed by screw or wire. A small fragment usually implies avulsion of the ulnar collateral ligament and if there are persisting symptoms this may require repairing. Dislocation of the inferior radio-ulnar joint may involve partial or total disruption of the triangular fibro-cartilage. Severe injuries of the lower radius may dislocate the distal radio-ulnar joint entirely. Careful reduction of the fracture, with every attempt to prevent later collapse and deformity of the lower radius, will usually reduce the dislocation with eventual restoration of rotation and comfort. However, if the joint remains deformed, or if it is painful and unstable, further surgery will be necessary. More rarely, there is recurrent dislocation of this joint which is a painful and alarming episode for the patient.

Ulnar variance

This condition is defined as a disproportion of the length of the ulna to the radius. It may by itself be symptom-free but may predispose to painful conditions. If shorter than normal it is said to be the underlying cause of Keinbock's disease (Fig. 5.3). Operations for lengthening the ulna or shortening the radius have been devised, but the etiology is not universally accepted. On the contrary, comparative lengthening of the ulna will cause its impingement upon the ulnar aspect of the carpus with early degenerative change and loss of ulnar flexion.

This is a feature of epiphyseal arrest of the lower radius (Fig. 5.4) and in hereditary diseases, such as Madelung's deformity. If the joint is not too seriously disrupted, shortening of the ulna can be achieved in its lower third by osteotomy and internal fixation; while if there is limited rotation of the forearm excision of the ulnar head (Darrach's operation) should be considered. Excision of the neck of the ulna is, however, to be preferred, as this allows the head to drop back into place with the establishment of a pseudarthrosis at the osteotomy site (Baldwin's operation) (Fig. 5.5). However, if the ulnar head is likely to remain unstable after this procedure, the soft tissues of the inferior radio-ulnar joint should be excised and

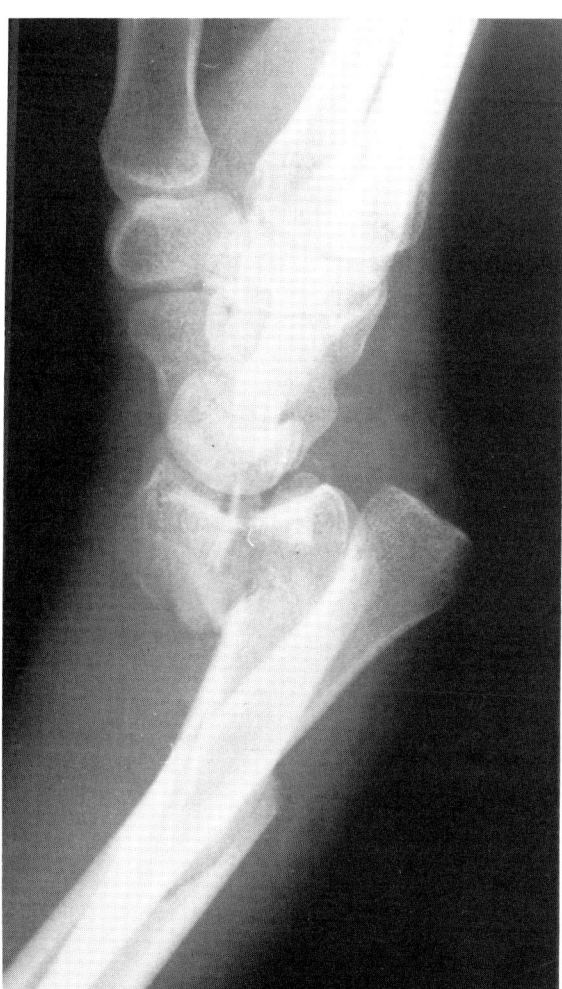

Fig. 5.2 Barton's fracture–dislocation with rupture of the inferior radio–ulnar joint.

52 MANAGEMENT OF PAIN IN THE HAND AND WRIST

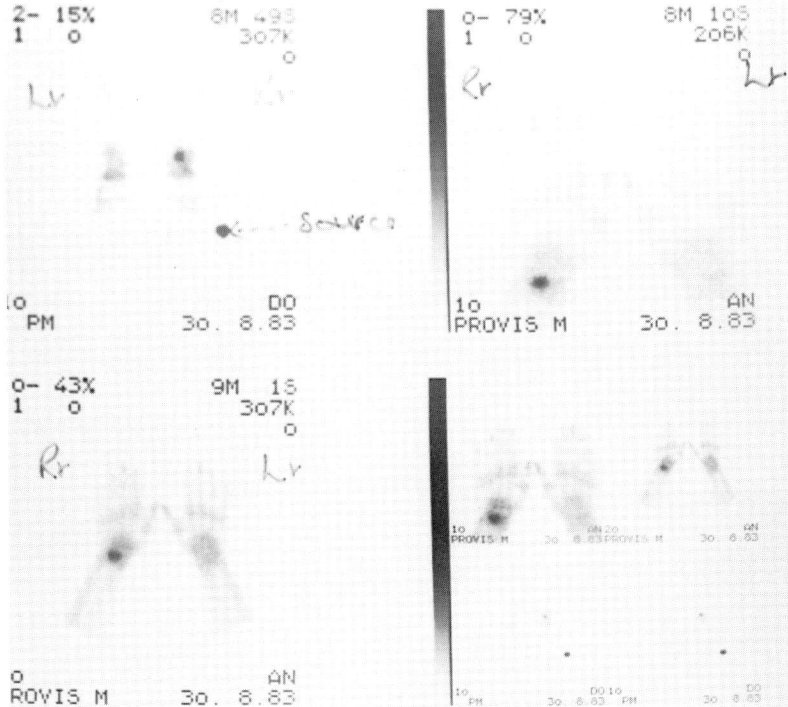

Fig. 5.3 Scintigraphy demonstrating uptake in the lunate in a case of Kienbock's disease.

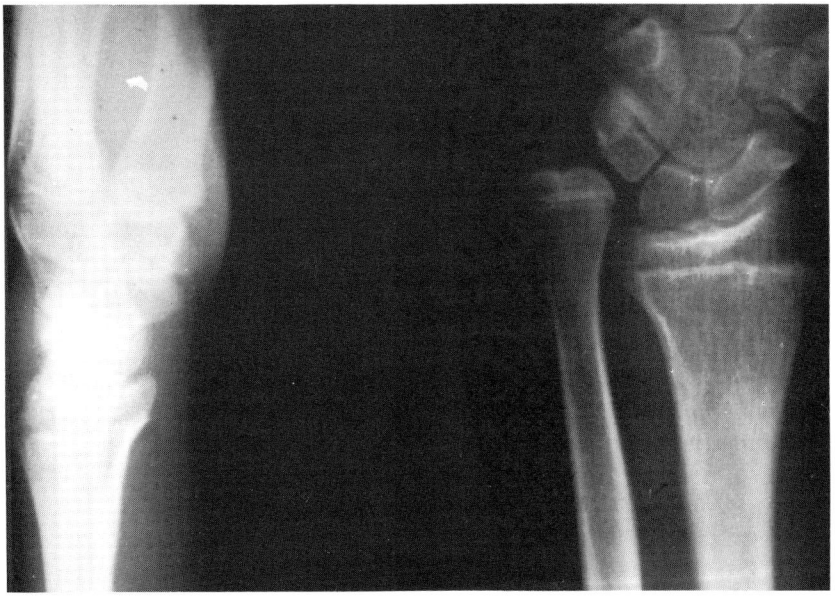

Fig. 5.4 Shortening of the radius from premature fusion of the lower radial epiphysis.

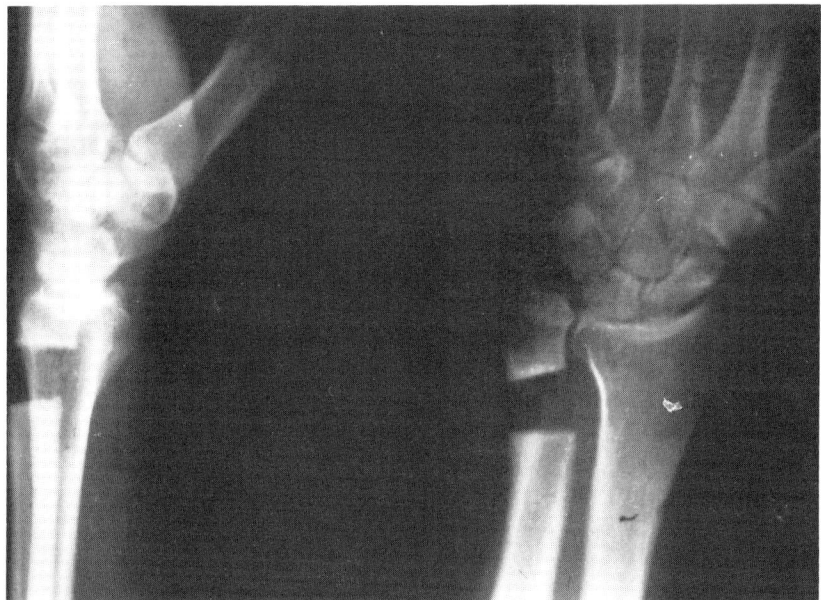

Fig. 5.5 Baldwin's operation.

the ulnar head transfixed to the radius by a compression screw bringing about ankylosis (Suave–Kapandji operation). One of the most difficult surgical problems is the unstable joint, where the ulnar head is persistently tender and prominent at the back of the wrist. Reduction of the deformity is achieved simply by pressure on the ulnar head but it will recur as soon as the pressure is released (piano key sign). Many operations have been described in attempts to stabilise this joint but they are often unsuccessful.

The triangular fibro–cartilage

Clicking, grating and transitory locking may occur in the ulnar region of the wrist when the triangular fibro-cartilage, either by its displacement, its tearing or degenerative change, produces uneven movement of the wrist. Operative arthroscopy may reveal the diagnosis and it is sometimes possible to remove fragments of fibro-cartilage, but excision of the whole articular disc should be performed with caution. Arthroscopy may reveal erosions on the ulnar head itself or on neigbbouring carpal bones and debridement may be necessary. Pains arising from the ulnar side of the wrist may be due to instability of the ulnar column of the carpus and this should be carefully excluded before operation on the triangular fibro-cartilage is contemplated.

Rheumatoid arthritis (see p. 59) is perhaps the commonest cause of pain in the ulnar side of the wrist with collapse of the carpus; the ulnar head becomes exposed and rotation of the forearm is painful and increasingly limited. Excision of the ulnar head may give a wonderful relief of pain. However, such an operation should be carried out with caution since excessive excision of the lower ulna may simply lead to instability of the ulna itself with pain and weakness of the forearm and hand. Rheumatoid disease may also cause sliding of the whole carpus down the slope of the radial articular surface so that it impinges against the ulnar head (the so called 'translocation') (Fig. 5.6). In these circumstances removal of the ulnar head will simply aggravate this deformity with further sliding of the carpus. Arthrodesis of the wrist onto the end of the radius with secondary surgery on the ulna is probably the wisest course.

Occasionally rheumatoid disease will lead to ulnar displacement of the extensor carpi ulnaris tendon with pain, clicking and instability of the inferior radio-ulnar joint, with further ulnar drift

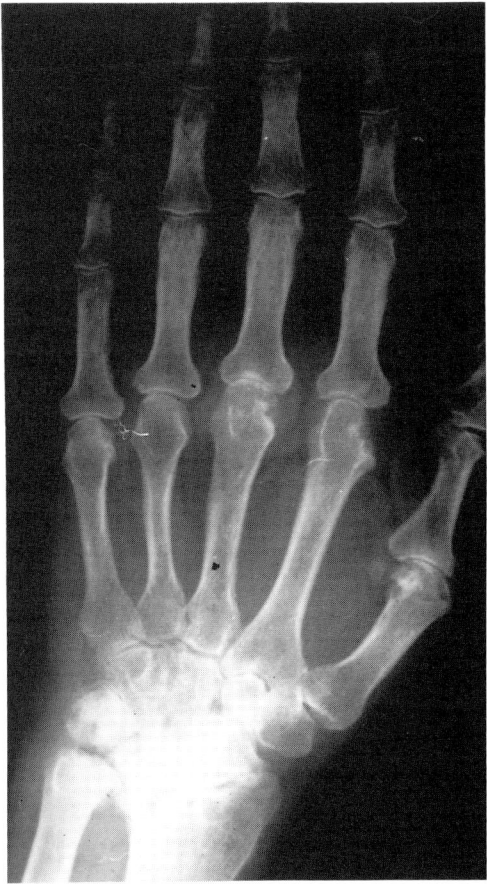

Fig. 5.6 Rheumatoid arthritis showing destruction of the proximal carpus, ulnar translocation with impaction of the ulnar head and involvement of the inferior radio-ulnar joint.

of the head. It is important to restore alignment of the tendon in its bony groove and stabilisation by some form of soft tissue sling.

FRACTURES AND DISLOCATIONS

Fractures around the wrist joint are extremely common and unless they are promptly and efficiently treated they will be a source of prolonged pain and disability. These fractures occur principally in two main age groups: young male adults exposed to violent trauma and elderly females when postmenopausal osteoporosis renders them more vulnerable to the effects of falls on the outstretched hand. Early radiographic examination with good quality films taken in four planes are essential. Careful and prolonged examination of these films may be necessary to analyse the nature of the deformity and displacement. Once a confident diagnosis is made reduction and efficient fixation should be carried out.

Colles' fracture

In the lower radius, Colles' fracture (Fig. 5.7) is by far the commonest injury and routine treatment consists of reduction of the fracture under general or local anaesthesia, followed by fixation in a padded plaster cast or plaster slab and bandage. Renewal of the cast is usually necessary after 10 days when the swelling has subsided. Unfortunately in the osteoporotic state there is almost invariably subsequent collapse of the lower radius with some return of deformity, although this is usually not incompatible with an excellent functional result. Many methods of fixation have been advocated in an attempt to prevent shortening but no one method has obtained universal approval. One well-recognised complication, which is often misdiagnosed, is rupture of the tendon of extensor pollicis longus at the level of Paget's tubercle. It is undecided whether this is an attrition rupture or segmental tendon ischaemia, but it occurs most typically at six weeks after Colles' fracture. It results in aching, tenderness and inability to extend the terminal phalanx of the thumb. It is very effectively treated by transfer of the tendon of extensor indicis into the frayed distal end of the ruptured tendon. Other injuries of the lower radius, such as Barton's fracture–dislocation, will require open reduction and internal fixation by an Ellis plate or similar device. The involvement and later treatment of the inferior radio-ulnar joint has already been discussed.

In the carpus itself the commonest fracture is that of the *scaphoid*. If there is clinical evidence of such a fracture (such as tenderness in the 'anatomical snuff box', weakness of grip and pain on compression along the line of the second metacarpal), immobilisation of the wrist and forearm is essential even if careful X-ray studies do not at first confirm the diagnosis. Even in the absence of a history of injury, X-ray examination may reveal a hitherto unsuspected fresh or old fracture of the

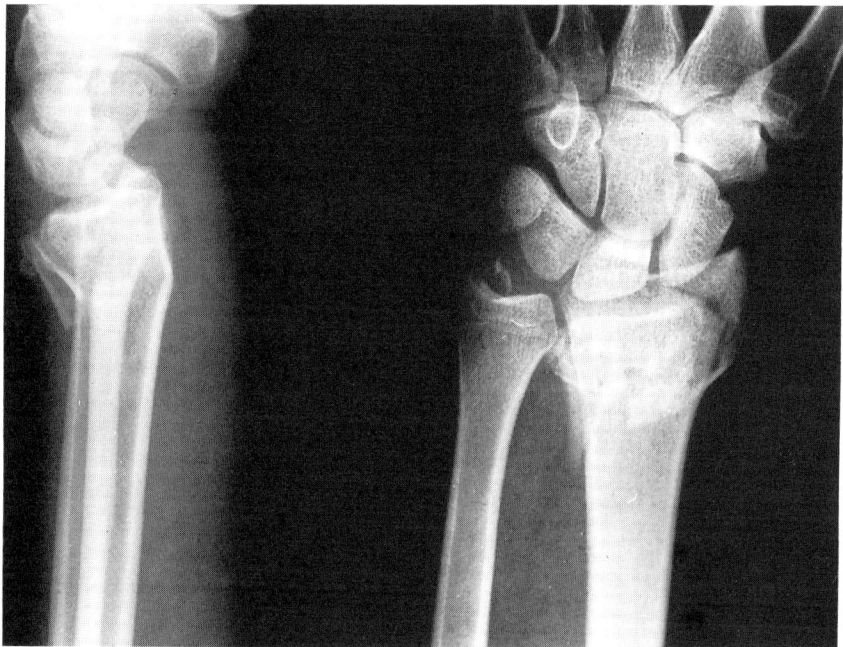

Fig. 5.7 Colles' fracture.

scaphoid. Treatment of the ununited scaphoid fracture may consist of internal fixation with or without grafting the fracture, but if carpal instability is associated with the fracture then wedge grafting is usually necessary to restore the length of the scaphoid, the alignment of the carpus and bony union.

Successful treatment of fracture-dislocation of the carpus depends upon accurate diagnosis, followed by closed or open reduction and internal fixation as necessary. Dislocation of the lunate is almost invariably accompanied by signs of median nerve contusion and if symptoms of tingling, sensory loss or motor weakness do not resolve within a few days, especially if accompanied by pain, rapid early surgical release is essential since recovery of nerve function is almost never complete after much delay.

Kienbock's disease (lunatomalacia)

This is a rare but well recognised source of aching pain in the wrist, usually appearing spontaneously and without a definite history of injury. The condition is typically seen in the second to fourth decades. There is usually limitation of wrist movement and localised tenderness over the lunate bone (which lies in the centre of the wrist between the chaplet creases).

The etiology of this condition is as yet uncertain. Some authorities regard ulnar variance as an important predisposition but very accurate X-ray views are necessary to confirm the comparative length of the radius and ulna. Others regard trauma as important either as a result of fracture (which may not have been observed) or repeated minor injuries resulting in intermittent ischaemia of the lunate.

X-ray examination shows the first indication of avascular necrosis by an increased density of the lunate (Fig. 5.8). Later stages show fragmentation and collapse. The final stage of healing results in a flattened lunate bone with very gross bony sclerosis; the whole process takes about 2 years. Once this process has commenced there is no certain way of stopping it, slowing the disease or reversing the changes. The prognosis probably depends upon the degree of intrusion by the capitate into the space between the scaphoid and triquetrum created by the lunate collapse. In the younger age

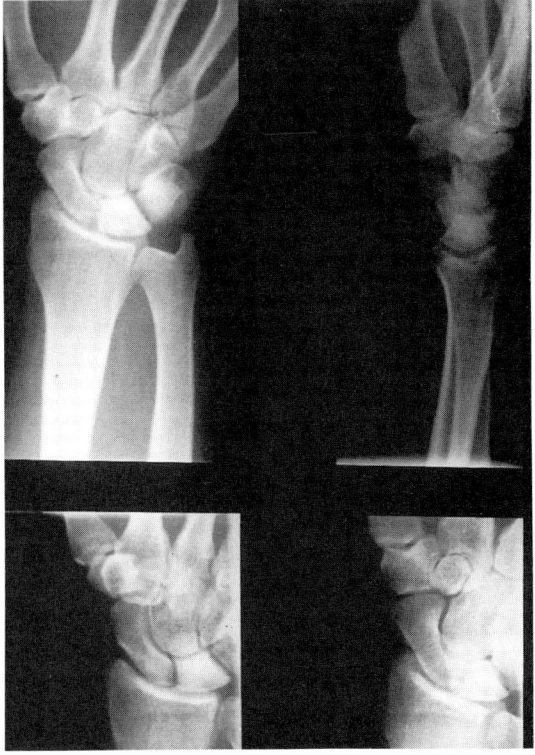

Fig. 5.8 Early Kienbock's disease showing density of the lunate without collapse.

group with only early changes, prolonged immobilisation in a plaster cast or splint may bring about relief and healing in the least distorted position and allows the patient to remain at work. In older age groups excision of the lunate alone may give relief of pain with some distortion of the carpus but the wrist will remain symptom-free for many years. Replacement of the lunate by a prosthesis (usually of silicone rubber) may preserve the normal carpal alignment (Swanson 1970). Unhappily there is a tendency for these prostheses to dislocate or themselves undergo wear or fracture. However, if such a prosthesis is removed the wrist may remain stable from the scarring that has taken place around it. In a similar way the diseased lunate may be replaced by other inert material, such as rolled up tendon. Where symptoms persist or there is perilunar arthritis (Fig. 5.9), early fusion of the wrist may be the best way of preserving hand function, comfort and a good grip at the expense of movement.

Nerve injury

One of the most distressing causes of wrist pain results from peripheral nerve involvement, either

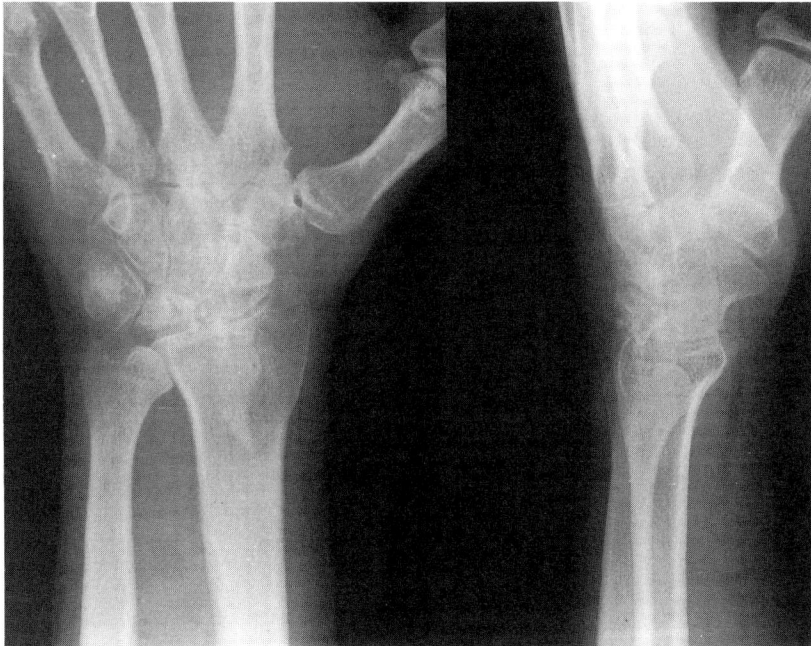

Fig. 5.9 Arthrodesis of the wrist with perilunar arthritis.

locally or referred from more centrally placed lesions. Cervical disc lesion may give intense pain in the forearm, wrist or hand and present a problem of differential diagnosis. There is, however, usually localised pain, tenderness and stiffness of the cervical spine depending on the level of the root compression (C5–6 is the commonest level). There is usually associated sensory disturbance in the forearm and hand. There may be muscle weakness and an X-ray film usually shows narrowing of one or more cervical disc spaces. Sleep is disturbed by pain in the neck and symptoms are usually relieved by a collar, cervical traction and other conservative therapies.

Axillary compression syndromes

Axillary compression syndromes giving rise to pain are usually associated with vascular changes, intrinsic muscle wasting or weakness in the hand and sensory disturbance down the inner side of the forearm and hand.

Nerve compression syndromes

Nerve compression syndromes in the arm are more likely to give rise to sensory and motor loss rather than pain. Symptoms of 'tennis elbow' are occasionally referred to the wrist area.

Carpal tunnel syndrome

Compression of the median nerve at the wrist joint, however, is perhaps the most frequent cause of pain in the wrist and hand. Compression of the median nerve may be brought about by swelling of the structures in the carpal tunnel (usually tendon sheaths), narrowing of the tunnel, bony outgrowths from the carpal bones or distortion of the articulations from injury or disease. The condition is most commonly seen in middle aged females and sufferers from rheumatoid arthritis. Symptoms are often aggravated or precipitated by persistent rhythmic use of the hand, such as knitting, but it is occasionally brought on by injury and is characterised by burning pain in the radial half of the hand with numbness and tingling. The symptoms are worse at night and relieved by shaking the hand, elevating the limb, immersing it in cold water, etc. Examination in the early stages reveals tenderness over the front of the wrist and sensory disturbance over the territory of the median nerve, that is to say the lateral three and a half digits. Later on there may be wasting of the thenar emience and weakness in abduction of the thumb. Phalen's test (holding the hand in full wrist flexion for 2 minutes) or the application of a sphygmomanometer cuff for the same length of time may precipitate symptoms. Once the diagnosis of carpal tunnel syndrome has been accepted, treatment will first of all be conservative and the patient should be persuaded to give up, for the time being, long periods of repetitive manual work. A night splint should be supplied which will hold the wrist in a little dorsiflexion; in mild cases this may be all that is necessary. If splintage fails to relieve symptoms a hydrocortisone preparation can be injected into the carpal tunnel to suppress inflammatory changes in the tendon sheaths, but this is not without risk since the median nerve may itself be damaged with permanent ill effects. In any event, not more than 3 injections should be made in the course of 2 weeks.

Surgery is, however, the most certain way of bringing about relief of pain and tingling. Sensory disturbance normally recovers but wasting of the thenar eminence is usually not restored in late cases, although muscle power may be greatly improved. It is therefore important to offer surgical relief before this stage is reached. The operation can be performed on a day patient under general or regional anaesthesia. A longitudinal sinuous incision is made over the front of the wrist and base of the hand as far as possible passing along the volar creases. It is important that the palmar branch of the median nerve, which usually arises in the centre of the wrist at the base of the palm, should be preserved, since its division will lead to persisting pain and the formation of a tender neuroma. Incision, therefore, may be made down the thenar crease and across the radial side of the wrist or, if it is thought necessary to explore the ulnar nerve, along the ulnar crease. The incision should extend sufficiently proximally to allow visualisation of the whole extent of the transverse carpal ligament and this should be completely divided; some surgeons remove a strip of this ligament to prevent its subsequent reforming. The median

58 MANAGEMENT OF PAIN IN THE HAND AND WRIST

nerve should be exposed and it may be freed from any constricting bands etc. but intraneural dissection confers no benefit. The emergence of the motor branch to the thenar muscles is extremely variable and it must on no account be damaged. Only the subcutaneous tissues and skin are sutured. The patient should gain immediate relief of symptoms with a return to full normal activities within 2 or 3 weeks. There is, however, a small group of patients who do not respond to surgery despite clear physical signs and EMG changes. This may result from inadequate surgical release, permanent intraneural damage or fixation of the pain in the psyche. The use of TCNS is worth considering, or reference to a pain clinic. Thus median nerve compression at the wrist must be carefully distinguished from referred pain from the neck, shoulder or other compressive lesions in the arm, elbow or forearm. *Surgery for symptoms which have no clear diagnostic physical signs is to be deprecated*; it is always wise to perform nerve conduction studies in doubtful cases.

Ulnar nerve compression

Ulnar nerve compression at the elbow will give rise to numbness and tingling on the inner side of the forearm and the inner one and a half digits with hypothenar wasting and weakness, but is rarely associated with pain. Anterior transposition of the ulnar nerve at the elbow or simply division of the arcuate ligament in the early stages will bring about complete relief of symptoms.

Laceration of the wrist

This may cause total or incomplete division of the ulnar and median nerves and if not diagnosed and promptly resutured will result in persisting pain, paraesthesia and tenderness with the formation of neuroma. There is some evidence to suggest that a small proportion of Sudeck's dystrophy is due to involvement of the median nerve at the wrist following Colles' fracture (see p. 54) and surgical release of the nerve may be beneficial.

Minor cutaneous nerves around the wrist may be divided by unwisely placed surgical incisions. The resulting tender neuroma gives rise to symptoms out of all proportion to the neurological deficit. The palmar cutaneous branch of the median nerve has already been mentioned and the other important nerve is the superficial branch of the radial nerve which is in danger in operations for the relief of de Quervain's disease. Rarer compressive lesions may give rise to pain, paraesthesia and weakness in the hand, such as a ganglion in Guyon's canal, or ulnar artery thrombosis at the base of the palm when the heel of the palm is habitually used for percussion.

Bony swellings around the carpus

Isolated exostoses and avulsions occasionally cause persisting symptoms of tenderness and swelling which distress the patient and are quite effectively cured by minor surgery. 'Bossed' carpus, dorsal lunate ridge and chip fracture of the dorsum of the triquetrum usually results from violent dorsi-

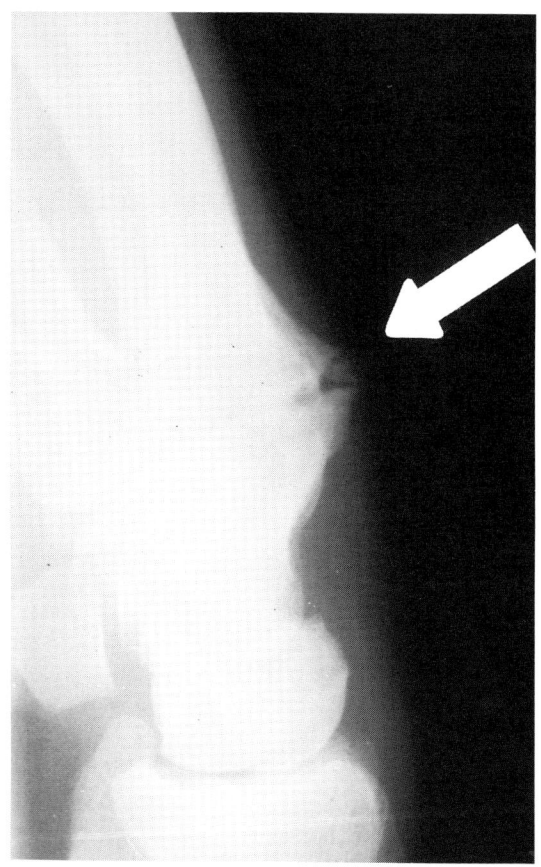

Fig. 5.10 Ununited styloid process of the third metacarpal.

flexion of the hand and may be recognised on lateral X-ray views of the carpus (Fig. 5.10). Ununited styloid process of the third metacarpal is occasionally seen in boxers. This may be safely excised or an attempt may be made to achieve bony union. On the flexor aspect, tenderness of the pisiform bone is sometimes seen in racquet players, and even localised osteoarthritis of the pisi–triquetral joint has been reported. These symptoms may be overcome by excision of the pisiform and repair of the structures inserted into it.

More rarely, a persistent tenderness and pain is localised to the volar radial aspect of the carpus. This may be due to irritation of the tendon and sheath of flexor carpi radialis where it lies in its groove on the trapezium as it passes deeply to its insertion. The tendon may even rupture. It is said to be most commonly seen in office workers and relief may be obtained by release or repair of the tendon.

DEGENERATIVE AND INFLAMMATORY DISEASES

These are a common cause of persisting wrist pain, only second in frequency to trauma. The effects are among the most crippling and relief of symptoms results in welcome restoration of function. Untreated inflammatory arthritis, associated with muscle spasm and joint effusions with softening of capsules and tendon sheaths, will lead inexorably to hideous deformity and total loss of function. Involvement of the inferior radio-ulnar joint results in loss of function in the forearm, often with secondary changes in the elbow and shoulder.

Rheumatoid arthritis

This diathesis includes rheumatoid arthritis in adults and children, lupus erythematosus, psoriatic arthritis, gout, pseudogout, scleroderma and many other diseases. Rheumatoid arthritis affects predominantly young adult females. Both wrists are usually affected with puffiness from synovial thickening and effusion with progressive loss of function. X-ray examination at this stage may well show progressive osteoporosis with narrowing of joint spaces. As the condition progresses there will be gradual destruction and erosion of the articular cartilage, softening of capsules and ligaments, and progressive collapse of the articulations of the wrist. In later stages the carpus may dislocate anteriorly at the radio–carpal joint with progressive fixed flexion. The carpus may also drift to the ulnar side of the radio–articular surface (ulnar translocation of the carpus) until there is impingement of the carpus upon the ulnar head.

Deformities at the wrist will account for some of the loss of function in the digits, with ulnar drift of the fingers and swan neck deformities.

Involvement of the inferior radio-ulnar joint will result in dorsal subluxation of the ulna with erosion of its head and dislocation of the extensor carpi ulnaris tendon. The deformed ulnar head may penetrate the dorsal wrist capsule and spicules of bone will cause progressive fraying and ultimate division of the extensor tendons (Vaughan-Jackson 1948), commencing in the little finger and moving progressively towards the radial side. Compression of the median nerve at the wrist occurs with thickening of flexor synovial sheaths and the articular capsules and carpal deformity; it is the commonest symptomatic cause of carpal tunnel syndrome.

Treatment

In the early stages rheumatoid arthritis is best treated by a physician with a special interest in the subject. Much depends on the pattern of the disease and whether it is intermittent or progressive in nature, although the cause of rheumatoid arthritis is not known and its cure is some way off. There is, however, an array of well recognised drugs which can suppress the activity, minimise pain and improve the general health of the patient. However, it should be realised that, accompanying conservative care, every attempt must be made to prevent the deformity of the wrist and hand by early functional splinting. This will relieve pain, prevent deformity and allow continued use of the upper limb. Physiotherapy and occupational therapy are of the greatest value in the prevention of deformity and preservation of function. Unhappily, there is hardly a department of physical medicine in the UK in which deformities of the hands are not seen which could have been prevented by earlier treatment or in which deformity

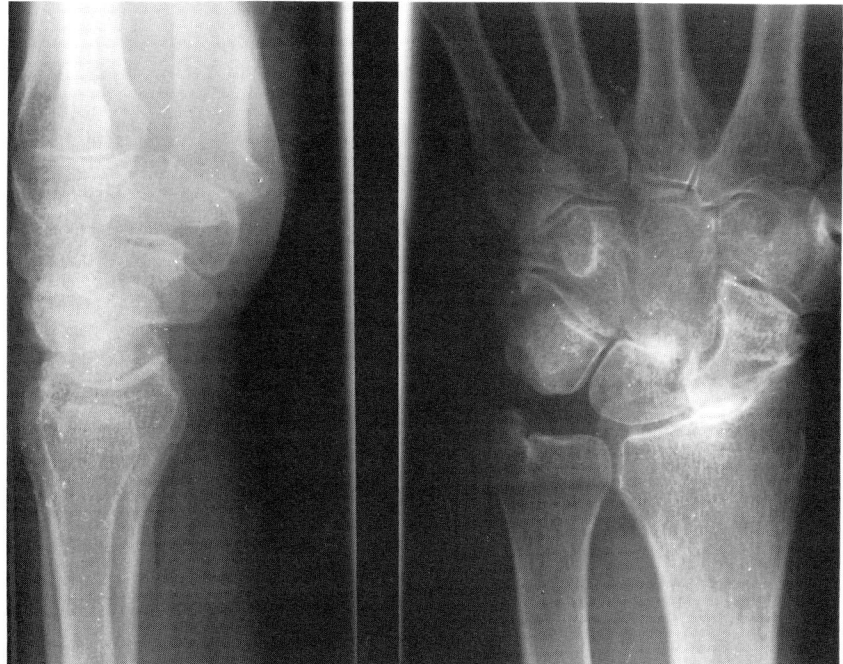

Fig. 5.11 Rare primary arthritis of the wrist in a man who used double-handed crimping pliers at work for many years.

is amenable to surgery. Drugs that help to alleviate the condition in the early stages comprise non-steroidal anti-inflammatory drugs, sometimes in company with intra-articular injections of corticosteroid. At a further stage gold, delta–penicillamine and systemic corticosteroids are considered by the physician. A period of rest and graduated activity in hospital is worth considering where treatment can be intensified and the general health and morale of the patient improved.

Reconstructive surgery may involve partial or complete resection of the ulnar head, synovectomy of the carpus and dorsal tendon sheaths. This is best performed through a straight dorsal incision with transposition of the dorsal carpal ligament beneath the extensor tendons. Reposition of the extensor carpi ulnaris and its stabilisation is often helpful. Rupture of the extensor tendons cannot usually be repaired directly and suture of the distal part of the tendon to an adjacent intact one can sometimes be successful; tendon transfers from the radial aspect or the flexor side will also restore useful extension. Overcoming ulnar drift of the carpus will improve the function of the fingers. Flexor tenosynovectomy may be carried out at the time of carpal tunnel release and unsuspected rupture of the flexor tendons may be appropriately repaired.

Finally, arthrodesis of the wrist (Fig. 5.9) may be the only measure which will stabilise the hand, relieve pain and restore function to the hand and fingers, and its effect is permanent. However, in a patient already severely crippled by joint disease, or where both wrists are affected, replacement arthroplasty would be an immense improvement. Unfortunately these operations have not proved to be of permanent benefit and further revision surgery is often necessary. The types available are the silicone wrist prosthesis of Swanson and the total wrist arthroplasties of Meuli (1980) and Volz (1978), which comprise metal implants with polythene hinged devices. There is little doubt that in time arthroplasty will become the standard treatment of the severely affected rheumatoid wrist.

Osteoarthritis

Primary osteoarthritis of the wrist (Fig. 5.11) is a remarkably rare condition considering the stress to which the wrist is continually subjected. Arthritic degeneration is most frequently seen after fractures and dislocations of the radius and carpus. It almost always follows unrecognised or untreated carpal instability. Partial arthrodesis may relieve discomfort at the expense of movement but some forms of intercarpal fusion may themselves precipitate degenerative changes in neighbouring joints. A painless pseudarthrosis may result from excision of the whole proximal row of carpal bones.

Infective diseases

Happily pyogenic infections of the soft tissues and bones of the wrist are now very rare. Before the advent of antibiotics, crippling effects of uncontrolled infection were the principal preoccupation of surgeons and concealed the many other deformities of the wrist and hand (Fig. 5.12). Nowadays, when it does occur, there is often a delay in diagnosis just because of its rarity and osteomyelitis of carpal bones will very rapidly destroy the joint with early dislocation. The best result to be hoped for is ankylosis of the wrist in a good position. Early treatment by antibiotics, splintage and surgical intervention will minimise the dreadful deformity which is the melancholy result of uncontrolled infection.

Tuberculous infection of the wrist is rare but compound palmar ganglion is characterised by a swelling in the palm of the hand and fluctuation under the transverse carpal ligament. Apart from general therapy, the fluctuant and thickened synovial bursa containing melon seed bodies should be widely excised.

Gout will also give rise to acute inflammation and swelling of the wrist with fulminating pain which does not respond either to antibiotics or analgesics. Indomethicin may give immediate and dramatic relief of pain but should symptoms persist serum uric acid levels should be estimated and uricosuric drugs given. A long term xanthine oxydase inhibitor might be necessary if serious attacks occur more than twice a year.

de Quervain's disease

This term describes pain, swelling and tenderness of the extensor-abductor tendon sheaths of the thumb. It is brought about by unusual or excessive use of the hand, especially in unskilled or anxious workers, often after a holiday or change of employment. It is almost entirely confined to women. There are two manifestations: the first is the classic 'chamois leather creaking' which can be felt when the patient moves the thumb, and secondly it is characterised by a nodule in the region of the radial styloid which will give rise to pain, clicking on movement and local tenderness. Some authorities believe that symptoms arise from the passage of the extensor pollicis longus muscle and tendon where it lies across the extensor tendons of the wrist. Unfortunately this condition is often arbitrarily diagnosed and is used for any painful condition around the wrist and thumb. The most effective treatment is, firstly, firm reassurance and the provision of a splint to immobilise the wrist in extension, perhaps including the thumb. The pa-

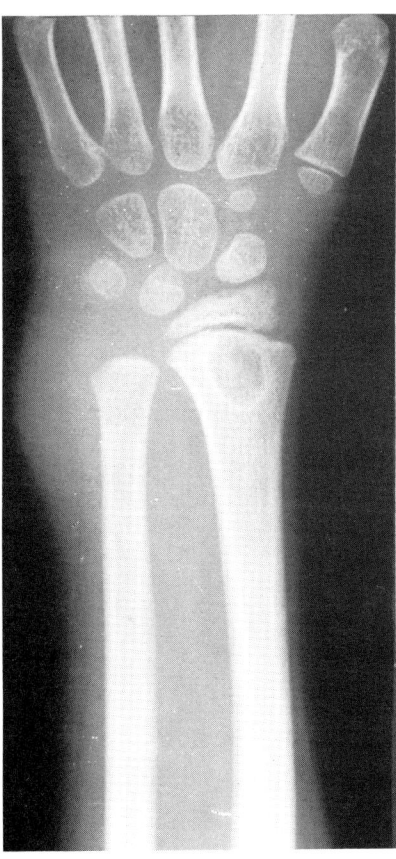

Fig. 5.12 Brodie's abscess in the lower radius of a child.

tient should be encouraged to remain at work. If this does not bring about rapid resolution, injections of hydrocortisone into the abductor tendon sheaths are usually effective. However, if symptoms persist, then release of the abductor–extensor tendons from their sheaths should result in a cure. There are cases where there are no significant physical signs and persisting symptoms are characteristic of a functional disorder.

Osteoarthritis of the carpo–metacarpal joint of the thumb

This is a disorder commoner in women and is sometimes called 'housewife's disease', since it is most frequently seen in this group: the presumption is that degenerative changes are brought about by domestic chores. It appears not to be related to injury and, in fact, Bennett's fracture-dislocation of the base of the first metacarpal surprisingly rarely results in a painful osteoarthritis. In the early stages the base of the thumb becomes more prominent, there is usually an element of subluxation present and active and passive movement give rise to unpleasant crepitus. Abduction of the thumb is lost, gradual stiffening takes place and in its last stages the thumb is ankylosed in a position of adduction, its metacarpal lying alongside the second metacarpal. As a result of this stiffening, there often develops a compensatory hypermobility of the metacarpo–phalangeal joint which becomes hyperextended and the ulnar collateral ligament becomes so lax that weak abduction and opposition is achieved at this level.

Treatment

In the early stages the condition can be alleviated by self-traction associated with strapping or bandaging in a figure-of-eight fashion around the base of the thumb and the distal carpus. A splint designed to hold the thumb in abduction allows useful movement to be retained; much comfort is obtained from various forms of heat, such as wax baths, short wave diathermy or ultrasound. Long-term relief may be obtained by repeated injections of corticosteroid into and around the joint and this may be combined with physiotherapy. Finally, surgery may be called upon to bring about permanent cure.

Arthrodesis. Arthrodesis of this joint is the obvious solution but unhappily the function of the hand is seriously limited by a thumb fixed in permanent abduction and opposition. The hand is certainly improved for pinch and power grip and writing, but it cannot be put on a plane surface or into a confined space, such as a pocket.

Excision of the trapezium (Gervis 1949). This has the merits of simplicity and there are many published series of satisfactory and durable results. However, a proportion of these thumbs undergo gradual deformity, dislocation and a loss of function. As a result of this uncertainty various *prostheses* have been designed but these are apt to dislocate, and increasingly complex surgical manoeuvres of tendon transfers have been devised in an attempt to retain the prosthesis and the thumb in its correct alignment. A simple 'space filler' which will hold the metacarpal base away from the distal pole of the scaphoid is probably the most satisfactory and a block of high density polyethylene cut to size and shape on the operating table may be inserted. Soft material to fill the gap, such as rolled up tendon or fascia, rarely dislocates; the deformity is prevented and function retained.

Osteoarthritic degeneration of the scapho–multangular joints will give aching pain and stiffness on the radial side of the carpus. It may not be immediately recognised but an X-ray will show a narrowing of these joints; for in the writer's experience this condition usually results from secondary degeneration following mild rheumatoid disease.

CYSTS AND TUMOURS

The commonest cyst seen around the wrist joint is the simple ganglion. This usually arises on the dorsum of the wrist, often appearing acutely as a tender swelling which gives rise to aching and stiffness of the wrist far in excess of the simple nature of the condition. Less often these cysts are seen on the volar surface in the region of the lower end of the radius; rarely, they compress the nerves in confined spaces, such as the carpal tunnel, or the ulnar nerve distal to Guyon's canal which will give rise to a motor lesion in the hand without sensory disturbance. A ganglion may occasionally distort the course of the radial artery. In the early stages the ganglion is unilocular and will transluminate and fluctuate, but in time a pseudocapsule will gradually form, become thickened and will present as a hard nodule. A ganglion may also penetrate over a long distance around the wrist joint. Occasionally, particularly in children, the ganglion may disappear spontaneously.

Etiology of ganglion is not entirely clear. It is best defined as a 'hydropic degeneration of connective tissue' which contains extracellular fluid (Carp & Stout 1928). Its contents closely resemble synovial fluid. Histologically, the ganglion is at first lined by a thin wall of columnar cells which later become squamous with daughter cells forming in the false capsule. There is usually 'a tail' leading down to a joint capsule or tendon sheath but communication with the joint cavity is rarely established. The ganglion probably arises in connective tissues subject to a great deal of movement as the result of one layer moving upon another.

In the early stages the fluid in a ganglion may be dispersed by puncture or compression but this is followed by a high rate of recurrence. The cyst may be aspirated and instilled with hyaluronidase (which is supposed to bring about increased tissue diffusion) but the most certain treatment is careful excision under a tourniquet with dissection of the cyst and its pseudocapsule, every attempt being made to include any deep protrusions.

Bone cysts and tumours

The bones of the wrist joint are subject to the same neoplastic and metabolic changes which are common to the whole skeleton but in its confined space (Fig. 5.13) such abnormalities may give rise to symptoms of aching or pain which would be symptom-free elsewhere. The so called *'unicameral'* bone cyst is occasionally seen in the proximal carpal row. Aching pain may be attributed to this cyst and it may require curettage and packing with bone chips.

Multiple cysts

Multiple cysts in carpal bones (Fig. 5.14) are occasionally seen in manual workers using vibrating

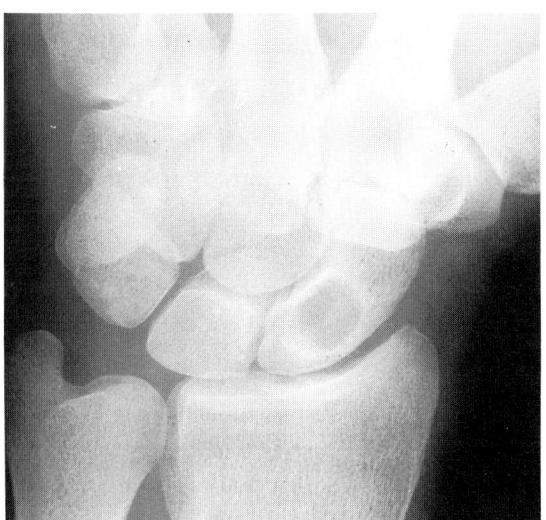

Fig. 5.13 Unicameral bone cyst in the scaphoid.

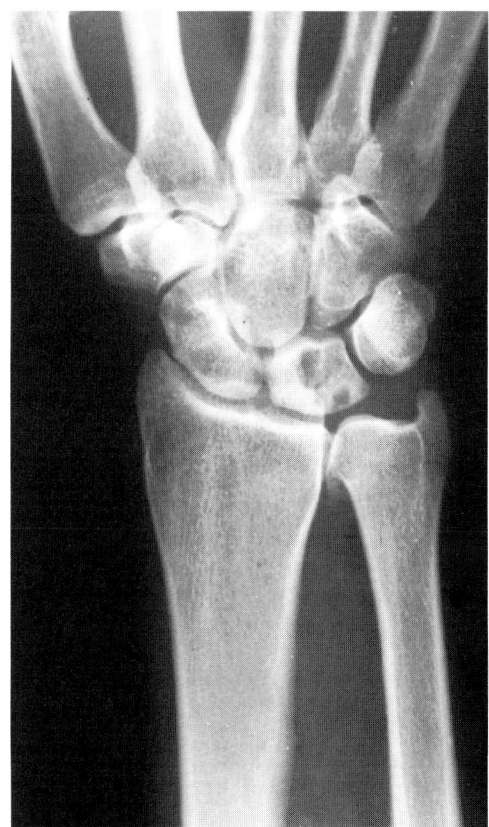

Fig. 5.14 Multiple cysts in carpal bones.

tools. These themselves are of no significance and probably arise from the extrusion of synovial fluid through fissures in the articular cartilage of the carpal bones with inhibition of endosteal bony replacement. Such cysts are not to be confused with erosions and protrusions of diseased synovial membrane of active rheumatoid arthritis or of gout or other metabolic diseases.

Osteoid osteoma

This is a perplexing condition only rarely seen in carpal bones, with pain in the wrist which is worse at night and relieved by aspirin, a therapeutic test. Characteristic X-ray appearance of osteoid osteoma is a clear circular area with sclerosed walls, in the centre of which is a dense 'nidus', but in the bones of the wrist the full radiological picture may not be present. The treatment consists of excision or curettage of the whole lesion. Osteoid osteoma is not to be confused with simple cortical islands which are frequently seen in carpal bones and which are of no significance.

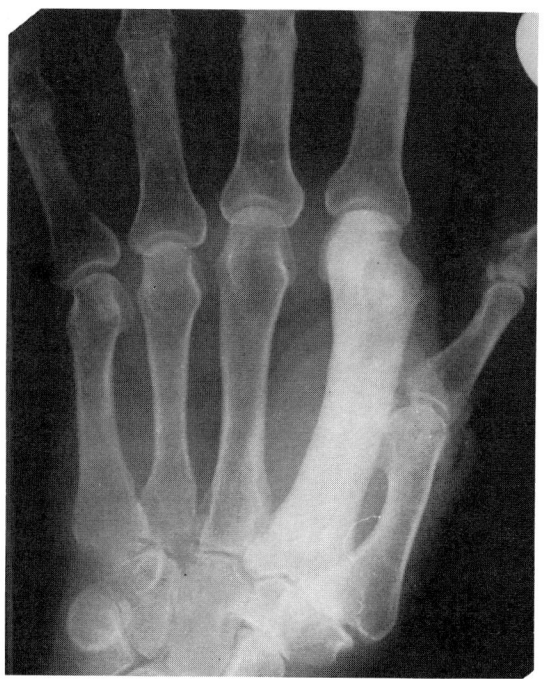

Fig. 5.15 Paget's disease of the second metacarpal giving aching pain in the wrist.

Pigmented villonodular synovitis

Sometimes called 'xanthoma of tendon sheaths', this is an occasional cause of swelling and pain in the wrist region and simple excision of the swelling cures the condition.

Amyloid deposits

These are sometimes seen in tendon sheaths and this is a rare cause of compression of the median nerve in the carpal tunnel.

Brodie's abscess

Brodie's abscess (Fig. 5.12) in the lower radius or ulna may give rise to perplexing symptoms but nowadays is very rare.

Paget's disease

Paget's disease (Fig. 5.15) is only rarely manifested in carpal bones or metacarpals.

Calcification

Calcification of soft tissues around the wrist is occasionally described and this usually disappears spontaneously or after a period of splintage.

Primary or secondary malignant disease

This occasionally occurs as a curiosity.

Synovial sarcoma

This may occur in tendon sheaths around the wrist joint. This condition is unhappily highly malignant and, although local excision may give rise to temporary relief, the patient may need to face amputation.

Osteoclastoma and osteosarcoma

Bone tumours, such as osteoclastoma or osteosarcoma, may affect the bone of the lower forearm but are excessively rare in the carpus itself.

FUNCTIONAL DISORDERS

In medical practice there is always a tendency to call a condition functional which you cannot diagnose. However, when repeated examination and investigations prove negative there remains a group of perplexing conditions which often give rise to quite severe disablement, usually totally resistant to treatment and not benefited or indeed aggravated by well meaning attempts at treatment, including surgery. These conditions are often associated with stress and anxiety, and not infrequently involve protracted medico-legal procedures for compensation. Speaking generally, once the practitioner is satisfied that there is no significant organic cause for the patient's complaints, he should firmly resist the blandishments of those who wish to capitalise on the latest fashionable social neurosis. However, it is of value to recognise the clinical picture and to understand the pressures and circumstances which motivate these syndromes – but not to offer specific palliation which simply acts as a reinforcement of the underlying functional disorder.

Secretan's disease

This is a condition seen usually in male manual workers. The back of the hand presents a thickened indurated swelling in which there appears to be serious loss of tendon function, particularly extension of the fingers, with much pain and tenderness and general serious loss of use of the hand. The patient remains absent from work, sometimes for many months, he may bring an action for negligence against his employer, he resists examination and resents attempts passively to move the fingers (Vander Elst 1975). The X-rays are always normal and there is no blood dyscrasia. There is sometimes a surgical scar where biopsy has been performed or a foolish attempt has been made to remove the swelling. No specific pathology is observed. Several independent investigators, after careful assessment, have come to the unanimous conclusion that this condition is self-inflicted. 'More of a job for Sherlock Holmes than Dr Watson' (Reischauer). Only resolution of the precipitating circumstances will bring about cure.

Painful wrists in schoolgirls

The child is usually brought to hospital by an anxious parent because of her persistent complaint of weakness of grip, inability to write or use the hand comfortably in sport. Examination reveals ill-defined tenderness, some resistance to passive movement but normal X-rays and blood count. On enquiry there is usually some emotional tension either in the family, with boy friends, at school or importantly anxiety over impending examinations. Sympathetic reassurance and a promise to re-examine the wrist in a few months' time usually result in spontaneous resolution.

Writer's cramp

This is a closely allied condition but seen in adults. Any attempt to use the hand is frustrated by the fingers and thumb being tightly clenched into the palm. These women find it difficult or impossible to write or draw, or in the teaching profession, are unable to write on the blackboard. Again, sympathetic reassurance and an explanation of the condition to enable the patient to get an insight into the condition usually result in cure.

'Overuse syndrome'

'Recurrent locomotor strain', 'repetitive strain syndrome' and several other synonyms are used to describe a condition of tenderness and weakness of the wrist, hand and arm. This is usually accompanied by a disproportionate degree of invalidism, absences from work and claims for financial compensation. It sometimes reaches epidemic proportions. This condition has been presented to the public and manual workers generally (including the unions) as a new medical discovery, as though previous generations had never suffered from 'overuse' of the hand and that there was something special about modern industrial conditions. Indeed this bizarre collection of symptoms has been known since time immemorial. The current syndrome has been defined as 'a condition of pain and loss of function in muscle groups and ligaments through excessive use'. The syndrome is often confused with de Quervain's disease (extensor-abductor tenosynovitis) and is referred to in industrial lay circles as 'teno'. Tenosynovitis appears as a diagnosis in the Schedule of Industrial Diseases. However the condition of 'overuse syndrome' rarely presents with any cardinal physical signs. It is said to be common in musicians, office workers using keyboards and factory operatives carrying out repeated rhythmic and tedious work on assembly lines (Fry 1988). There are a number of different although allied manifestations with a common factor of tension and anxiety. Musicians are usually intelligent enough to have some insight into their discomfort and will understand that the unnatural postures required to play various musical instruments over long periods may prove to be uncomfortable. A dedicated performer whose achievements are not matched by his or her ambition may often subconsciously resort to a supposed physical disability to explain lack of success and to conceal frustration and disappointment. Prolonged rest seems to be the common factor in bringing about relief. In other manual workers symptoms are out of all proportion in relation to the physical signs and the more treatment is offered the more the disability becomes fixed in the sufferer's mind. The melancholy clinical picture finally emerges of a patient complaining of persisting pain in the wrist and hand even though the arm is immobilised in a plaster cast from the elbow to the finger tips and supported in a sling. He will have undergone a variety of injections, manipulations, physiotherapy and even surgery without the slightest relief.

The writer was invited to examine the workers in a chicken factory in the West Country where complaints of pain in the hand and wrists had reached epidemic proportions. Examination of the women in the assembly lines revealed a few cases of incipient tenosynovitis, there were a few cases of paraesthesia from direct nerve compression in the palm but nothing was found which minor modification of working conditions would not quickly correct.

It is my personal view, supported by the great majority of hand surgeons, that this is the latest in a series of fashionable diagnoses, with an element of verisimilitude, which allows the vulnerable personality to opt out of stressful conditions without loss of face or social stigma. It takes its place in history with 'slipped disc', ulcers, neurasthenia, nervous exhaustion, 'going into a decline', attacks of 'the vapours' etc.

Sudeck's post-traumatic dystrophy

This is a distressing condition seen in the wrist and hand, most commonly following Colles' fracture. It is not possible to say what part stress and anxiety play in the onset of this condition but it does not seem to affect those patients with a robust temperament. The severity of the injury and the subsequent treatment seems to bear no relationship to its onset. It affects predominantly middle aged females. The prodromal symptom is complaint of severe pain in the wrist even after a good reduction of the fracture and immobilisation in a satisfactory plaster splint. The wrist and fingers become progressively stiffened with the early onset of secondary changes in the elbow and shoulder. The wrist is held stiffly, with the fingers out straight, and there is much resistance to attempted active or passive movement. The skin is purplish, shiny, atrophic and sweating. X-ray examination will show early onset of patchy rarefaction proceeding to gross osteoporosis. The relentless pain is relieved only by strong analgesics while high elevation of the limb in a warmed atmosphere is helpful. On the supposition that this condition is caused by a disturbance in the autonomic nervous system most treatment is directed towards the interruption of the sympathetic nerve pathways (see Ch. 6). The condition usually resolves within 12 months with relief of pain but some residual stiffness which may be permanent, depending upon efforts made to keep the wrist and fingers mobile during the active stage. It has been suggested that the condition arises from median nerve compression in the carpal tunnel and that early surgical release is advocated, but this is by no means the cause in many cases. Remineralisation of the skeleton slowly takes place leaving a characteristic coarsely trabeculated medullary bone.

THE PAINFUL WRIST: PROBLEMS AND SOLUTIONS 67

APPENDIX 1: AFTER DESTOUET, GILULA & REINUS

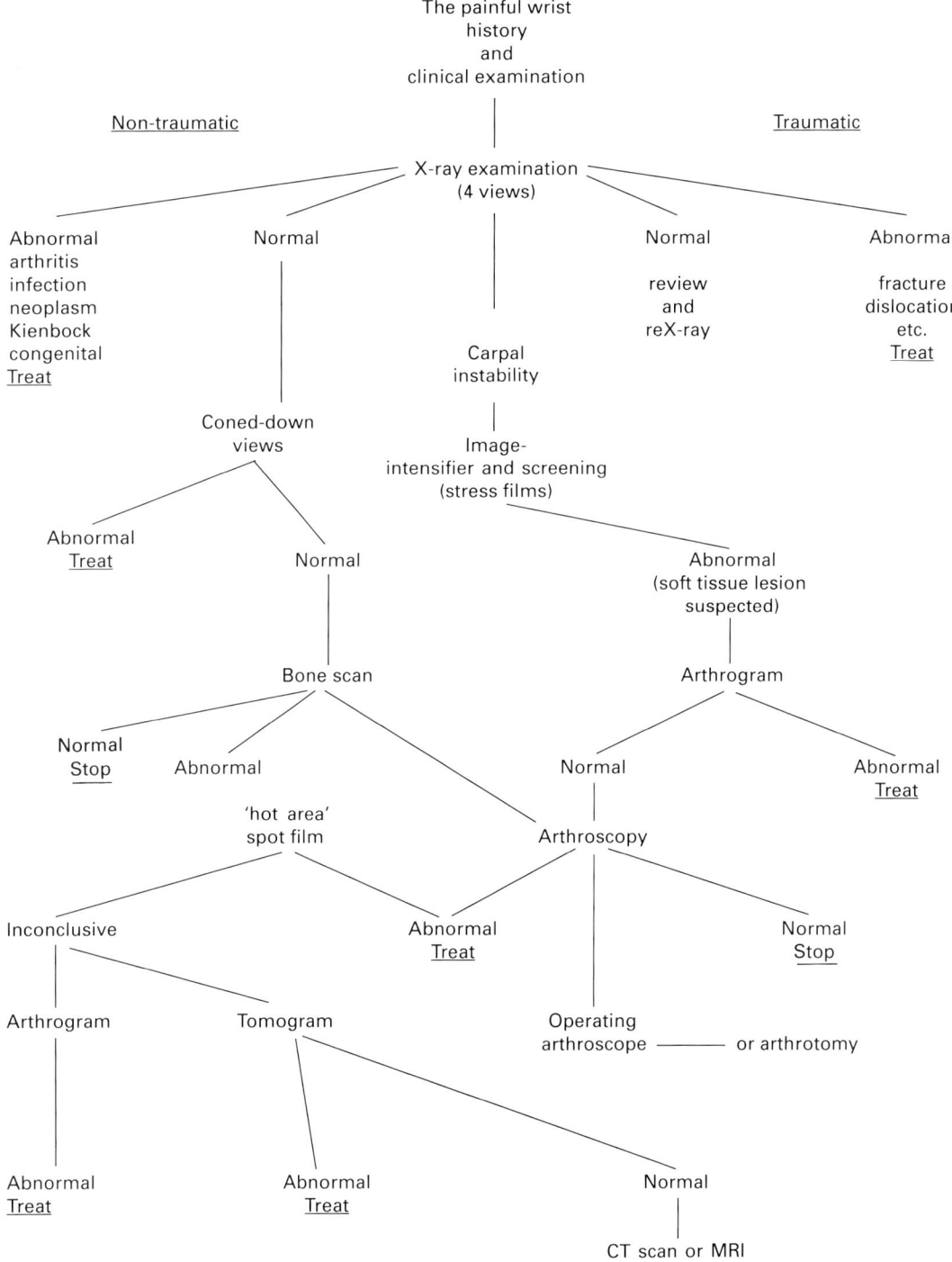

REFERENCES

Baldwin W I 1921 Surgery of the hand and wrist. In: Jones Sir R (ed) Orthopaedic surgery of injuries. Hodder and Stoughton, London, p 241

Carp L, Stout A P 1928 Surgery Gynaecology and Obstetrics 47: 460

Darrach W 1912 Anterior dislocation of the head of the ulna. Annals of Surgery 56: 802

Fisk G R 1970 Carpal instability and fractured scaphoid. Annals of the Royal College of Surgeons of England 46: 63

Fry H J 1988 The treatment of overuse syndrome in musicians. Journal of the Royal Society of Medicine 81: 572

Gervis W H 1949 Excision of the trapezium for osteoarthritis of the trapezio-metacarpal joint. Journal Bone and Joint Surgery 31B: 537

Leroy Young V, Kraemer Bruce A, Pin P et al 1989 Fluctuation in grip and pinch strength among normal subjects. The Journal of Hand Surgery 14A: 125

Linscheid R L, Beabout J W, Dobyns J H et al 1972 Traumatic instability of the wrist. Journal of Bone and Joint Surgery 54A: 1612

Mayfield J K 1988 Pathogenesis of wrist ligament instability. In: Lichtman D M (ed) The wrist and its disorders. Saunders, Philadelphia

Mayfield J K 1956 Mechanism of carpal injuries. Clinical Orthopaedics 45: 149

Meuli H C 1980 Arthroplasty of the wrist. Clinical Orthopaedics 149: 118

Moberg E 1958 Objective methods for determining the functional value of sensibility in the hand. Journal of Bone and Joint Surgery 40B: 3, 454

Reischaver quoted by Vander Elst E 1975

Seddon H (ed) 1954 Peripheral nerve injuries. Medical Research Council Report 282. HMSO, London

Swanson A B 1970 Silicone rubber implants for the replacement of the carpal scaphoid and lunate bones. Orthopaedic Clinics of North America 1: 299

Vander Elst E 1975 The thick hand. In: Stack G, Bolton H (eds) Proceedings of the second hand club 1956–1967. British Society for Surgery of the Hand, London

Vaughan-Jackson O J 1948 Rupture of extensor tendons by attrition at the inferior radio-ulnar joint. Journal of Bone and Joint Surgery 30B: 528

Volz R G 1978 Total wrist arthroplasty. Clinical Orthopaedics 128: 180

Watson H K, Hempton R F 1980 Limited wrist arthrodesis. 1: The triscaphoid joint. The Journal of Hand Surgery 5: 320

FURTHER READING

Watson-Jones R 1982 Fractures and joint injuries, Wilson J N (ed), 6th edn. Churchill Livingstone, Edinburgh

C. B. Wynn Parry

6 Painful peripheral nerves and the painful stiff hand

The vast majority of injuries to peripheral nerves affecting the hand do not cause significant pain. The recovery stage after suture of nerves is often associated with paraesthesiae – which may persist for many months or years particulary after median nerve suture at the wrist. However it seldom causes the patient to seek medical advice. All that is required is reassurance that this is part of the recovery process and that the myelin sheath takes a long time to mature. We liken the situation to lack of insulation in electric cables and the patients then readily understand why disorders like mild electric shocks persist. These symptoms are always worse in cold weather and it is wise to counsel patients to wear gloves and to avoid putting their hand into the refrigerator. If patients continue to complain and hope for some amelioration we advise progressive desensitisation, first by the physiotherapist, and then by the patient at home. This takes the form of gradually increasing sensory stimuli to the affected area with brushes and soft textures, progressing to harder textures, e.g. cotton wool, lint and later fine sandpaper. Rubbing the hands together regularly can often reduce the symptoms temporarily.

Potent causes of painful nerves are the entrapment neuropathies. The median nerve is commonly compressed at the wrist in the carpal tunnel and the ulnar nerve at the elbow. The brachial plexus can be compressed at the root of the neck in the so called thoracic outlet syndrome and various tumours can compress the nerves along their course, e.g. ganglions, lipomas, schwannomas, and neurofibromata. The site of compression is usually clear clinically although electrical studies may be necessary to confirm the localisation of the lesion.

ENTRAPMENT NEUROPATHIES

Carpal tunnel syndrome

No special clinical or electrical tests are required to make the diagnosis in a patient who wakes in the early hours with paraesthesiae in the median distribution, relieved by hanging the hand out of the bed. Sometimes the pain can spread across the whole hand, up the arm and even up to the shoulder. In these circumstances the condition may be confused with cervical spondylosis causing nerve root irritation spreading down the arm or even with severe rotator cuff lesions. Indeed all these conditions may co-exist and lower the threshold of sensation to one another. Patients often complain that they cannot hold a newspaper with their elbows flexed. None of the clinical signs descriptive of this condition such as Phalen's test or the Tinel have been shown on critical examination to be consistent enough to make a reliable clinical diagnosis. If there is any doubt clinically then electrical studies are mandatory before operation. It may be argued that this is a simple operation from which no harm can come but there is growing evidence that there is a quite definite morbidity from this operation, particularly if it is done by less than skilful operators. It is not unknown for junior surgeons to be assigned this procedure and various complications can ensue, the most serious of which is division of the palmar cutaneous branch (Kessler 1986).

Management

Many patients respond to simple measures such as a resting splint in the neutral wrist position at night and the prescription of a diuretic for those whose symptoms are most troublesome at or around the time of the period. Similarly, in the later stages of pregnancy, symptomatic treatment should be provided as the condition is most likely to resolve completely after delivery. A popular treatment is the injection of steroid into the carpal tunnel but Donal Brooks (personal communication) has repeatedly confirmed that at operation crystals of hydrocortisone can be found around the nerve years after injection and may be a potent cause of continuing irritation. We are not persuaded that steroid injection should be a routine treatment: we recommend it only if surgery is contraindicated and simple measures have failed, and then we always use soluble steroid rather than suspension to avoid persistent irritation.

At the stage that the patient usually presents to the surgeon there is no wasting, very little weakness, and usually no clear sensory loss although there may be some diminution to touch at the fingertips. A series that we conducted correlating the clinical and electrical findings with the pre-operative findings and post-operative course showed that in no case of 30 patients studied was there alteration in the sensory function test as judged by the ability of the patient to recognise textures and objects blindfold. When there is wasting of the thenar eminence and obvious sensory loss the diagnosis is all too obvious and the opportunity for treatment has been missed, usually by many years. The condition is very often bilateral and it is common for the electromyographer to demonstrate quite definite abnormalities on the asymptomatic side. The possibility that the symptoms of carpal tunnel may be the precursor of a generalised peripheral neuropathy must always be kept in mind. It is well recognised that the early signs of generalised peripheral neuropathy show at sites where the nerve is likely to be compressed and this implies the median nerve at the wrist, the ulnar nerve at the elbow and the lateral popliteal at the knee. For this reason, careful electromyographers will invariably test the ulnar nerve by measuring the sensory action potential in the fifth digit and if there is any doubt the sural nerve action potential.

Similarly, central lesions can masquerade as the carpal tunnel syndrome, particularly cord compressions, e.g. syringomyelia and tumours. One of the commonest presentations of patients who have had carcinoma of the breast and irradiation thereafter is of progressive paraesthesiae in the hand due to compression of the plexus at the root of the neck. We have seen many patients in whom the carpal tunnel has been decompressed as it had not been appreciated that the condition was caused more proximally. It is quite common for elderly patients to have some wasting of the thenar eminence. This is well shown in the studies Rembrandt made in his paintings of old people. It is also common to find some wasting of the thenar eminence in patients with carpo-metatacarpal osteoarthritis. In such patients EMG is particularly helpful, for it will distinguish by demonstrating normal sensory conduction that the wasting is not due to a local nerve lesion. The symptoms of carpal tunnel syndrome are often variable and may remit and relapse over many years. It is here that serial EMG studies are particularly helpful. Latterly very sophisticated and refined tests have been developed for demonstrating slight abnormalities of nerve conduction at the wrist (Mills 1985). A routine for such patients is to measure the sensory action potential of the index or middle finger. If this is diminished in amplitude compared with normal and with the other side, and the latency is delayed, then conduction studies and possibly electromyography of the abductor pollicis brevis are undertaken. If there is a delayed latency at the wrist, then this confirms the diagnosis. If these studies are normal and yet the symptoms are highly characteristic, then the palm to wrist test described by Mills is particularly helpful. Here recordings are made over the median and ulnar nerve at the wrist with surface electrodes and the median and ulnar nerves are stimulated in the palm at the same distance from the 2 recording sites. There should of course be little or no difference in the latencies and if the latency is more than 0.5 milliseconds for the median nerve, this is clear evidence of compression at the wrist. The clinician must always be alert to the possibility of carpal tunnel syndrome being symptomatic rather than idiopathic. The commonest causes are rheumatoid arthritis, post-fractures, particularly Colles' fracture, and myxoedema. The case of rheumatoid arthritis is particularly important. In many instances painful paraesthesiae characteristic of carpal tunnel syndrome may be lost in a mêlée of generalised rheumatic symptoms with painful swellings of the wrist, MP and PIP joints.

It is vital not to miss the possibility that a part at least of the patient's symptoms are caused by compression of the median nerve in the carpal tunnel by exuberant tenosynovitis with rheumatoid tissue infiltrating the tendon sheaths. Inflammation of the flexor tendons as a cause of symptoms in rheumatoid arthritis is often overlooked and pain in the hand, particularly on functional activities, is ascribed to inflammation of the MP and PIP joints. For months or years before the overt appearance of joint swellings the tendons may be inflamed and cause severe symptoms. There is a tell-tale swelling in the palms and at the wrist and a boggy feel on pressure. When one can demonstrate full passive movement of the joints with relatively little pain but lack of full active movement, then there is a high index of suspicion that the condition is due to inflamed flexor tendons. Careful questioning may then reveal that the patient is experiencing symptoms suggestive of early compression of the median nerve. Electrical studies will then confirm this and decompression of the carpal tunnel and of the flexor tendons can relieve the compromise of the nerve and deal with the tendon problem at the same time. Barnes & Curry (1967) found that 49% of 45 patients with rheumatoid arthritis had electrical evidence of median nerve compression. Polley & Lipscomb (1966) found that of 1200 cases of carpal tunnel syndrome 29% had rheumatoid arthritis. A surprising number of tendons are found to be ruptured and there is no doubt that there should be a much greater awareness of the problems presented by the tendons in rheumatoid arthritis. The incidence of tendon involvement is much higher than realised. Brewerton (1957) and Souter (1979) found that some two-thirds of the patients they studied had tendon involvement both in the fingers and the thumb. Flatt (1974) has pointed out that the incidence is probably even higher, for it is not easy to examine the tendons overlaid as they are by firm skin, fascia and the retinaculum. Tenosynovitis is often found unexpectedly to be quite marked at operation for carpal tunnel syndrome. If after six months' adequate conservative treatment the synovitis has not settled, then operation to decompress the tendons and nerve should be advised. The author holds strong views also on the importance of early synovectomy of MP joints to prevent subsequent deformity.

We entirely agree with Freyberg (1969) who argues that if synovitis causes the destructive changes which in turn cause the dysfunction and deformities, operation should be advised before erosions are obvious and deformities begin. In 100 patients he studied at 13 year follow up, 61% had important deformities with functional problems. It is generally felt that there is a 50% chance after 10 years that deformities and functional loss will occur and that these may well be prevented.

Unfortunately most patients are seen far too late and the early signs of impending trouble are missed. It has been well established that recurrences are rare after synovectomy provided the operation is undertaken before erosions appear. The surgeon's role in offering relief of pain in this disease by removing inflamed tissue which is compromising nerves, joints and tendons, cannot be over emphasised. We believe he can prevent damage by early surgery as well as by improving function and he should be given the opportunity to see patients at a much earlier stage than at present. There may well be diminution of range of movement after such procedures although pain is almost always relieved. As Flatt (1974) has pointed out, movement does not improve fully until 6 months after surgery so the end result should not be assessed until then. The very recent work of Brown & Brown (1989) is particularly pertinent here. They studied patients with persistent synovial swelling, in whom medical treatment had failed to relieve the signs and symptoms, for more than 6 months and their criteria for surgery were reduced active movement in the presence of significant flexor sheath swelling and greater passive range of movement than active. 173 patients were submitted to tenosynovectomy. In 50% who were operated on for prophylactic reasons there was clear evidence of tendon invasion. At follow-up 70 months after operation only one invaded tendon and one normal extensor tendon had ruptured. These authors convincingly argue that operation must have interfered with the natural progression of the disease and that prophylactic tenosynovectomy is strongly recommended, both to relieve pain and to prevent further deformity. Moreover they show that there was no definite way to determine preoperatively which patient had synovial invasion of tendons, although patients with more active disease or marked localised disease recalcitrant to medical treatment were more likely to have extensive involvement. Surgeons with the most extensive experience of rheumatoid surgery are all agreed that a very high priority should be given to early tendon surgery. At the Royal National Orthopaedic Hospital in London, the second commonest operation on the rheumatoid hand was tenosynovectomy, replacement arthroplasty being only marginally ahead.

There are a variety of circumstances in which the peripheral nerves can be involved in rheumatoid arthritis. By far the commonest are the entrapment neuropathies, carpal tunnel at the wrist in which the nerve is compressed by flexor synovitis or by inflammation of the wrist joint itself, inflammation and swelling of the elbow joint causing compression of the ulnar nerve at the elbow and rarely involvement of the posterior interosseous nerve at the elbow. Secondly the digital sensory nerves can be involved in a somewhat random way (Pallis & Scott 1965). Here the patient complains of numbness and tingling and sometimes pain in 2 or more fingers; examination reveals that the condition is confined to branches of the digital nerves. Prognosis here is good for eventual resolution. Thirdly, generalised polyneuropathy can be a feature of severe rheumatoid disease. Here the patient will feel paraesthesiae and pain in both hands and often in the feet and conduction studies will show that there is slowing of conduction in many nerves. Finally cervical myelopathy is a most important cause of paraesthesiae and pain in the hands. This may well be confused with generalised peripheral neuropathy or with localised entrapment neuropathy such as bilateral carpal tunnel syndrome. The demonstration of normal sensory conduction and denervation in small muscles in the presence of marked sensory abnormality will indicate that the lesion must be proximal and attention will be directed to the cervical spine. Many surgeons will not operate on a patient with rheumatoid disease until they are satisfied that the cervical spine is stable and electrical studies can be most helpful in assessing this type of problem.

Median nerve at the elbow

Occasionally the median nerve can be trapped between the two heads of pronator teres at the elbow. Patients characteristically feel pain from the elbow radiating down the forearm into the hand, on rotation or holding the arm in the flexed position. In established cases there should be weakness of the flexor pollicis longus and the flexor profundus to the index finger. Tenderness can be felt at the elbow and pressure reproduce the paraesthesiae and pain down the forearm into the hand. Measurement of the amplitude to supramaximal stimulation both at wrist and elbow recording over the abductor pollicis brevis may well show evidence of a conduction block.

A demonstration of denervation in the long flexor of the thumb or the index finger or in pronator quadratus will be helpful confirmatory signs.

Ulnar nerve compression

At the wrist the ulnar nerve can be compressed in Guyon's canal by ganglions, lipoma and sometimes in occupational disorders. It may affect either the superficial or the deep branch or both and thus symptoms can sometimes be clinically confusing and electrical studies will be helpful in indicating the level of the lesion. Electromyographers will always bear in mind the possibility of a Martin Grueber anastomosis in which fibres leave the median and cross to the ulnar nerve at midforearm level or vice versa. By far the commonest cause of pain in the hand due to ulnar nerve compromise is from pressure on the ulnar nerve at the elbow. Unfortunately there is still a tendency for surgeons to explore the ulnar nerve at the elbow and transpose it too readily. There is clear evidence in the literature that causalgia and local hyperaesthesiae around the scar are not uncommon sequelae of operations on the ulnar nerve at the elbow and it is our view that surgery to decompress the ulnar nerve should only be undertaken if there is unequivocal evidence clinically of the site of lesion backed up by hard electrophysiological data, with a satisfactory reason for the compression, e.g. an abnormal bed following fracture or swelling due to arthritis. The so called idiopathic varieties are usually due to pressure by Osborne's band and simple decompression is all that is required.

We have seen such distressing sequelae of ulnar nerve transpositions where there has been inadequate reason for the operation to be strongly of the view that this should only be done where the indications are absolute and incontrovertible. Patients are not uncommonly referred for electromyography with the diagnosis of a compressive lesion of the ulnar nerve at the elbow when the patient has quite clear sensory abnormalities in the forearm. Clearly this cannot be localised to the elbow and it must be more proximal. Compromise of the ulnar nerve at the elbow is usually associated with paraesthesiae, numbness and altered sensation rather than pain. *Pain* along the inner side of the forearm with paraesthesiae in the little and ring fingers, is much more likely to be due to compromise of the nerve at the thoracic outlet or in the cervical spine. Electrical studies are particularly helpful in localising the level of the lesion. In a patient with abnormal sensation in the ulnar distribution the demonstration of a normal action potential in the little finger is virtually certain evidence that the lesion is not in the ulnar nerve at the elbow. The following protocol is adopted in our unit for studying ulnar nerve dysfunction: measure the sensory action potential for the little finger on both sides; measure the nerve action potential stimulating at the wrist and recording above the elbow on both sides; record the action potential with surface electrodes over abductor digiti minimi and stimulate with supramaximal shocks at wrist and elbow to detect any decrement at the elbow indicating a conduction block; sample first DIO and/or ADM to determine evidence of denervation, particularly fibrillation potentials and giant units; record in flexor carpi ulnaris and stimulate the ulnar nerve above the elbow to determine a prolonged latency and compare with the other side. Always measure the sensory action potential in the median nerve and if abnormal make sure that this is not due to a co-existing carpal tunnel syndrome and in such cases always measure the sural action potential to make sure that this is not a generalised neuropathy.

Thoracic outlet syndrome

Few clinical orthopaedic conditions have given rise to more confusion than this syndrome. Pain is felt in the shoulder radiating down the arm, with paraesthesiae in the fingers. Characteristically the symptoms are made markedly worse by carrying objects in the affected arm. There are a variety of causes which have been described, the classical cervical rib, the scalenous anticus syndrome, in which a band of the scalenous muscle compresses the neurovascular bundle at the root of the neck, and tight fascia are the commonest. The various anatomical anomalies that may give rise to compression of the neurovascular bundle in the root of the neck are well described in *Campbell's Operative Surgery* (1987) where a full list of references are given. A variety of tests are described but none of them is sufficiently consistent to allow a firm diagnosis to be made. In Adson's test the patient takes a deep breath, holds it, raises up his chin, and turns it towards the side of symptoms. A positive test involves obliterating or reducing the radial pulse.

In the costo–clavicular manoeuvre, the patient shrugs the shoulders backward and downward and takes a deep breath. Again the radial pulse will be obliterated. The problem is that in many normal people both these tests produce reduction in the radial pulse. In Wright's hyperabduction manoeuvre the arms are held above or behind the head with the elbows flexed and this should reproduce the symptoms if the tendon of pectoralis minor is compressing the bundle or it is compressed between the clavicle and the first rib. Pain around the shoulders radiating down the arms is a very common condition, particularly in women who have a lot of lifting and carrying to do or develop a poor posture crouched over a typewriter or VDU. Many such patients have poor musculature around the shoulder and there is no doubt that shoulder raising exercises and attention to postural exercises can markedly relieve such symptoms. We believe that this syndrome is over-diagnosed, and many unnecessary operations, often with disastrous effects are undertaken. It is unfortunate that a paper was published suggesting that there was a typical electromyographic picture of slowing of nerve conduction across the root of the neck. The findings on which this interpretation was based have now been challenged and accepted as wrong. Experienced electromyographers internationally agree that there are no clear cut diagnostic criteria electrophysiologically for this condition. The value of electromyography is in excluding other conditions which may masquerade as the outlet syndrome, in particular paraesthesiae in the hand caused by the carpal tunnel syndrome or ulnar nerve compression at the elbow. We have over the last 10 years been carrying out electrical studies for our hand surgeon who has made a particular study of this condition. In only two patients referred to us have we been able to demonstrate an abnormality suggestive of proximal compression and in both, denervation was found in the small muscles of the hand in the presence of normal motor and sensory conduction. In such circumstances if the symptoms are extremely distressing and the patient has not responded to simple conservative measures, exploration may well be justified but it is mandatory to carry out arterial studies, particularly digital subtraction angiography to make sure that the symptoms are due to vascular compression.

When the patient presents with pain arising from the shoulder, radiating down in the forearm into the hand, with weakness and sensory disorder in the hand and evidence of circulatory compromise with colour changes and in whom the arterial studies are positive, exploration is clearly indicated. In the early stages of this condition there are no neurological signs, no wasting, weakness is usually only symptomatic of pain and the diagnosis can only be made on the classical symptoms. At a late stage the lesion described by Gilliat et al (1970) with wasting of the thenar eminence and paraesthesiae in the ulnar distribution with normal sensory action potential in the median nerve but a reduced action potential for the ulnar nerve with or without denervation in the small muscles, obviously indicates a compressive lesion and usually a cervical rib. However, orthopaedic surgeons rarely see such a phenomenon; they are concerned with the early stages of the condition in which the patient complains of painful paraesthesiae and weakness in the hand and there are no overt physical findings. Neurologists are, of course, more likely to see patients with marked wasting and sensory loss, and a failure to realise the different clinical material that these two specialties will see has led to the belief that the diagnosis of the thoracic outlet syndrome can only be made when there are marked neurological changes. In an admittedly confusing situation we believe that the diagnosis is best made on a very characteristic long-standing history of pain in the shoulder, radiating down the inner arm into the fingers; the pain is worse on carrying, with symptoms often reproduced by deep pressure over the thoracic outlet on the affected side and with relief by elevating down the inner arm into the fingers; the supraclavicular fossa. It must be remembered that there is a definite morbidity from surgery in this area and that even successful surgery by no means always results in resolution of symptoms.

Cervical spondylosis

Osteoarthritis of the apophyseal joints can cause pain referred down the arm with painful paraesthesiae in the hand. The mere demonstration of degenerative changes on X-ray does not imply that these are the cause of symptoms. Well over half the population over the age of 40 have clear cut radiological changes in the cervical spine and the vast majority are symptom-free. The diagnosis of cervical spondylosis as causing root pressure symptoms in the arm and hand should only be made if moving the neck away from the site of pain increases the pain and moving towards the site or traction relieves the pain. Other causes of paraesthesiae and pain in the hand must be excluded particularly the entrapment neuropathies, and thoracic outlet syndrome.

Radicular pain is one of the most distressing of all pains to which man is heir. Physiotherapy can be helpful but in our experience traction almost invariably makes the pain worse and in acute and severe cases the only possible way of obtaining relief is by prolonged immobilisation in a well fitting collar with adequate analgesia. Patients who have suffered weeks of severe pain affecting sleep can be almost invariably totally relieved of their symptoms after 48 hours rest in hospital. At a later stage when the acute symptoms have subsided, gentle active exercise to the neck and isometric exercises to build up the stabilising power of the neck muscles are indicated. In the chronic stage where one can demonstrate limitation of movement in one direction and tenderness over a particular apophyseal joint, mobilisation by Maitland's techniques by the physiotherapist is indicated.

Often injections of trigger spots with local anaesthetic and steroid can be very effective. If there are multiple trigger spots we routinely use needle acupuncture and if this fails, electroacupuncture. We have been most impressed with the value of acupuncture in its various techniques for patients with chronic neck pain, in contradistinction to patients with intractable back pain, where it is only rarely helpful. In patients with persistent severe pain along the distribution of one root who have been unaffected by conservative measures, decompression can be most rewarding. Neurosurgeons may well ask the help of the electrophysiologist to establish, first, that the symptoms are not due to distal entrapment neuropathies, and secondly, that there is denervation or slowing of reflex time in the particular root affected.

Brachial plexus palsy

One of the most devastating effects of traction injuries of the brachial plexus is the severe pain felt by a high proportion of patients after avulsion injuries. In a series of 108 patients described by the author (Wynn Parry 1980) with known avulsion lesions of one or more roots of the plexus, 98 suffered significant pain. Subsequently the same author described 540 patients with traction lesions of the brachial plexus in whom 149 were known to have avulsion of one or more roots and 90% suffered severe pain (Wynn Parry 1984). We did not see any patient with a post-ganglionic lesion suffering significant pain. Causalgic pain, however, can occur in the later stages of recovery in patients in whom grafting has been effected, when the nerves begin to reinnervate the upper arm and forearm. The existence of pain in a completely anaesthetic limb has been known for many years and was christened 'anaesthesia dolorosa'. It has been as much a puzzle to the medical profession as it has to patients how a totally anaesthetic limb can be the seat of such very severe pain. Prior to the experimental work that has made clear the cause of this pain, patients were regarded as either mentally disturbed or depressed for no one could understand how this phenomenon could arise when there was no afferent input to the spinal cord. Loeser & Ward (1967) and Anderson et al (1971) showed that deafferentation leads to profound changes in the spinal cord. Loss of input to the spinal cord results in spontaneous firing of cells in laminas 1 and 5 which gradually increase with time. Study of the experimental records shows an enormous amount of spontaneous firing of high frequency. Two different types of spontaneous discharge are seen: a constant barrage of high frequency activity interspersed with periodic much higher frequency, short duration, paroxysmal discharges. This is entirely mirrored in the clinical situation where patients suffer 2 characteristic types of pain: one, a constant burning, crushing pain, usually felt in the hand or forearm; secondly, periodic paroxysmal shoots of pain lasting a second or two with frequency varying from several times a minute to a few times a day. Not only do deafferented cells start firing spontaneously and continue for years if not indefinitely, but abnormal circuits develop with collateral sprouting at that level.

Wall & Devor (1981) have shown that deafferented cells after a time begin to respond to inputs to which they were normally not sensitive. There are thus a variety of changes centrally which lead to abnormal circuits and abnormal firing states. Albe Fessard & Lombard (1981) showed that after cutting the roots of the brachial plexus in rats abnormal spontaneous firing was seen in the dorsal horn and that after a time this activity might diminish and disappear altogether, only to reappear at much higher levels particularly in the thalamus. This therefore explains how patients' pain can persist indefinitely. Interestingly, these authors showed that electrical stimulation above the level of the avulsion could markedly diminish the amplitude and amount of the spontaneous discharges. They also showed that application of transcutaneous stimulation prior to the experimental lesion might curtail or prevent the development of spontaneous firing altogether. It is thus clear that by applying transcutaneous stimulation at the outset there is a possibility that the development of pain may be prevented. Similar pain is felt after amputation – the so-called phantom pain – and after complete division of the spinal cord. There is some controversy about the incidence of phantom pain. It is usually given as between 5 and 10%, but Sherman et al (1980) have recently shown that it is much higher, particularly in the first 6 months after injury. They found that some 50% of patients had significant pain although most lost this by 6 months after injury. It is well known that the likelihood of developing phantom pain is much greater if there has been significant pain for any length of time before the amputation, as in, for example, peripheral vascular disease. The incidence in spinal injuries is not known but it is certainly higher than is usually believed.

Many patients have told us that they are loath to discuss this with their doctor as they fear they may be thought mentally disturbed by describing pain in an anaesthetic area. What is quite certain is that pain is far commoner in avulsion lesions of the plexus possibly because there is much more damage caused by the disrupting effect of the traction injury than in a clean cut with an amputation or a spinal injury. Excessive gliosis consequent on severe traction may lead to many more abnormal cells firing spontaneously

The onset of pain was immediate in 40% of the author's series but in 11% the pain did not arise until 3 months after injury. In a high proportion, of course, it was impossible to state exactly when the pain began as many patients has head injuries and suffered disturbances of consciousness for some weeks after injury.

It is astonishing how consistently patients describe their symptoms. Most refer to a severe burning quality as if a kettle of boiling water was being poured on their hand or as if red hot pokers were being applied to their skin. In many cases there is a superadded element of severe electric shocks. A high proportion also describe a crushing effect as if the hand or forearm is being compressed in a vice or being slowly tightened by some screw mechanism until it reached bursting point, but it is the paroxysmal shooting pain that is the most difficult to tolerate. Patients after a time become able to cope to some extent with the constant pain but the paroxysmal shooting pains come without any regularity and thus the patient is unable to anticipate them. Often they cry out, seize their arm or bend their neck into their chest, turn away or sometimes even have to leave the room. It is this paroxysmal shooting pain that becomes most wearing and ultimately leads the patients to seek drastic methods of help such as the DREZ operation. Characteristically this pain is much worse in cold and wet weather and is improved in dry warm weather. Several of our patients have found that their pain disappeared completely when they holidayed in a warm climate, but it has to be dry – the humid climates, such as in the Far East, do not relieve the pain. Intercurrent infection and stress always exacerbate the pain and patients can often predict when they are about to suffer an attack of influenza by an exacerbation of their constant pain.

The most consistently significant way of controlling pain is by mental distraction. Almost all our patients tells us that if they can be totally absorbed in some meaningful task at work, or a challenging hobby, they can forget the pain or it can become very much less obtrusive. Paradoxically it is when such patients relax after a hard day's work that the pain hits them with a vengeance and it may make social life intolerable. We have recently analysed 409 patients with known avulsion lesions of the brachial plexus. In 51% the pain settled within 3 years, in 29% the pain was present for longer than 3 years but had become acceptable and did not seriously interfere with their ordinary life. In 19% the pain had been severe for many years and was seriously disrupting their life. In only 1% had there been no pain at any time. 27 patients (0.6%) had to have recourse to the DREZ operation.

208 patients were seen in whom the pain completely settled – 60% within one year (27% within 6 months), 81% within 2 years and 96% by the end of the third year. The natural history of the condition, therefore, seems to be that within one year over half the patients will lose their pain or be able to control it so as to be able to live a reasonably normal life and that most will have lost their pain within 3 years. It is important to appreciate

Table 6.1. Brachial Plexus Lesions
Type of lesion in those with severe pain
(n = 52)

30%	complete C5 – T1
18%	C8 – T1
20%	C7 – T1
15%	C6 – T1

the natural history of this condition so as not to recommend drastic procedures such as dorsal root entry zone lesions within the first 3 years, for there is a high chance that patients will spontaneously lose their pain or be able to come to terms with it.

52 patients were seen who had had pain for many years. We analysed the nature of the lesion in these patients and Table 6.1 shows the result. In 39 there was no pain or pain was never a problem, and again we analysed the level of lesion to see if there were any significant findings. There was no difference in the type of lesion in those patients who had very severe pain or with little or no pain. We had expected to find that patients with total lesions were unlikely to have no pain but this was not the case, for 60% of the patients who had no pain had complete lesions involving C5 to T1.

Of those patients we studied in whom the pain was still severe many years after the injury, nearly half had had the pain for more than 20 years. The single most effective modality to relieve this pain has proved to be transcutaneous electrical stimulation. This was tried in 158 patients and was effective in 100. We studied the length of time patients had suffered pain before they responded to TNS: surprisingly, however long there have been symptoms, there may still be a dramatic response to transcutaneous stimulation. One fifth of the patients had had symptoms for more than 5 years. The nature of the lesion was not particularly significant in the response to treatment although there was some evidence that total lesions were less likely to respond, for in our series 23 patients with total lesions responded to TNS whereas 34 did not.

The technique of application of transcutaneous stimulation is all important. Far too often pain clinics hand the patient a stimulator with scant instructions on how to use it. Many have been told to try it for half an hour or an hour daily or even only 3 times a week. We have had extensive experience of the use of this modality and we insist on admitting our patients to our rehabilitation ward where our physiotherapists experiment with different placings of the electrodes with different repetition rates, durations and frequencies of the stimulator for varying periods of time (Frampton 1982). It is our custom to insist that patients use the stimulator at least 8 hours a day and try at least 4 different positions and variable settings of the parameters. We are amazed to find that patients have been advised to put the electrodes on areas where there is inadequate or even complete absence of sensation. The rationale of the use of this modality depends entirely on obtaining maximum afferent input above and below the level of the spontaneous firing in the spinal cord. It is believed that TENS acts both pre- and post-synaptically but in avulsion lesions it will clearly act to prevent transmission of nociceptive impulses to the higher centres. The beauty of this treatment is that it is non-invasive, entirely safe and can be used indefinitely. It is also considerably cheaper than regular analgesics. Occasionally patients form allergies to the electrode jelly and one must experiment with different types of jelly and different types of electrodes. One cannot, of course, use the stimulator in patients with a pacemaker but otherwise there are few if any contraindications.

The standard drugs are singularly unhelpful in this type of pain. Some patients find codeine preparations take the edge off pain but interestingly enough, the narcotics are useless. In 18, carbamazepine was of significant help for the paroxysmal shooting pains. If patients have periodic attacks of paroxysmal pain with relatively long pain-free intervals we prescribe the carbamezapine syrup rather than regular medication with tablets. We use the standard medical dosage schedule for carbamazepine, i.e. 100 mg twice a day, doubling at the end of the week and increasing up to 1200 mg maximum dose. A few patients responded to triptafen, a combination of an antihistamine and an antidepressant and there is no doubt that the antidepressants can be helpful in central pain, not for their antidepressant properties but for their effect on serotonin production. It is, of course, essential to explain to patients that this compound is being used for its pain relieving properties and that one does not regard the patient as being depressed. The patients' confidence in their doctor may be seriously undermined if they discover they are being given antidepressants and believe that the doctor feels that they are mentally disturbed.

Fortunately there are a very large majority of patients who find relief from pain by intensive work or demanding hobbies. It is therefore of paramount importance to ensure that these young people are offered retraining or get back to work as soon as possible. A resettlement officer is an integral part of our rehabilitation team at the Royal National Orthopaedic Hospital. His role is to make contact with the employer, keep him in touch with the patient's medical progress and enquire into the work situation so that it can be adapted to the patient's requirements. Most employers will be delighted to keep a place open for their employee provided they are kept informed of progress. We have an 80% success record in returning these patients back to work or to retraining as a result of the efforts of our resettlement officer.

For those patients who fail to respond to an intensive rehabilitation programme including prolonged and proper application of TENS, trial of the various drugs, trial of a significant period at work or with demanding hobbies, and the pain is still devastating their life, there remains the operation of dorsal root entry zone coagulation as described originally by Nashold and his co-workers in Duke University, North Carolina (1976). The rationale here is to destroy that part of the spinal cord where the actual abnormality arises, i.e. to destroy those deafferented cells which are the seat of spontaneous discharges and therefore pain. It is unlike most neurosurgical procedures for pain in that it does not divide tracts for it is now known that division of spinothalamic and mesencephalic tracts are doomed to failure. Within months pain returns often much worse than before – for dividing tracts produces more deafferentation, more spontaneous firing and therefore more pain. The DREZ lesion, however, is based on a different rationale. Nashold & Osdahl (1979) have reported on an 8 year follow up on a series of some 70 patients with a 60% relief of pain (see Ch. 10).

We have experience of 35 patients, the operations being carried out by Mr David Thomas (Thomas & Sheehy 1983) at the National Hospital, Queen Square, London. Again, there is a 60% relief rate but it must be stressed that there are serious complications. In one of our cases long term impotence was produced and in 2 impotence for 6 months. In 5 there was weakness of the ipsilateral leg and in 2 of these it was severe. In 2 there were considerable problems with neck instability and chronic pain. In 9 there were mild sensory disturbances on the trunk and in 3 of the contralateral arm. In 6 there was severe temporary weakness of the leg which improved with time and rehabilitation.

In our series therefore there were no complications in 19, in 9 there were motor complications, in 4 sensory complications and motor and sensory complications together in 4, including clumsiness, ataxia and severe post-laminectomy pain. We are unfortunately now seeing patients in whom the pain has recurred after some years, and it is for these reasons that patients must be psychologically robust before we recommend this procedure for they may have to cope with the possibility either of no relief of pain at all after a severe operation, or the return of the pain some years later. It is therefore imperative that patients regard this procedure as the last resort and are not recommended for it until at least 3 years after the injury, to cater for the natural history of the condition. We always interview the spouse of the patient and both the patient and the spouse must be desperate for surgery. The doctor must be persuaded that the pain is destroying both the patient's and the family's life. Certainly no patient should be referred for a DREZ lesion unless he has had a very extensive assessment as an inpatient and been seen by all members of the rehabilitation team. We have a number of patients desperate with pain but who, when the whole matter was explained in detail to them and they were given an intensive rehabilitation programme including a fitness programme, and prolonged counselling from our clinical psychologist, accepted that they must come to terms with the pain and were able to manage without having recourse to the operation.

Because of the radical nature of the DREZ operation and the fact that some patients have suffered severe locomotor disability thereafter, some have claimed that they would have preferred the pain rather than suffer these complications. It is as well to make a tape recording of the patients' description of the pain and of the effect it is having on their lives, with comments from the relevant spouse, so that it is recorded that they will go through anything in order to get rid of the pain. Wherever possible it is important for the patient to see somebody who has had this procedure. We cannot emphasise enough the importance of a comprehensive assessment and rehabilitation programme before submitting the patient to this operation. The right person to recommend it is the physician not the surgeon for once the patient sees a neurosurgeon he is very likely to be offered an operation. This is, after all, what the surgeon is trained to do and it is not reasonable to expect him to go through a prolonged preoperative assessment procedure – this should be the responsibility of the physician. A refinement is to carry out sensory evoked potentials to demonstrate whether there have been subtle long tract signs before operation so that the surgeon can be reassured that he has not in fact damaged tracts as a result of the surgery.

When the nature of the operation is explained to them many patients fight shy of such a destructive procedure and decide that they will continue to try and cope with their pain. Some of them are frightened at the idea of operating directly on their nervous system. Interestingly, many years ago we tried the effect of a thalamic stimulator on 5 patients: 2 were a success, 2 were a failure and 1 had no effect. We offered this treatment to several patients, many of whom said that they could not bear the thought of a surgeon operating on their soul! One thing, though, that patients do find helpful is to know that there is still something else at the end of the line and they have not reached a final stage in which nothing more can be offered. Even if they have decided not to have the DREZ operation, the fact that there is something else there if they become totally desperate is psychologically a great boost to them.

Over and over again we hear from patients that reaching and maintaining a reasonable standard of physical fitness does help them to cope with the pain much better.

One of the more extraordinary phenomena in this field of brachial plexus lesions is the report from Narakas & Henz (1988) and Bonnard & Narakas (1985) that neurotisation and nerve grafting can very markedly reduce or even abolish the severe avulsion pain. This has been confirmed by our group although it is by no means invariable.

It is difficult to understand how neurotisation, the transfer of intercostal nerves to the distal stump of the median, or musculocutaneous or putting the accessory into the suprascapular, can affect pain after an avulsion lesion. It may be that increased afferent input around the area where there is spontaneous firing in laminas 1 and 5 of the dorsal horn may be just sufficient to damp down the transmission of the abnormal impulses. It is however an undoubted fact that some people do achieve relief of pain by nerve grafting procedures. It would be a brave surgeon who would operate in this regard solely for pain and if grafting procedures are being considered the fact that the patient has severe pain is an added reason for attempting to improve function.

One of the most important points in management is explaining in detail to the patient exactly why he has the pain, its nature, the natural history and how important it is for he himself to try and control it by distraction. Even though an explanation may not affect the actual disorder itself it certainly allays the patient's fears and anxieties that he is mentally disturbed and an appreciation of the nature of the beast is often very therapeutic. It is also a great help to a patient to meet others with like disabilities, to compare notes and realise that he is not the only person in such trouble. This is one of the many reasons why the intensive rehabilitation ward is so useful, as these patients can meet together, work together and play together. From time to time we have patients who have gone completely to pieces as a result of the pain and they are given a remarkable psychological boost by other patients helping them to come to terms with it. It is a great help, for example, for somebody in the first few months of the disorder to see patients two or three years on who have mastered their pain or in whom it is very little trouble. They can also learn little tricks of the trade from other patients as to how they cope with their pain. Some find that if they allow the pain to break over them like a wave and allow it to reach its zenith they can relax afterwards and the pain may be kept at bay for some time. Others try and fight the centre

80 MANAGEMENT OF PAIN IN THE HAND AND WRIST

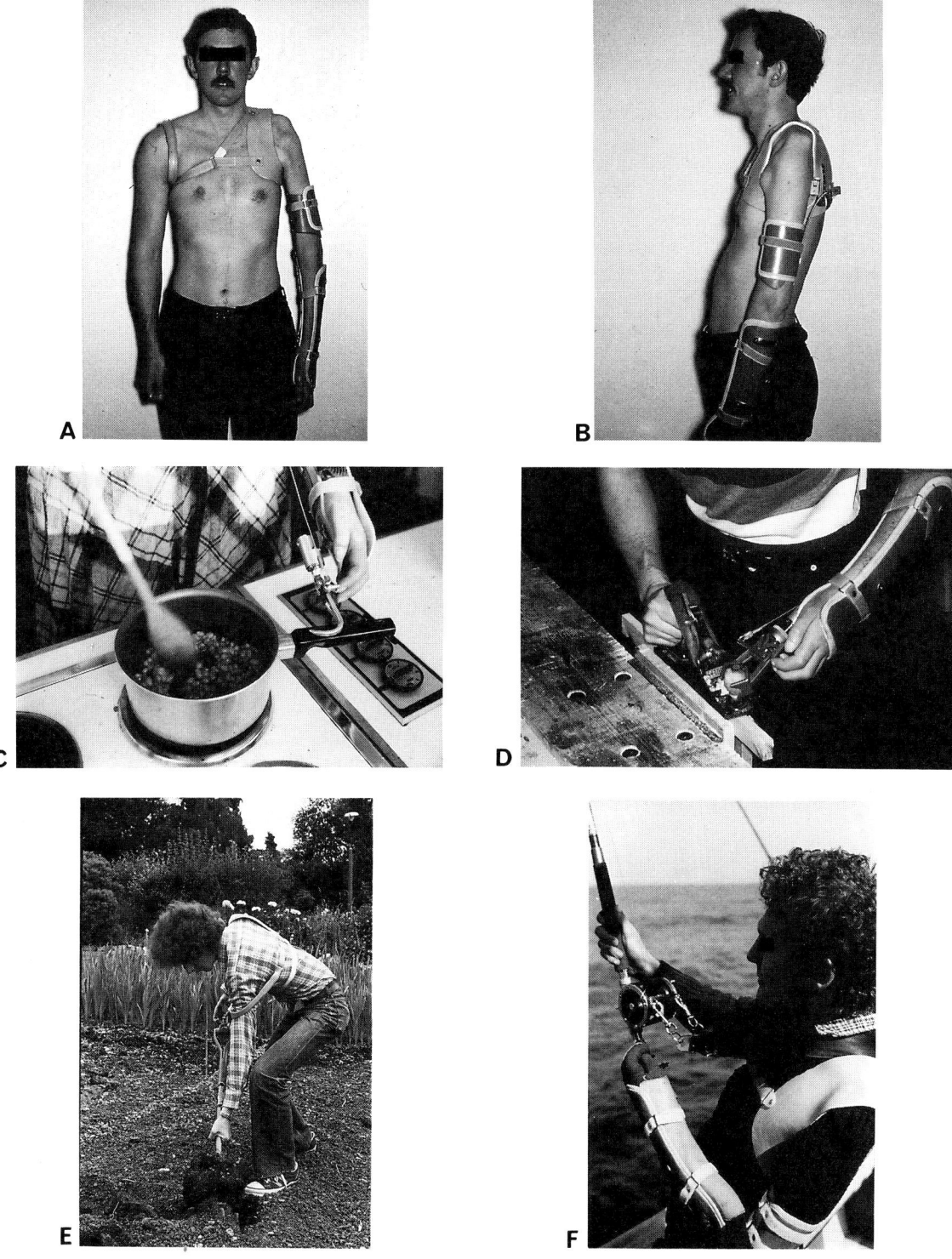

Fig. 6.1 Flail arm splint for total paralysis after brachial plexus lesions: (a) (b) Splint. (c) Split hook. (d) Universal tool holder. (e) Attachment for holding spade. This patient was a full time professional gardener. (f) Attachment for fishing.

of the pain, as it were, to stop the wave reaching its maximum height but most patients find it better to allow the pain to take them over and then relax thereafter.

We did try the effect of hypnosis from a professional hypnotist but this proved very disappointing. We had 7 patients with severe pain who found no benefit at all from autohypnosis. Relaxation techniques are always worth teaching as many patients find that it helps them to adjust to their pain and to give their body the best chance of fighting it.

We have emphasised the great importance of helping these patients to return to work or to meaningful hobbies in order to obtain maximum distraction and to this end some years ago, we introduced functional splinting, in particular for patients with total paralysis of the limb. The idea is to provide as it were an artificial arm over the patient's own arm. The splint consists of a shoulder supporting piece, an elbow-locking device so that the patient can put his elbow into one of 5 different positions; and a forearm trough on the wrist support into which the standard appliances for an artificial limb can be slotted (see Fig. 6.1). The terminal device can be either operated by the other hand or by the shoulder harness from the contralateral arm as in a standard artificial limb. The splint becomes as it were a mobile vice and allows patients to put objects into the terminal appliance in order to hold things and support them. The most popular devices are the split hook and universal tool holder. A wide variety of trades are made much easier by this device. These include spray painting, welding, engine fitting, painting and decorating and gardening.

Figure 6.1e shows a patient wearing the full flail arm splint being able to carry out his profession as a full time gardener. This patient became so adept at the use of the splint that he was in no way disabled and could carry out every activity that an able bodied person was able to do. Many patients do not require the splint at their work, particularly if it is a clerical type of job but do find it useful for their hobbies, particularly 'D-I-Y activities', fishing, golf and even cricket. A well trained skilled orthotist can devise an appliance to cater for almost any needs and often patients think up ingenious devices themselves.

This is another advantage of the inpatient intensive rehabilitation service, where the occupational therapist, orthotist and the patient can work out together solutions to functional problems. In patients who have C5/6/7 palsies with paralysis of elbow flexion, elbow extension and wrist and finger extension, the elbow lock splint with or without a wrist support can be provided. Finally, in the rare patients in which there is either sparing or full return of elbow function, e.g. in a C8/T1 lesion, then the forearm element of the splint alone need be provided so that the patient can flex and extend his elbow himself.

The splints are ready made, coming in 3 standard sizes, and the orthotist by adjustment can make the splint fit almost anyone. It is however a skilled procedure and we have noticed that a number of units are disappointed in the use of this splint and on enquiry it has been found that the splints have been supplied without proper fitting and training. We insist that all our patients are admitted, for it takes some 10 days for the fitting and proper training of the patient in the use of the splint. At a recent follow up of over 100 patients who had been provided with the full flail arm splint, 70% were using them either at work or at hobbies or D-I-Y activities. Furthermore, employers are often reluctant to take on employees with a totally paralysed arm and much more willing if the patient can show that he has some function using a splint. There is no doubt that the provision of functional splinting has revolutionised the management of these unfortunate patients and has enabled many of them to return to work and thus distract themselves from pain or to pursue meaningful and demanding hobbies with the same effect. We have had a number of housewives with brachial plexus lesions and the splint, with the various attachments, has allowed them to cook and run their household.

CASE HISTORIES

Case history 1 (BJC)

Total brachial plexus palsy 5 years ago.

'The pain is present all the time on a scale of 1 to 10, about 5–6 with occasional bursts of 9–10 which last between 10–15 seconds. I have noticed that a day or so before the symptoms of a cold or flu come out, the bursts of pain become much more frequent. I don't use the stimulator anymore because I found it becoming less effective. When I first used it, it did nothing for the constant pain but it did halt the sharp peaks of pain. I take 2 DF118 to sleep each night, which last until the early hours when I just doze on and off.'

Case history 2 (KW)

Total brachial plexus palsy in a woman in which the pain appeared 2 months after onset. The stimulator was of great help in the early stages. Two years later she reported as follows: 'I have very little pain on the whole, i.e. I have no pain for a few weeks then I'll have a day or two when it is painful. Most significant amount of pain happens when I have my period, although pain doesn't happen every period. If any one period pain starts then it will usually continue for a few days (intermittent pains, not constant) whereas if I have pain at some other time (other than when I have my period) it only lasts for that day. Before the accident I never had any bad periods and my actual period still causes no bother. I have several distinct types of pain and I can usually tell how long it will last and whether I ought to take pills. When pain is severe in finger and thumb then I'll take pills, otherwise I tend not to.'

Case history 3 (PGK)

Complete lesion 2 years ago.
Severe pain 3 weeks after injury with shooting pains lasting 10–20 seconds several times a day. He reports: 'Psychologically I feel that I want to move my arm and clench my fist but can do neither. My mind tells me that I can, yet physically it is impossible. One of my favourite hobbies is fishing and in this weather my arm and hand gets very cold. About 3 days after this, then I get really severe pains, and this can be almost constant for 8–12 hours. Otherwise pain is periodic, maybe 2 or 3 times weekly, but only for short bursts.'

Case history 4 (JB)

He reports 6 years after the injury:
'Since the date of the accident the pain has become tolerable but it still affects me. I still feel the hand and more important the wound, also the elbow. At times the elbow and hand contort in different positions not the normal positions of relaxed arms and hands as they should be, for instance, I felt my hand upon my shoulder as if it was stuck on. I can move my fingers and wrist, my fingers are always in the gripped position but I can move them slightly. I feel my hand all the time, I am used to it. When I do get the bad pains I clutch my shoulder and arm – this doesn't get rid of the pain but now I feel you are trying to do something about it. When the pain comes on the wrist twists itself inwards and I can't stop that.'

Case history 5 (SH)

Seven years after the accident, he found that the stimulator was a great help. His comments in reply to a standard questionnaire are:
'The stimulator has removed all severe pain, both spasmodic and continuous, although I stated a 90% improvement on the previous page, I feel that I could create a situation of almost 100% if I wore the stimulator on a regular basis instead of when the pain felt imminent. The form has been answered with conditions that prevailed before wearing the stimulator because most of the questions do not now apply, such is the effectiveness of the stimulator in my case.'

Case history 6 (JMCA)

One year after total lesion:
'The stimulator helped when the pain was constant but now that the pain is periodic the stimulator doesn't work. Regarding alcohol I find that if I have quite a lot to drink I get more pain in my arm the following day. It seems to help at the time of drinking but I suffer for it afterwards.'

Case history 7 (MAA)

Reporting 3 years after the accident:
'I personally found that in the early stages of pain after my accident, I could delay or lessen the pain by massaging or moving the fingers on my affected hand with my good hand. I feel I have learnt to control the pain much better nowadays but there are 3 things that nearly always give extremely severe periodic shooting pains: (1) very cold or unsettled weather (could it be something to do with atmospheric pressure?); (2) illness, particularly when I feel run down, as with 'flu; (3) tiredness: if I have been working hard during the day and I relax by say, watching television, I find I often get severe pain.'

Case history 8 (AH)

Twenty years after the accident, he gives a graphic account of the pain:
'In the summer of 1979 I tried the electrical stimulator for the first time. It seemed to work until the onset of winter when the severe bouts of pain became so frequent and so prolonged that I would black out with the intensity. The sensation felt can

only be described as starting with very intense pins and needles sensations shooting from the wrist to elbow, on to the shoulder joint. All joints of the limb seemed centres for severe pain. After 5–10 minutes the pain becomes scalding pain, and feels like plunging the arm in boiling water. When this occurs I usually black out. I consider that if I have to stop doing any concentrated work or activity twice or more in any hour the pain gets worse and I then have to resort to drugs. Some days I get only 4 short periods (1–2 minutes) of pain where the intensity is beyond a level where it can be ignored. This is the average and the only thing I find is that one becomes used to feeling pain constantly at low levels and ignoring it.

Causalgia

Causalgia means burning pain and was a term originally invented by Weir-Mitchell to describe the very severe pain felt in some patients with partial nerve lesions following gunshot wounds in the American Civil War. His book *Gunshot Wounds and other Injuries of Nerves* was published in 1872 and the clinical description of patients with this severe pain has never been bettered. A short time after injury and in some cases within hours a severe burning pain would develop in the hand or foot according to which nerve was involved, median or sciatic. This was followed graphically by what Weir-Mitchell described as hyperaesthesiae and we would now describe as allodynia, that is the abnormal response of light touch to the skin by severe pain. He noted marked colour changes with cyanosis and mottling of the skin, often eruptions of the skin so that it might mimic a number of skin diseases, often swelling of the joints mimicking rheumatoid arthritis, severe dystrophic nail changes with pitting, coarseness and overgrowth, loss of hair in the distribution of the affected nerve, in time spread to other nerves such that some months after damage to a median nerve the patient would notice allodynia and spontaneous pain in the distribution of the ulnar nerve, in severe cases spreading to involve the entire arm.

At a later stage a fine tremor or complex spontaneous movements could develop in the affected limb spreading at a much later stage to the contralateral limb. He noted that these symptoms might well subside with time but were liable to recur with subsequent illness. He pointed out the chronicity of the condition for in many patients the symptoms would last indefinitely. Weir-Mitchell's son was also a neurologist and he followed up 22 of his father's patients 27 years after injury and found that half of them were still suffering very severe pain (Mitchell 1895).

Thus he was able to trace 6 patients with median and ulnar nerve lesions, of which 3 were still suffering severe pain; 4 patients with sciatic lesions, of which 2 were suffering severe pain and 5 patients with gunshot wounds to the brachial plexus, all of whom were still suffering severely. Characteristically there is both spontaneous pain and pain following nonnociceptive stimuli. It is almost invariably associated with partial lesions and it is very unusual in total lesions. Clearly there needs to be a significant amount of afferent input in order to produce the symptoms. Experimental work referred to elsewhere in this volume has shown that it is a hypersensitivity of the large diameter afferent fibres to circulating adrenergic substances that is responsible and it is not a disorder of the sympathetic nervous system itself. This condition is one example of sympathetic dependent pain (as is reflex sympathetic dystrophy or Sudeck's atrophy), a term describing the relationship of the symptoms to the sympathetic nervous system but not necessarily incriminating the system as abnormal. Wallin et al (1981) have shown that in a patient with causalgia who responded dramatically to transcutaneous stimulation, recording of electrical activity in the sympathetic fasicles showed no change before and after treatment. Clearly the immediate onset of pain in many of these patients must imply a central mechanism for there is not time for the peripheral results of nerve damage so well described by Wall and others to appear. In the more chronic case, there will be both peripheral and central effects. Peripherally there is the spontaneous firing from the neuroma and sprouts from regeneration and abnormal sensitivity to circulating noradrenalin (Scadding 1984). Local ischemia may cause the nerve to become an ectopic generator (Ochoa and Toebiork 1981). There are, of course, the widespread rapidly developing central changes as a result of partial deafferentation described by Wall & Devor (1981), the response of deafferented cells to inputs to which they do not normally respond, abnormal sprouting and the development of spontaneously firing neurons in the dorsal horn following deafferentation. In Chapter 2, Roberts argues convincingly that the involvement of the sympathetic nervous system is due to disinhibition at spinal level.

Why should a small proportion of patients after peripheral nerve damage show this extraordinary phenomenon? All nerves repair by formation of a neuroma but in only a small proportion does this neuroma become severely painful, giving spontaneous burning pain and allodynia. Why, too, after division of the nerve with temporary relief of pain does the pain often return and exactly in the site where the pain was present before? (Nordenboos & Wall 1981). Clearly there must be a central template of pain awaiting to be aroused when afferent input returns. It is the large soft swellings that are the most painful. These are loaded with fine, immature, inadequately sheathed and highly sensitive sprouts. Farcot (1985) has reported on 230 patients in which nerve suture was carried out – 70% within one year, mostly in the first 6 months. 50 showed mild hyperaesthesiae, 15 allodynia and hyperpathia and in 4 symptoms were very severe. The type of injury was not important and there was no suggestion of a causalgic diathesis. The literature is full of references, particularly in reflex sympathetic dystrophy to the type of patient likely to develop this syndrome, who is nervous, immature and neurotic. We strongly refute this theory. Patients with chronic pain of this sort develop reactive depression and as soon as their symptoms are relieved they become quite normal. There is therefore something between a 5 and 7% incidence of causalgia after nerve injuries – it is far more likely to develop in partial lesions and in those nerves with a large sensory component. This is why they are commonest in median and sciatic nerves lesions. The ulnar nerve, however, is also prone to this condition particularly in patients who have repeated transpositions for suspected ulnar neuritis at the elbow.

These patients classically develop allodynia and hyperpathia in a wide area round the scar at the elbow, such that they are quite unable to wear clothing next to the skin. In both causalgia and reflex sympathetic dystrophy there are common features. Both show spontaneous burning pain with allodynia and/or hyperpathia. Both have trophic changes in the soft tissues and nails, both show colour changes. One of the striking features in patients with chronic causalgia are the changes in the fingers. The skin loses its wrinkles and becomes smooth, hairless and sometimes pink and blotched and always showing marked reduction in its size. Often sensation is relatively well preserved and once the pain is relieved one can see how sensory function becomes almost normal as judged by the ability to recognise textures and objects blindfold. Weir-Mitchell recognised this and described it as follows: 'It was common in many of the cases of burning pain to witness a condition in which a touch was interpreted or felt as pain. In such incidents localisation is often perfect and the sense of touch not lost but practically defective by reason of the overwhelming influence of the pain.' It cannot be over-emphasised how chronic this condition can be when untreated, although as can be seen later over 70% of our patients obtained complete or substantial relief of symptoms by vigorous treatment. 30% are left with chronic intractable pain and of these who do respond a significant proportion recur and need to be followed up indefinitely.

It must also be emphasised how patients may respond either by surgery or to conservative treatment with marked relief of pain for a short period of time. It is well recognised that after nerve grafting symptoms may abate completely only to return when afferent input returns. It is therefore essential that surgeons and physicians alike follow up these patients indefinitely and are not hoodwinked into thinking that their efforts have been successful by too short a follow up period.

The classical case is that of Josh H. Corliss, late private of B Company, 14th New York State Militia, aged 27, a shingle dresser enlisted April 1861. 'At the second battle of Bull Run, 29 August 1862, he was shot in the left arm 3 inches above the internal condyle and the bullet emerged 1.25 inches higher. He was ramming a cartridge when hit and thought he was struck on the crazy bone by some of the boys for a joke. Resection of the median nerve was no good. A week after he was shot in the right arm, he was weak and could not feed himself. By April 1864 he was better, he had pain in the median distribution but excessive pain in the ulnar. He kept his hand strapped in a rag, dampened with cold water and covered with oil silk. Moisture was more essential to him than cold, he kept a bottle of water about him with a wet sponge in his right hand, and kept water in his boots. It was as if a rough bar of iron was thrust to and fro through the knuckles and a red hot iron placed at the junction of the palm and thenar eminence with a heavy weight on it and the skin rasped off his finger ends. The rattling of a newspaper, a breath of air, the step of another across the ward, the vibrations caused by a military band or the shock of the feet in walking gave rise to increase of pain. He insisted an observer wet his hand before touching him – cold weather eased it, heat made it worse.'

Involuntary movements are a feature of severe chronic pain but are curiously overlooked in the literature. Most of our patients with chronic causalgia and chronic reflex dystrophy develop abnormal involuntary movements. These are never a simple tremor but a complex coordinated system of movements indicating that there must be a lesion at spinal level at least. It is not at all uncommon to see similar movements develop at a later stage in the contralateral limb. Weir-Mitchell describes one of his cases: 'For a long time after the injury he had lateral twitching and feeling as if his toes were crawling on top of another.'

Case report:

Colonel JCP, aged 41, an officer of the 139th Pennsylvanian Volunteers of good character, was shot in the right wrist. At once he became singularly excited and felt as if he were crazed. Under sudden influence of these sensations, he ran along the line of his regiment, only half conscious. Amputation of the forearm was carried out, middle and lower third. Three months later, quivering of the stump commenced, extending to all muscles of the forearm except extensors, and by the close of the second month, it had spread to biceps, triceps and deltoid. The scar was dissected out, for a few days he did better and then relapsed, as happened after use of other remedies. On 1 March 1865, his forearm was incessantly in motion, whether asleep or awake. Every 20 minutes or sooner, the forearm was suddenly flexed and more rarely thrown across the chest or upwards and outwards. This did not interfere with voluntary movement, and increased if attention was drawn to it. There was no tenderness of the stump. He continued to serve. On 25 March 1865, he was wounded in the left side. From then on, the arm ceased to jump as it had.

One of the characteristic features of this condition is that, although light touch is virtually unbearable, the patient can tolerate firm pressure by gripping the affected part firmly, which can often relieve the pain. Some people find that rubbing vigorously above the level of the pain can be helpful. In both circumstances one imagines that the large afferent fibres are being stimulated and gating off the nociceptive traffic centrally. In severe cases, these patients cannot bring the affected limb into use at all for the slightest touch, breath of air, or vibration causes an exacerbation of pain. They then develop stiffness in the affected digits. There is a characteristic picture, for example, in median nerve causalgia, of the index and middle fingers being kept straight and activities being only carried out by the unaffected fingers. The patients are almost always worse in cold, wet weather.

Reflex sympathetic dystrophy (RSD)

At least 22 different descriptions have been given of the condition of severe burning pain following trivial injuries or minor fractures with swelling of the part, spontaneous pain and allodynia progressing in time to a stiff useless hand or foot. Sudeck (1900), who was a radiologist, described the X-ray appearances as an acute atrophy of bone associated with swelling, pain and loss of function and described it originally in the foot. Three stages, acute, sub-acute and chronic are recognised but in practice the condition is acute with severe swelling, spontaneous burning pain, allodynia and marked colour changes in the skin followed in the chronic stage by an atrophic, stiff, useless, frozen but usually not painful hand or foot. The nosology of this condition and the probable mechanisms are described fully elsewhere in this volume. Clearly any theory has to take into account the surprisingly speedy development of symptoms following relatively trivial injuries. The very worse case we have ever seen followed in a man who accidentally knocked his hand against a wall whilst playing ball with his small son. A hairline fracture in the head of one metacarpal developed but subsequently he developed a very severe dystrophic painful condition in which the entire hand was completely immobile and allodynia spread involving the whole hand up to the mid forearm. In another of our patients repeated attempts to deal with a stiff finger after damage to the flexor tendons and the digital nerve involved operations and multiple amputations. This resulted in allodynia and spontaneous burning pain affecting the whole of the forequarter of that limb. We are impressed with Roberts' theory of disinhibition of sympathetic neurones centrally, fully described in Chapter 2. We do not subscribe to the view that the definition of reflex sympathetic dystrophy or causalgia is 'that pain that responds to the sympathetic blockade', for many of our patients do not respond. Moreover Burnstock (1983) pointed out there are at least 16 transmitters in the sympathetic nervous system and that ATP may be much more important than noradrenalin. Failure to respond to blocking noradrenalin may by no means mean that the condition is not associated with supersensitivity and sympathetic drive. As Janig & Koffman (1984) have pointed out, there are probably 8 different sympathetic nervous systems involving different systems in the body. Clearly the whole condition is very much more complicated than originally thought but clearly also there are many patients who respond to blocking of the sympathetic nerve and the sympathetic nervous system must play an important part in one way or another.

Among the conditions described that can give rise to this disorder are soft tissue injuries, fasciitis, ligament injuries, arthritis, fracture dislocation, immobilisation in plaster, deep venous thrombosis.

Recovering brachial plexus lesions and nerve root lesions can also be responsible including accidents, tumours, and spinal cord trauma. Idiopathic cases can arise where there is no evidence of trauma at all and occasionally it may follow prolonged immobilisation. Central lesions fully described in Chapter 4 can cause classical RSD.

Investigations of this condition, particularly for research purposes, must involve pre- and postsynaptic block signatures to show the change in hand function, and careful recording of changes in sensation. Skin temperatures are measured by thermography, and sweat tests, skin blood flow, ice response of skin blood flow, possibly a bone scan and certainly X-ray investigations should be carried out in all cases.

A characteristic feature of Sudeck's atrophy or RSD is the osteoporosis that can follow quite quickly after the injury, and is of course the salient feature in the original description of the condition by Sudeck himself. Less often realised is that osteoporosis almost invariably follows causalgia and most of our patients with causalgia following nerve lesions develop marked osteoporosis, first in the digits affected by the nerve and later perhaps spreading to the whole hand or foot. There may be a relation between another condition – acute idiopathic osteoporosis of bone, in which patients develop severe swelling, pain and osteoporosis in a hand or foot without preceding trauma. The condition is usually self-limiting but may give severe symptoms for several months. It is important to insist that the condition of reflex sympathetic dystrophy is only applied to those conditions with the classic features of spontaneous pain, allodynia, swelling, colour changes in the skin, trophic lesions in the tissues and osteoporosis. No purpose is served by describing anyone with a stiff painful hand after injury as having Sudeck's atrophy, as periodically appears in the literature. Extravagant claims are made for treatment regimes in Sudeck's atrophy, but careful scrutiny of the papers reveals that these are not true Sudeck's atrophies at all but simply stiff and painful hands following injury or prolonged periods in plaster.

TREATMENT

The management of causalgia and reflex sympathetic dystrophy will be discussed together for we are convinced that the underlying mechanisms of both conditions are alike. The symptomatology is virtually the same as are the end results of untreated cases. The natural history of reflex sympathetic dystrophy is as gloomy as causalgia. The biggest series was reported from the Mayo Clinic in 1981 (Subbarao & Stillwell 1981): 17% of 86 patients followed up had poor results. The majority of their patients still had pain in the shoulder or hand at follow-up 14 months after injury, 35% were officially disabled. Everyone dealing with these conditions agrees that the earlier treatment is started the more likely it is to be successful, not only in relieving severe pain but in preventing development of subsequent deformities. Some of the worse deformities of the hand that we have seen have followed untreated Sudeck's atrophy. Clearly surgical attempts to improve range of movement by capsulotomy and ligament resection are fraught with the danger of the patient developing Sudeck's atrophy again. In this regard we urge our surgical colleagues always to give a guanethidine block following operation if somebody who has developed causalgia or Sudeck's atrophy in the past requires surgery at a later stage, in the hope that the condition can be prevented. We know only too well how liable these conditions are to recur with subsequent illness or following surgery (Livingstone 1943).

The dramatic effect of sympathetic block was first shown by Barnes (1954) in his experience of patients with peripheral nerve injuries in the Second World War. Unfortunately in many patients the pain recurred as severely as before, some months after sympathectomy and the effects of stellate block were only temporary in most cases. However Barnes had shown quite clearly that the condition was reversible and that the sympathetic nervous system must play an extremely important part. Subsequently Hannington Kiff (1974) showed that guanethedine was a potent means of providing prolonged sympathetic block, was more efficient and of course more convenient than stellate block. Stellate block requires an experienced anaesthetist and is not without dangers.

Guanethedine block can be entrusted to a competent house physician or surgeon and can of course be repeated as often as necessary. Guanethedine depletes the tissue stores of noradrenalin and leads to prolonged blockade lasting many hours or even days often with increase in circulation and a feeling of warmth. That the involvement of the sympathetic nervous system is more complicated than would seem is shown by the fact that patients may often have profound vasodilatation without any relief of pain. Most patients do not respond to one or two blocks with more than a very temporary abatement of the pain, say 10 minutes to half an hour at the most. We have learnt that we were far too timid in our approach in the past and we now give at least 6 blocks on alternate days before we regard sympathetic blocking treatment as ineffective. All our patients are treated as inpatients so that they can have the benefit of repeated blocks on alternate days and intensive desensitisation by physiotherapists and occupational therapists after the blocks and intensive rehabilitation on the non blocking days. The aim of treatment after all is to abolish the pain and then allow the patient to cooperate in an intensive rehabilitation programme.

All these patients will have stiff joints, weak muscles and poor functioning limbs and the sympathetic block must not be regarded as an end in itself but simply a means to provide adequate rehabilitation.

The technique is as follows: the upper limb is occluded by a tourniquet and the pressure raised to 300 mg mercury for the upper limb and 500 mg for the lower limb. The pressure is recorded. An intravenous cannula is inserted as near as possible to the hyperpathic area. The dorsum of the hand is preferred when possible to allow the patient freedom for activities and desensitisation. Another cannula is inserted into a vein in the other arm in case injections of drugs are required for resuscitation.

1% lignocaine is administered, 5 cc in the upper limb and 10 cc in the lower limb. 20 mg in 20 cc of guanethidine is then injected slowly into the affected arm for the upper limb, 30 mg in 20 cc for the lower limb.

The tourniquet can be distressing in the lower limb and in such cases – 5–10 mg i.v. diazepam is given.

The nurse checks drugs and records the blood pressure every 15 minutes and for 2 hours afterwards. After 20–30 minutes the tourniquet is slowly released and the cannula removed. Observation is continued for 2 hours. It is hoped that substantial reduction in pain and hyperpathia will be experienced at least for a few hours after the injection and during this time the opportunity is seized to desensitise the area by stroking, rubbing and encouraging activities in physiotherapy and occupational therapy to restore power to weak muscles and range of movement to stiff joints.

The lowest dose possible is used so that the patient can be as cooperative as possible in active movements and desensitisation in the pain free period.

The usual pattern of response is for pain to be reduced for a few hours after the third or fourth block, though in some cases dramatic responses are seen after the first or second block.

Up to 6 blocks are given every 48 hours – if there is no response to 6 blocks the technique is abandoned and stellate blocks are considered.

Rehabilitation will involve intensive exercise to regain range of movement in stiff joints and build up power in weak muscles and occupational therapy to provide realistic functional activities such as carpentry, metal work, craftwork, cooking and household activities. Clear objectives are set and objective measures of outcome are recorded weekly so that progress can be seen by both patient and rehabilitation team (Withrington & Wynn Parry 1984b). There is little or no place for drug treatment in this condition. Sometimes if the patient has severe paroxysmal shooting pains, carbamazepine or its analogues can be helpful, but most patients find the side effects too troublesome. In patients with severe chronic pain triptafen is occasionally of help, (a combination of an antihistamine and an antidepressant). In circumstances where the guanethedine block is inappropriate, e.g. patients with cardiac problems or who have not responded before, or who have responded unfavourably with prolonged hypotension, then serial stellate ganglion blocks are used, but after these the same intensive rehabilitation programme must be adopted.

Transcutaneous stimulation is most likely to be effective in patients with symptoms suggestive of ongoing nerve discharges, i.e. with painful paraesthesiae. In our series, no patient with pure allodynia and hyperpathia responded to transcutaneous stimulation but in those patients with spontaneous pain and painful paraesthesiae, TENS helped one quarter. It is certainly well worth trying it in all patients on the off chance that it may be effective for it is non-invasive, relatively cheap and may possibly reinforce the effect of sympathetic blockade. Several of our patients come in for repeated blocks and when they do they usually bring their stimulator saying that they find it helpful in severe exacerbations of pain.

Wall & Sweet (1967) were the first to report that electrical stimulation could relieve pain in humans and Wall & Gutnik (1974) showed that this worked experimentally, both by reducing or silencing the spontaneous discharges from the neuroma and by reducing transmission of nociceptive activity centrally. Transcutaneous electrical nerve stimulation has now become a routine part of the management of painful nerve disorders. It is logical to use electrical stimulation in patients who suffer predominantly from paraesthesiae and hyperaesthesiae.

In those patients in whom transcutaneous electrical stimulation produced a significant relief of pain, a stimulator is provided for home use. Far too often patients are improperly instructed in the use of this most valuable treatment. In our view it is essential that the patient wears the stimulator for many hours a day for weeks on end. The effect is cumulative and the best results are obtained by its prolonged use. Our physiotherapists are highly skilled in the application of this treatment, and they will experiment with different positions of the electrodes and different settings of pulse width, repetition rate and frequency over a period of 1–2 weeks. The majority of patients prefer a high rate of stimulation in the 60–100 herz range (Frampton 1982). There is some evidence to suggest that continuous high frequency electrical stimulation is effective through endorphin release centrally, whereas the brief, painful low frequency impulses (which a few patients prefer) alert the central inhibitory systems (Melzack & Wall 1983). Acupuncture however in our hands has proved disappointing and seems unhelpful in severe pain states.

RESULTS

We here present the results of our experience over the last 10 years (Wynn Parry & Girgis 1989).
Effect of serial guanethedine blocks for hyperpathia and allodynia (n = 78).
40 females, 38 males.

Lesions treated

Median nerve lesions at the wrist: 25
 13 release of carpal tunnel
 12 traumatic
Digital nerve lesions: 21
 20 crush
 1 Dupuytren's contracture
Ulnar nerve lesions at the elbow: 12
 11 traumatic and 1 tumour
Foot: 8
 7 post-surgical (hallux valgus, equinovarus, tuberculosis (4),
 1 sprain
Ulnar lesions of the wrist: 3
 all traumatic
Knee: 3
 2 trauma
 1 popliteal cyst
Superficial radial nerve: 2
 both post du Quervain's surgery
Branchial plexus lesions: 2
 post-ganglionic
Post-herpetic neuralgia: 2.

During 1979–1986, 696 guanethedine blocks were administered. The maximum number given to one patient on one admission was 31, and on recurrent admissions, 39.

The least number was a patient in whom instant relief resulted with one block but with recurrence 8 months later requiring 3 more blocks.

All 78 patients had temporary relief of pain for a few minutes – presumably through the effect of ischaemia or local anaesthetic. Thereafter patients either showed relief for some hours or an increasing period of relief after subsequent blocks, or no relief at all.

In 11 patients there was no effect until after the 5th block when steady improvement with subsequent blocks was noted, the period of relief increasing with each block.

In 5 patients there was no effect in spite of 9 blocks and they were therefore discontinued.

We have assessed our results as *excellent* – complete relief of allodynia and hyperpathia, *good* – improved by over 50%, *moderate* – some relief but less than 50%, and *no effect at all*.

Excellent 23–30%
Good   23–30%
Moderate 15–20%
No effect 17–20%

We have analysed the effectiveness of blocks in relation to the nature of the lesion.
In those 23 with excellent results:
 9 of 13 had carpal tunnel release (69%)
 8 of 21 digital nerve damage (38%)
 3 of 3 ulnar nerve lesions at the wrist
 2 of 11 ulnar nerve lesions at the elbow.
In those in whom there was no effect from the blocks:
 7 of 8 had lesions of the foot
 6 of 12 had lesions of the median nerve at the wrist
 2 of 2 had superficial radial nerve lesions
 2 of 21 had digital nerve damage.

We conclude that ulnar nerve lesions at the elbow fare badly, reinforcing the view that surgery for transposition of the ulnar nerve at the elbow should only be considered when there is clear cut clinical and electrophysiological evidence of progressive damage to the nerve. We conclude that lesions of the foot fare badly and that nerve lesions as a result of crushing fare worse than a clean cut.

Among the 23 with excellent results, 16 did not recur while 7 recurred between 6 months and a year.

Among the 23 with good results, 18 recurred between 2 and 4 months while 5 did not recur.

Thus, patients who obtain an excellent response are most likely to remain pain-free and there is an increasing recurrence rate when the initial response is less satisfactory.

It is our practice to continue blocks until either complete abolition of pain is achieved, or until 3 successive blocks fail to achieve further relief.

We analysed the length of time patients had suffered symptoms before commencing treatment. In those with excellent results, the mean duration of symptoms was 2.5 years (1 month–7 years). In those where there was no effect the mean duration of symptoms was also 2.5 years (1–7 years).

There seems therefore to be no relation between the length of time of symptoms and the response to treatment and one need not be put off by chronicity of pain when deciding on sympathetic blockade.

SURGERY

It would seem logical when confronted with a patient with a large painful neuroma whose symptoms are so severe that function is seriously impaired, to consider resection of the neuroma and grafting. Unfortunately a very high proportion of such patients develop pain some 3 months after surgery. We are all too familiar with patients who have had repeated transposition of the ulnar nerve for ulnar neuritis of the elbow, each procedure resulting in a return of pain after an interval and the pain often being worse than before. If the nerve is bound down by scar it might seem logical to release it and carry out an external neurolysis and indeed in some circumstances this can be most effective but the surgeon must not be disappointed if the pain returns. We must always remember that in any longstanding cases there will be profound central effects of the nerve damage and pain has an unpleasant habit of recurring despite the original trigger being removed (Noordenbos & Wall 1981). Weir-Mitchell recommended nerve resection as being the definitive treatment and records 23 patients in which he had performed resection. In 2 there was no relief and 4 partial relief and in 17 immediate relief, but in 5 of these the pain returned later. A fascinating case history of Weir-Mitchell draws several interesting morals which are summarised at the end of his case report.

Case history 9

A. F. Swann, aged 34 captain C Company. He was a stout, robust man. On 28 May 1864 he was hit by a bullet 2 inches below head of radius affecting median nerve. Severe causalgia.
5 July Removed 3 inches median nerve. No relief.
Huge doses of morphine: 10 grains/day
June 1870. 6 years later.
His condition was most deplorable.
Pain intensified by any excitement indescribable with a fever of 2–3 hours' duration.
27 June 1870: 14 ounces of ether applied and an hour passed before he became quiet. 3 inches median nerve removed.
As soon as he passed from under the influence of ether, he declared that the pain had left him but he could not sleep.
Weir Mitchell sent him to a quiet country home and directed the full use of ale with a generous diet. No medicine of any kind was afterwards necessary. The important points, Weir Mitchell says, were:

1. Unceasing and great severity of pain for 6 years.
2. Entire freedom since operation.
3. Vast amount of morphine, 6–20 syringes a day for 6 years.
4. The rapid recovery.
5. The operation undertaken in opposition to the freely expressed opinion of all the medical gentlemen here and elsewhere who had been consulted after the failure of Dr. Bliss's operation.

Painful digital nerve lesions can respond to surgical treatment. Tupper & Booth (1976) reported 32% of excellent results after one resection in 172 patients and 32% excellent after 2 resections with a decreasing success after second operations. Snyder (1961) reported on 150 surgical procedures for painful neuromas which include resiting the nerve into bone or muscle, cutting it, crushing it, sheathing it, boiling it, freezing it and treating it with a variety of chemical agents. The whole question of neuromas is discussed in Chapter 7, but although results are better than in causalgia affecting main nerves they are still disappointing for the same reasons as already discussed, namely the central effects of peripheral damage and the ongoing effects in the periphery so well described by Wall.

In our series, 71 operations had been carried out in 50 patients specifically for pain and this included re-suturing, grafting, transposition, and neurolysis. In only one of them was the pain substantially relieved. Rolfe Birch (personal communication) who has worked extensively in this field, believes, as does the author, that one is allowed one attempt to improve the situation surgically, e.g. by neuroma resection and grafting. If this fails then further surgical attempts should be abandoned. Furthermore, surgery in this field is for the expert only. Continuity must be restored whenever possible. If this is impossible the nerve must be cut cleanly and allowed to retract. Internal neurolysis is avoided at all times. Finally surgeons must follow up their patients indefinitely for in so many the pain recurs months or years afterwards.

The painful stiff hand

A considerable problem in rehabilitation is the

management of the painful, stiff hand. Whatever the cause the end result is the same – the inability of the patient to use the hand for any functional activities and the vicious circle sets in; the less it is used, the stiffer it becomes and the more painful attempts thereafter to try and use it. The following are the major causes of the painful stiff hand other than Sudeck's atrophy and the end result of long-standing causalgia which have already been discussed.

Skin

The skin can become bound down and tight, restricting movement of tendons and free movements of joints. This is particularly manifest after burns. Skilled plastic surgery can produce amazing results from desperate looking situations but usually a period of rehabilitation is required to loosen up the injured soft tissues. Here regular sessions twice a day of gentle oil massage with intensive active exercise can soften the scarred tissues and encourage pliability of the moving parts. Static splints to maintain the correction obtained by the physiotherapist can be useful but need to be very carefully applied and padded. Aids to daily living are most important here and the occupational therapist can provide various devices to facilitate function of the hand, particularly feeding, dressing and household activities (Wynn Parry 1981). Any form of heat which includes ultrasound is contraindicated in this situation and it is here that the physiotherapist's manual skills are most important. Gentle, gradually progressive massage will loosen up the scarred structures and gradually encourage stretching of the skin and the underlying structures.

As in all severe injuries the best results are obtained by an intensive full-time progressive programme using exercises, physiotherapy, occupational therapy and recreational activities over a period of weeks.

Crush injuries

Here it is not so much the damage to the bone as the surrounding soft tissues that is all important. Bleeding occurs into the deep structures in the palm resulting in organisation, fibrosis, contracture and a stiff, frozen, painful hand. These crushing injuries are commonly seen in industrial injuries and in motor accidents. Often when the patient presents for rehabilitation, the hand and indeed the arm itself may be swollen. Until this swelling has dispersed there is no hope of obtaining satisfactory range of movement and power. We have been constantly amazed at the success of Donal Brooks's regime which is to admit the patient to the ward, elevate the arm in a sling with a roller towel and keep the arm there for 7–10 days, at the end of which even the most chronic oedema can resolve. As soon as the oedema has dispersed then an intensive programme, as already described for tendon contractures, is started. This will include progressively deeper oil massage, gentle stretches and plaster splints to maintain that correction (see Fig. 6.2). An intensive active programme of exercises and occupational therapy is vital. A remarkable improvement in function can be obtained even in desperate cases by this intensive programme (Wynn Parry 1981).

Tendons

A common feature after multiple tendon injuries is the adherence of the flexor tendons to the skin, to themselves and to the underlying deep structures, resulting in a fixed flexion deformity at the PIP and TIP joints. In severe cases this can also cause flexion contracture at the wrist. This situation often follows an injury where the patient puts his hand through a window and divides all the flexor tendons, both arteries and both nerves. Even after painstaking primary suture there can be a massive induration at the wrist with the flexion deformity described. This is particularly likely to occur if the wound is infected. The surgeon may be reluctant to proceed to tenolysis if he has already operated a few weeks previously and of course if there is infection it is contraindicated for at least 6 months. Therefore conservative treatment is required if the hand is not to become permanently stiff and the tendons permanently shortened.

The technique of oil massage, with slow stretches and serial plasters has proved its value. Intensive daily treatment is essential for success. In our units, the physiotherapist gives 2 or 4 ses-

92 MANAGEMENT OF PAIN IN THE HAND AND WRIST

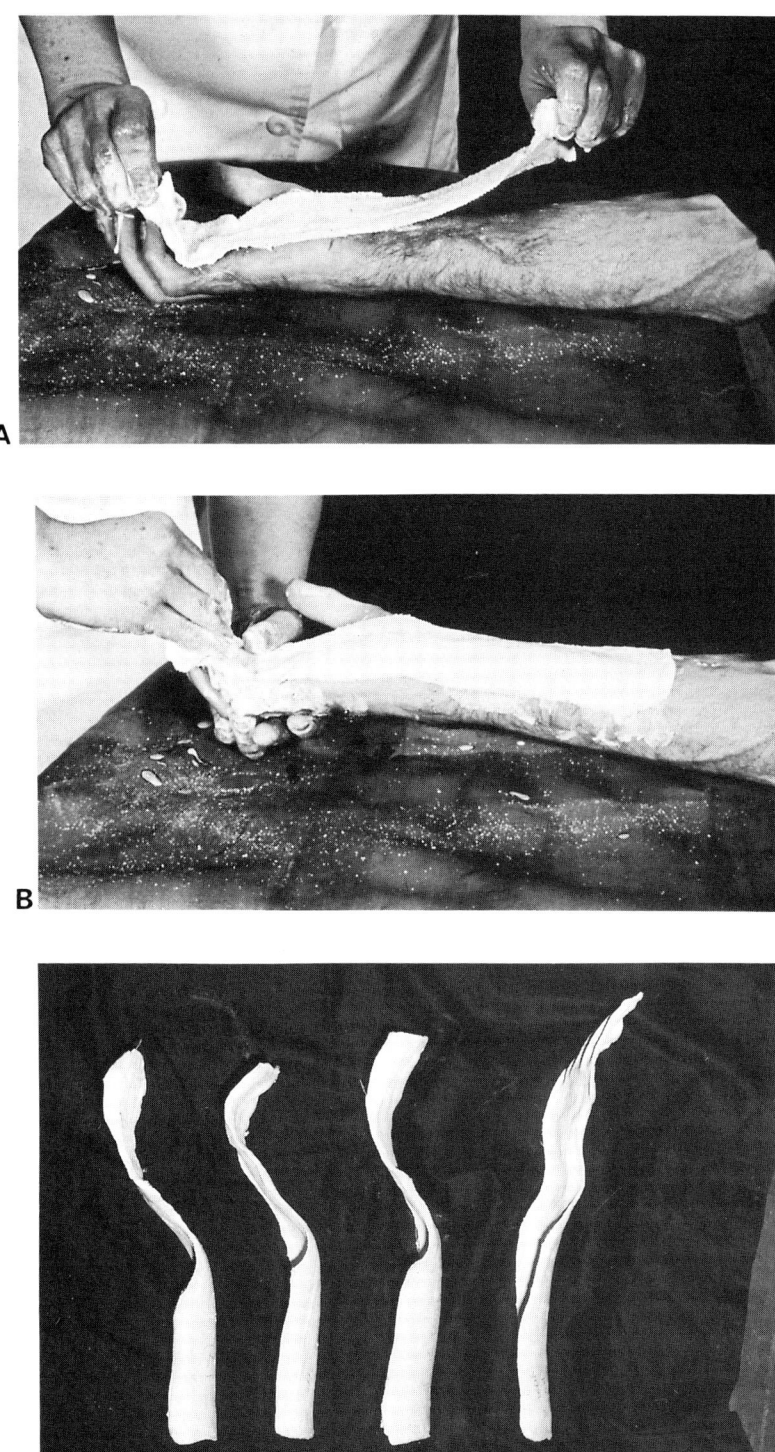

Fig. 6.2 Technique of serial plasters to correct deformity after crush injuries: (a), (b) application of plaster; (c) serial plasters over a period of 6 weeks to show progressive correction.

sions of 10 minutes of oil massage to loosen the indurated structures and follows this by very slow gentle stretches supporting the wrist and MP joints to try and lengthen the contracted structures. After each session a light plaster splint is applied which maintains the correction obtained – it is not in itself a corrective splint (see Fig. 6.2). As correction is achieved the splint is changed and this may require a new plaster splint 2 or even 3 times a week. Once a week the splint is kept, dated, and over a period of time the correction is vividly seen, in a manner not so obvious by photography or making measurements, the accuracy of which is difficult when the anatomy is as distorted as it often is. Over a period of 4 to 6 weeks even the most severe flexion contractures of the fingers can be corrected and the tendons restored to almost normal function. The technique is fully described and examples given in Wynn Parry (1981). After each session of physiotherapy the patient proceeds to the occupational therapy department, where he uses his hand actively in a variety of crafts and recreations. The emphasis must be on active contraction of the flexor tendons and not on activities which simply regard the hand as a holding instrument whilst the shoulder and elbow are exercised. Our occupational therapist has devised a number of means in which the tendons are forced to be active and these include the use of secateurs and pliers, a jig for making coathangers out of steel, which requires firm pressure with the fingers to be aligned correctly and a variable pressure handle for printing and guillotining paper (Wynn Parry 1981).

PIP joints

Individual PIP joints can become painful and stiff after a variety of conditions, particularly sprains. This results in capsular thickening and restriction of movement. A programme of application of ice, intensive active movements and slow stretches with application of individual plasters can result in excellent return of function. An intra-articular injection of steroid in recalcitrant cases can often make the physiotherapist's task easier.

These techniques of massage, slow stretches, splinting and an intensive exercise programme can be applied to any condition where there is a stiff and painful hand, provided the sensation is intact.

Scleroderma

This very distressing condition is untreatable as yet. No drugs or local treatment have yet been shown to be effective on a long-term basis. Gentle massage into the skin with oil can improve the feeling of the skin and encourage what movement is possible but there is no place for intensive massage, stretching or splinting in this condition.

Dupuytren's contracture

This condition is rarely painful and physiotherapy, except post-operatively, is not required. There is no evidence that regular physiotherapy can reduce the scarring. Surgery is the only way this can be achieved. Occasionally, digital nerves can be trapped in the Dupuytren's tissue giving tingling and painful numbness in the affected digit. Only surgical release is effective here.

Dystonia

A rare and puzzling condition known as dystonia can sometimes present to a hand clinic. The nature of this condition is obscure but following some quite often trivial injury, the patient may develop a progressive deformity of the fingers, often in a very bizarre fashion. This may spread to the contralateral limb. Patients have been seen with severe flexion of the fingers into the palm such that excoriation of the skin develops; sometimes it is noted that fingers begin to cross each other; sometimes hyperextension deformity occurs in one finger and a flexion deformity in the other. The bizarre nature of the clinical presentation should alert the examiner to the possibility of a dystonic condition. Clearly there is some profound central disorder (spasmodic torticollis is an example) and simplistic attempts to correct deformities can lead to disaster. A general anaesthetic often reveals that the majority of the deformity is correctable passively, although in long-standing cases there will be a combination of marked contracture and contraction. If there is complete relief of the deformity under anaesthetic, then the hand should be splinted in the corrected position and kept there for some weeks. When the plaster is taken off a splint must be ready to apply immediately. In rare cases surgical correction may be required, if it can be clearly demonstrated that there is a major element of permanent contracture.

Botulinum toxin has been used in severe cases with some success (see Ch. 4).

Shoulder–hand syndrome

This curious condition presents clinically with a swollen, stiff painful hand and a stiff and painful shoulder. It is a condition sui generis and there is usually no precipitating feature. The patient develops gradually increasing stiffness and pain in the shoulder which can be very acute and notices at the same time that the hand becomes stiff, swollen and painful. In time the condition is indistinguishable from the late stage of Sudeck's atrophy and a frozen shoulder. The central phenomena associated with this condition are fully described in Chapter 4. It is important not to confuse the stiff and painful shoulder after a stroke with this condition. The shoulder usually responds to intra-articular steroid and a progressive intensive active rehabilitation programme with hydrotherapy and exercises. The hand will respond to the standard treatment for reflex dystrophy. If there is allodynia then guanethedine or stellate blocks are used with an intensive progressive rehabilitation programme to restore range of movement of the stiff joints and increase power.

Prolonged rehabilitation is essential.

SUMMARY OF DRUGS IN THE TREATMENT OF CHRONIC BENIGN PAIN

The epithet benign in no way minimises the appalling distress felt by patients with painful non-malignant disease, but it serves to remind us that whereas powerful narcotic drugs are strongly indicated in patients with only months to live, in disorders where the pathological process is not life threatening, such as phantom pain, brachial plexus avulsion, and causalgia, recourse to addictive drugs should not be made except in very exceptional circumstances.

There are, however, circumstances in which narcotics, i.e. the opioids are admissible for short periods, although they are surprisingly ineffective in the most severe pains dealt with in this volume – deafferentation pains seem very resistant to the major opioids.

As Budd (1987) points out, the incidence of dependence is lower than generally believed and if an opioid is the only agent capable of offering a reasonable quality of life, it should be used. Hopefully, the indications will be rare – many patients are treated with opioids without having been through an intensive well structured rehabilitation programme and exposed to a variety of non drug modalities. Only in the event of all measures described in this volume having failed would we consider prescribing an opioid.

Major opioids

morphine 15–20 mg
diamorphine 5–10 mg

Both with effective duration of 4 hours. Response is variable and doses must be adjusted until adequate pain relief is achieved.

Minor opioids

Codeine 30–60 mg 3–4 h
Dihydrocodeine 40–60 mg 3–4 h
Dextropropoxyphene 65–130 mg

Duration 6–8 hours. Occasionally Buprenorphine, which is given as 0.2–0.6 mg sublingually, is helpful, but we have been disappointed in its use.

Non-steroidal anti-inflammatory agents (NSAID)

These are indicated whenever there is an inflammatory component to the disease process – classically in the rheumatic disease, rheumatoid arthritis and its variants and ankylosing spondylitis.

It is now recognised that osteoarthritis has an inflammatory component and that periodic flares with acute pain present as an inflammatory episode superimposed on the degenerative process. Use of a NSAID is therefore highly appropriate.

There is a large selection from which to choose and each prescription is a very individual process. It may be necessary to try several before the right drug for that particular patient is found.

The author favours naproxen, ibuprofen, feldene and paracetamol for the rheumatic diseases, indomethacin and voltarol for osteoarthritis.

Antidepressants

It is now well recognised that the antidepressants, through their serotonin sparing effect can be most valuable in central pain. It is important to explain that these compounds are being used for their central pain relieving properties and not as an antidepressant. Confidence can be rapidly destroyed if the patient believes that his doctor thinks he is depressed and that it is all in the mind.

With the vast publicity given these days to all things medical, patients know about most of the medicines in use and will have friends or relatives who are taking these compounds.

We particularly like triptafen, a combination of aminotriptyline and perphenazine. If ineffective it is worth trying the other standard antidepressants.

In the case of shooting paroxysmal pains, an anticonvulsant is tried.

Tegretol – carbamazepine is the first choice in doses of 100 mg bd, building up at weekly intervals to a maximum of 1200 mg. Side effects are unfortunately common and unacceptable, but when it does suit a patient it can be invaluable.

If ineffective, it is worth trying sodium valproate and the benzodiazepines.

Claims have been made that the serotonin precursor, tryptophan, given daily for an extended period can help patients with chronic pain and increase the effectiveness of TNS.

We have not been impressed and have given up its use having tried it in pain from plexus avulsion and phantom pain.

Most patients with severe pain from nerve damage (causalgia, deafferentation, plexus avulsion, phantom pain) do not respond to any analgesics. Those that do, find that paracetemol and codeine are the most likely to help but relief is rather mild and distraction by involvement in work or absorbing hobbies, together with TNS, is much the most effective treatment.

Functional paralysis (hysterical paralysis)

In some patients with intractable pain there may be a partial or even complete paralysis of part or whole of the limb. This is most commonly seen in patients with intractable back pain, where not only may the patient have backache and sciatica, but inability to move any muscle below the knee. Electrical stimulation reveals that this is a functional block, there being normal response to electrical stimulation in all the muscles supplied by the nerve stimulated. We have seen a number of patients with painful functional paralyses of the upper limb. This may follow an injury in which the patient presents for all the world as if with a traction lesion of the brachial plexus. The realisation after some time that there is no wasting and no trophic changes, will lead the examiner to suspect a functional block. If on stimulation of the nerves at Erb's point, at the elbow and at the wrist, normal, strong contraction is demonstrated in all muscles, a confident diagnosis of a functional block can be made.

The term 'conversion hysteria' is often used to describe this, but we feel that this is counterproductive. These patients are not in any way hysterical. Something extraordinary has happened in the central nervous system as a result of injury or severe pain, and the transmission of the nerve impulse peripherally is blocked. We are all familiar with the expression 'paralysed with fear' and similar mechanisms seem to be at work. The fact that one cannot demonstrate structural or biochemical abnormalities does not mean that the patient is malingering.

We have been able to show by an extensive rehabilitation programme with intensive exercise, biofeedback and the setting of progressive goals and a great deal of encouragement and support that such patients can regain full function in a matter of weeks and that as function returns, so the pain diminishes (Withrington & Wynn Parry 1984a).

MANAGEMENT OF CHRONIC PAIN

Many of our patients have become demoralised by chronic pain and have lost hope and confidence, believing that they will never be active housewives or useful employees again. The benefit of an intensive rehabilitation programme is as much in restoring confidence and helping these patients to develop a positive approach as in anything else. Here the clinical psychologist can be most helpful in explaining the various issues involved in chronic pain, helping patients to cope and firmly giving them the responsibility for taking charge of their own life. The role of clinical psychologists in chronic pain cannot be over emphasised. It is impossible to imagine a successful pain programme being run without their support. Many patients have become physically unfit through enforced inactivity and a programme for general fitness is always insisted on and in itself can help patients to accept chronic pain and take a more positive approach. There is an immense amount of truth in the saying 'mens sana in corpore sano'. On discharge all patients are given a programme to follow, with objectives, and are urged to record the amount of pain and also the amount of activity that they have been able to carry out. In patients whose pain we have been unable to help, benefit may result from a pain management programme, for one can at least try to reorientate the patient's attitude to achieving goals and improving lifestyle, despite continuing to suffer pain.

Such patients will tell us that they are now more active and are more involved in life and although the pain is still present they are prepared to accept it. In such cases, surprisingly enough, as the years go by, the pain may slowly diminish. It is as if the spontaneous unwanted electrical discharges both peripherally and centrally will eventually abate if the patients can bring their central inhibitory pathways into play by distraction and a positive approach to living.

PAIN MANAGEMENT PROGRAMMES

Despite an intensive programme of rehabilitation, including all the modalities described, there remain a small but significant number of patients with severe intractable pain.

Such patients present severe problems, for their whole lives and those of their spouses and immediate family circle are seriously disturbed.

It is for such patients that the pain management programmes originally described by Fordyce (1968) and increasingly used in rehabilitation centres in North America and the U.K. were described.

The rationale of this pain management programme was quite different from previous programmes in that it was not concerned with reducing pain but in achieving physical activity and reducing medication.

To quote Fordyce, 'behaviour is all that can be observed and measured as representative of the other's unknowable experience'.

Original tissue damage may cause persistence of pain, for this is reinforced by contingencies in the patient's environment. A fear of return to work or involvement in activities which might increase the pain leads the patient to become progressively more dependent. The end result is a patient with a set of learned behaviours – inactivity at home and much display of suffering. Eventually the patient unconsciously (or rarely consciously) manipulates his family and environment to such an extent that he is the centre of attraction. Fordyce et al (1981) showed that pain behaviour may be little, if at all, related to inferences about underlying noxious stimulation. In a study of 150 patients with chronic back pain who were asked to record a pain diary and assess their pain on a 0–10 scale, it was found that there were few relationships to consumption of medication or utilisation of health care. The diary recorded levels of activity or frequency of engaging in commonplace activities that were not related to recording of pain. In chronic pain, a questionable relationship exists between what people say about their pain and what they actually do, and therefore any assessment of pain must include analysis of the patient's behaviour. Fordyce's revolutionary approach involves the aim of treating the behaviour consequent on pain and not the pain itself. Behavioural methods, he has pointed out repeatedly, do not have as their principal objective a modification of nociception or direct modification of experiences of pain.

The aim is to improve the patient's lifestyle by increasing his activity and reducing his dependence upon medication. A vital component is the involvement of the family, so that they understand the rationale of the programme, disregarding complaints of suffering but praising and rewarding achievements such as increased activity or reduced medication. Anderson (1977) has summarised the objectives of a behavioural modification programme ... 'to increase physical activity to

Table 6.2 Timetable of Pain Management Programme at Royal National Orthopaedic Hospital.

	Monday	Tuesday	Wednesday	Thursday	Friday
Morning	Staff Meeting	Keep Fit	Keep Fit	Discussion with Psychologist	Alexander Technique
		Relaxation	Alexander Technique	Swimming	Keep Fit
		Pharmacist	Social Work Group		Weekend Assignments
Afternoon	Week 1 Introduction + Medical Registrar	Personal Targets OT.	Lecture from Physiotherapist	Autohypnosis	
	Assessments	Lecture from Nursing Staff	Swimming	Personal Targets OT.	
				Work paid or voluntary	

normal levels appropriate to the age and sex, to reduce or eliminate medication, to return the patient to a satisfying lifestyle with his family, to change family interactions so that there is less need to use pain to control the relationships, to eliminate the dependency on the medical profession, to change attitudes to health care and thus decrease pain complaints'.

In our service, patients are admitted for a four-week inpatient programme which is organised and supervised by the clinical psychologist. The clinician introduces the course by explaining the modern theories of pain, why the patient has the pain and the ways in which he is to be helped to cope with the pain and live as normal a life as possible. Thereafter the course is supervised by the clinical psychologist and the doctor plays no further part. This is particularly important as continual involvement with the doctor suggests to the patient that there is yet some drug or manoeuvre which can help; the patient must learn that it is up to him to learn coping strategies himself and to be no longer dependent on help from the medical profession.

The course is carefully structured, alternating exercise programmes, games, outdoor activities, relaxation sessions, group discussions and individual counselling. The aim is to increase the patient's physical fitness, to overcome anxieties and fears of the effects of his condition; to discuss modifications at work, hobbies and recreations, and to learn specific coping strategies when pain becomes severe (see Table 6.2).

Modern clinical psychology has a whole range of techniques in this respect and its contribution is central to successful rehabilitation in chronic pain. Throughout, achievement of goals is praised and rewarded while complaints of pain are disregarded. Thus, behaviour is gradually changed from dependence and complaining to a positive approach and reliance on self and not on others.

Linton (1986) has reviewed the results of 30 published pain management programmes. In all, a high proportion of success was achieved. Involvement of the family is vital – otherwise all the gains from the programme will be jeopardised by a too caring family who continue to reinforce learned illness behaviour. Thus, counselling of the family and their direct involvement in the programme is a sine qua non (Bond & Hughes 1987).

SUMMARY PROTOCOL OF PATIENTS WITH INTRACTABLE NERVE PAIN (CAUSALGIA AND RSD)

Full review of the clinical situation.
Is there any indication for definitive surgery?
If surgery has been undertaken in the past specifically for pain and has been ineffective, avoid temptation to operate again.
Full assessment of the patient's functional status and psychological approach to their pain.
Discussion wherever possible with the family so that a clear picture can be gained of the effect that

the pain is having on the patient's life and on those around him or her.

Review of previous therapies – has sympathetic blockade been given in an effective manner, i.e. regular guanethedine blocks rather than one a month?

Has there been an adequate rehabilitation programme as a back up?

Have transcutaneous stimulators been used effectively?

Encourage inpatient admission for full assessment and intensive treatment over a 2- or 3-week period allowing the patient home at weekends to put into practice what he has learnt during the week.

A full general medical assessment – if satisfactory proceed to guanethedine blocks on alternate days.

Desensitisation immediately after intensive care by both physiotherapist, occupational therapist and nursing staff.

Encouragement of the patient to make use of the painfree period by as much activity as possible.

Provision of a stimulator if there is an element of painful paraesthesiae or spontaneous pain.

Occupational social and psychological counselling to help the patient get back into a normal life and understand the nature of his pain and pain–coping strategies.

The help of a clinical psychologist is invaluable.

Review of the work situation or the situation at home to maximise functional abilities.

Alteration of work situation, adaptation of tools, aids to daily living.

A positive, ongoing programme with recorded outcome measures and goals on discharge.

Regular review indefinitely.

REFERENCES

Albe Fessard D, Lombard M C 1981 Use of an animal model to evaluate the origin and protection against deafferentation pain. In: Bonica J et al (eds) Advances in pain research and therapy, vol 5. Raven, New York, pp 691–700

Anderson L S, Black R G, Abraham V, Ward A A 1971 Neuronal hyperactivity in experimental trigeminal deafferentation. Journal of Neurosurgery 35: 444

Anderson T P 1977 Behavioural modification of chronic pain. Clinical Orthopaedics and Related Research 29: 96–101

Barnes C G, Currey H L P 1967 Carpal tunnel syndrome in rheumatoid arthritis. Annals of Rheumatic Disease 26: 226–233

Barnes R 1954 In: Seddon H J (ed) Peripheral nerve injuries. Medical Research Council Special Report Series no 282. HMSO, London

Bond M R, Hughes A M 1987 Psychological aspects of chronic pain. Journal of International Disability Studies 9: 23–26

Bonnard C, Narakas A 1985 Syndrome douloureux et lesions traumatique du plexus brachial. Helvetica Chirurgica Acta 52: 621

Brewerton D A 1957 Incidence of tendon injuries in rheumatoid arthritis. Annals of Rheumatic Disease 16: 1183

Brown F E, Brown M L 1989 Long term results after tenosynovectomy to treat the rheumatoid hand. Journal of Hand Surgery 13A: 704–708

Budd K 1987 Drug management of chronic benign pain. International Disability Studies 9: 30–33

Burnstock G 1983 Autonomic neurotransmitters and trophic factors. Journal of the Autonomic Nervous System 7: 213–217

Campbell's operative surgery 1987 Crenshaw (ed), 7th edn. Mosby, St Louis

Farcot J L 1985 Symposium on causalgia, organised by French Society for Pain, Strasboug

Flatt A E 1974 The care of the rheumatoid hand, 3rd edn. Mosby, St Louis

Fordyce W E, Fowler R S, De Lateur B 1968 An application of behaviour modification technique to a problem of chronic pain. Behaviour Research & Therapy 6: 105–106

Fordyce W E, McMahon G, Rainwater S, Jackins S, Questad K, Murphy T, DeLateur B 1981 Pain complaint – exercise performance relationship in chronic pain. Pain 10: 311–321

Frampton V 1982 Pain control with the aid of the transcutaneous stimulation. Physiotherapy 68: 77–87

Freyberg R H 1969 In: Early synovectomy in rheumatoid arthritis. Excerpta Medica Foundation, p 98

Gilliat R W, Lequesne P M, Loque V et al 1970 Wasting of the hand associated with a cervical rib or band. Journal of Neurology & Psychiatry 33: 165

Hannington Kiff J 1974 Intravenous regional sympathetic blockade. Lancet 1: 1919

Janig W, Koffman W 1984 The involvement of the sympathetic nervous system in pain. Arzneimettel-Forschurng-Drug Research 34: 1066–1073

Kessler F B 1986 Complications of management of carpal tunnel syndrome. Hand Clinics (Philadelphia) 2: 401–407

Linton S J 1986 Behavioural remediation of chronic pain. A status report. Pain 24: 125–14

Livingstone W K 1943 Pain mechanism. A physiological interpretation of causalgia and its related states. McMillan, New York

Loeser J D, Ward K H 1967 Some effects of deafferentation on neurons of the CAT spinal cord. Archives Neurology (Chicago) 17: 629–636

Melzack R, Wall P D 1983 The challenge of pain. Penguin, Harmondsworth

Mills K R 1985 Antidromic sensory action potentials from palmar stimulation in the diagnosis of carpal tunnel syndrome. Journal of Neurology, Neurosurgery & Psychiatry 48: 250–255

Mitchell J K 1895 Remote consequence of injuries of nerve and their treatment. Lippincott, Philadelphia

Narakas A O, Henz V R 1988 Neurotisation in brachial plexus injuries. Indication and results. Clinical Orthopaedic and Related Research 237: 43–56

Nashold B S, Urban B, Zorab D S 1976 Phantom pain relief by focal destruction of the substantia gelatinosa of Rolands. In: Bonica J J, Fessard A (eds) Advances in pain research and therapy, vol 1. Raven, New York

Nashold B S, Ostadahl R H 1979 Dorsal root entry zone lesions for pain relief. Journal of Neurosurgery 57: 90

Noordenbos W, Wall P 1981 Implications of the failure of nerve resection and graft to cure chronic pain produced by nerve lesions. Journal of Neurology, Neurosurgery & Psychiatry 44: 1066–1073

Ochoa J, Torebiork H E 1981 Paraesthesiae from ectopic impulse generation in human sensory nerves. Brain 103: 835–53

Pallis C A, Scott J T 1965 Peripheral neuropathy in rheumatoid arthritis. British Medical Journal 1: 1141–1147

Polley F, Lipscomb P R 1966 Les affections rhumatismales et le syndrome du canal carpien. Section of Medical and Orthopaedic surgery, Mayo Clinic and Mayo Foundation, Rochester, Minn. Médécine et Hygiène (Genève) 24/731: 408–409

Roberts W J 1986 A hypothesis on the physiological basis for causalgia and related pains. Pain 24: 297–312

Scadding J W 1984 Ectopic impulse generation in damaged peripheral axons in abnormal nerves and muscles as impulse generators. In: Ochoa J, Culp W (eds) Abnormal nerves and muscles as impulse generators. Oxford University Press, Oxford

Sherman R A, Sherman C G, Gall N G 1980 A survey of current phantom limb pain treatment in the US. Pain 8: 85–99

Snyder C 1961 The surgical handling of tissue. Proceedings of 7th Annual Convention. American Association Equine Practice, Texas

Souter W A 1979 Planning treatment of the rheumatoid hand. The Hand 2: 3–16

Subbarao J, Stillwell G K 1981 Reflex sympathetic dystrophy syndrome of the upper extremity: analysis of total outcome of management of 125 cases. Archives of Physical & Medical Rehabilitation 62: 549

Sudeck P 1960 Uber die akute entzundhiche knockenatrophic. J Arch Klin Chir II: 147

Thomas D G T, Sheehy J P R 1983 Dorsal root entry zone lesions (Nashold's procedure) for pain relief following brachial plexus avulsion. Journal of Neurology, Neurosurgery & Psychiatry 46: 924–928

Tupper J W, Booth D M 1976 Treatment of painful neuromas of sensory nerves in the hand. A comparison of traditional and newer methods. Journal of Hand Surgery 1: 144

Wall P D, Gutnik M 1974 Properties of afferent nerve impulses originating from a neuroma. Nature (London) 248: 740–743

Wall P D, Devor M 1981 The effect of peripheral nerve injury on dorsal root potentials and on transmission of afferent signals into the spinal cord. Brain Research 2209: 95–111

Wall P D, Sweet W H 1967 Temporary abolition of pain in man. Science 155: 108–9

Wallin H, Torebjork E, Hallin R 1951 Preliminary observations on the pathophysiology of hyperalgesia in the causalgic pain syndrome. In: Zotterman Y (ed) Sensory function of the skin in primates. Pergamon, Oxford, p 4489

Weir-Mitchell S 1872 Injuries of nerves and their consequences, reprinted 1965. Dover Publications, New York

Withrington R H, Wynn Parry C B 1984a Rehabilitation of conversion paralysis. Journal of Bone & Joint Surgery 635–637

Withrington R H, Wynn Parry C B 1984b Painful disorders of peripheral nerves. Postgraduate Medical Journal 60: 869–875

Wynn Parry C B 1981 Rehabilitation of the hand, 4th edn. Butterworth, London

Wynn Parry C B, Girgis F 1989 Management of causalgia. Journal of International Rehabilitation Studies. Int Disabil Studies vol 11 15–20

Wynn Parry C B 1980 Pain in avulsion lesions of the brachial plexus. Pain 9: 41

Wynn Parry C B 1984 Management of pain after avulsion of brachial plexus. Journal of Neurosurgery 15: 960–965

W. B. Conolly

7 The management of traumatic neuroma in the hand

DEFINITION
A neuroma is a non-neoplastic tumour arising from the central end of a cut nerve. It is a physiological (natural healing process) but usually abortive attempt at spontaneous axon repair after damage to a peripheral nerve. As the nerve fibres or axons grow out from the cut end they become incorporated in a mass of scar tissue derived from the supporting tissue of the nerve.

HISTORY
Odier used the term amputation neuroma in 1811. In 1829, Wood described the pathology of neuroma. Weir Mitchell described neuromas and other effects of injury to peripheral nerves in 1872. In 1920, Huber & Lewis published their experimental work detailing the mechanism of neuroma formation.

More recent reviews of neuroma have been by Sunderland (1978), and Badalamente (1985).

PATHOLOGY

Cause

A neuroma may be caused by an open or closed injury. An open injury may be from trauma or from a surgical procedure itself.

A closed injury may be by crushing, stretching or compression of the nerve.

Injury may also occur from an injection into the actual substance of a nerve, e.g. local anaesthetic or corticosteroid into the median nerve at the wrist in a patient being treated for carpal tunnel syndrome.

Pathogenesis

After injury to a peripheral nerve, the proximal severed nerve fibres undergo retrograde degeneration to the level of the next proximal node of Ranvier. The nerve cell body undergoes chromatolysis and begins to make new ribose nucleic acid (RNA) to support the repair process for axonal regeneration. Fine axonal sprouts grow from the cut end of the nerve, where they are met by a tangled mass of fibroblasts and regenerating Schwann cells. If these sprouts fail to enter the endoneural tubes of the distal part of the cut nerve they form

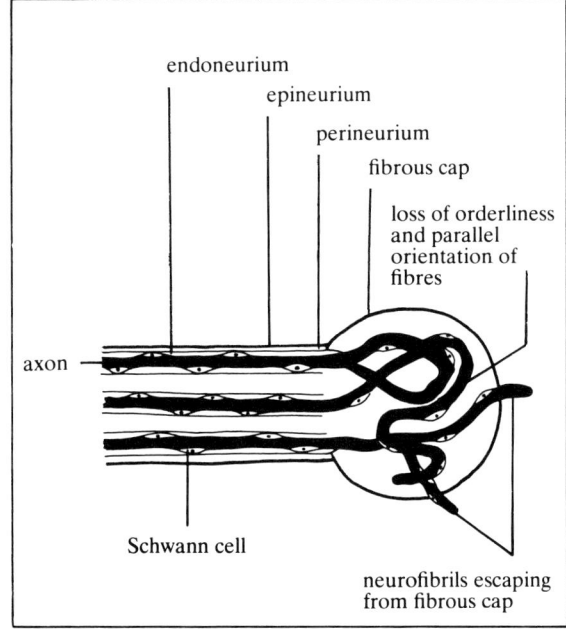

Fig. 7.1a Diagram of a neuroma. (Reproduced from *A Colour Atlas of Hand Conditions* by W. B. Conolly with kind permission of Wolfe Publishing).

TRAUMATIC NEUROMA IN THE HAND 101

Fig. 7.1b Photomicrograph of a neuroma demonstrating disorganised tissue composed of axons, fibroblasts, Schwann's cells and blood vessels.

a neuroma (Fig. 7.1). The neuroma contains poorly vascularised connective tissue infiltrated with large numbers of sprouts of the parent axons. The neuroma may be encapsulated in a fibrous sheath or it may be firmly attached to surrounding structures by fibrous adhesions. The terminal sprouts become most active about 30 days after nerve section. The growth and direction of the axons are influenced by the barrier of the fibroblasts and the Schwann cells. Their irregular branching forms whorls, spirals and convolutions. Most are contained in a disorganised mass or nodule of connective tissue. Though most become encapsulated, a few escape attempting to reach the distal stumps of the cut nerve. It is the nodule at the end of the nerve stump which is the neuroma. Progressive fibrosis converts an originally soft nodule into a firm hard one. Badalamente et al have identified myofibroblasts in neuromas.

CLASSIFICATION

Neuromas may be classified as follows (Sunderland 1978):

1. After complete division of the nerve
   a. Amputation stump neuroma (Fig. 7.2). Because there is section of the nerve and all adjacent tissue at the one level, the nerve stump lies in a composite tissue bed. Such terminal bulb neuromas are more liable to fibrosis from the healing stump tissues and more liable to repeated trauma from the knocking of the stump, increasing the fibrosis and sensitivity of the neuroma.

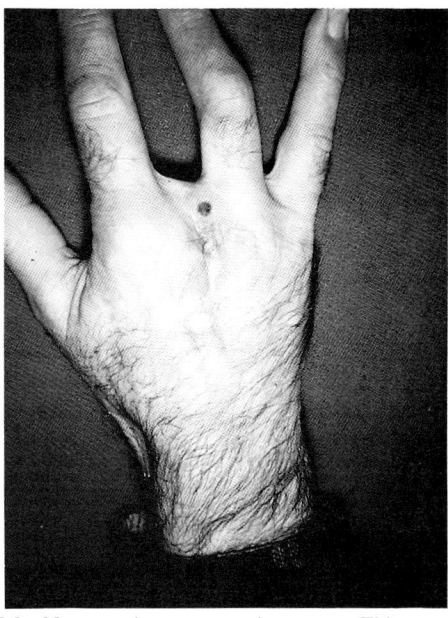

Fig. 7.2a Neuroma in an amputation stump. This 50-year-old upholsterer had severe pain on any contact in the area of the neuroma. (Reproduced from *A Colour Atlas of Hand Conditions* by W. B. Conolly with kind permission of Wolfe Publishing).

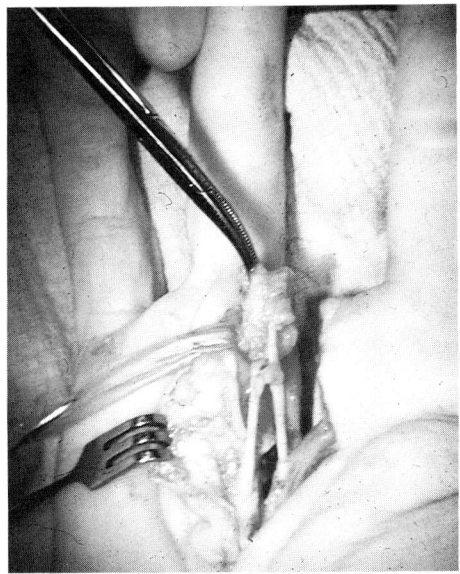

Fig. 7.2b Findings at operation. Resection of the neuroma and electrocoagulation of the nerve stump gave him 30% relief of pain. (Reproduced from *A Colour Atlas of Hand Conditions* by W. B. Conolly with kind permission of Wolfe Publishing).

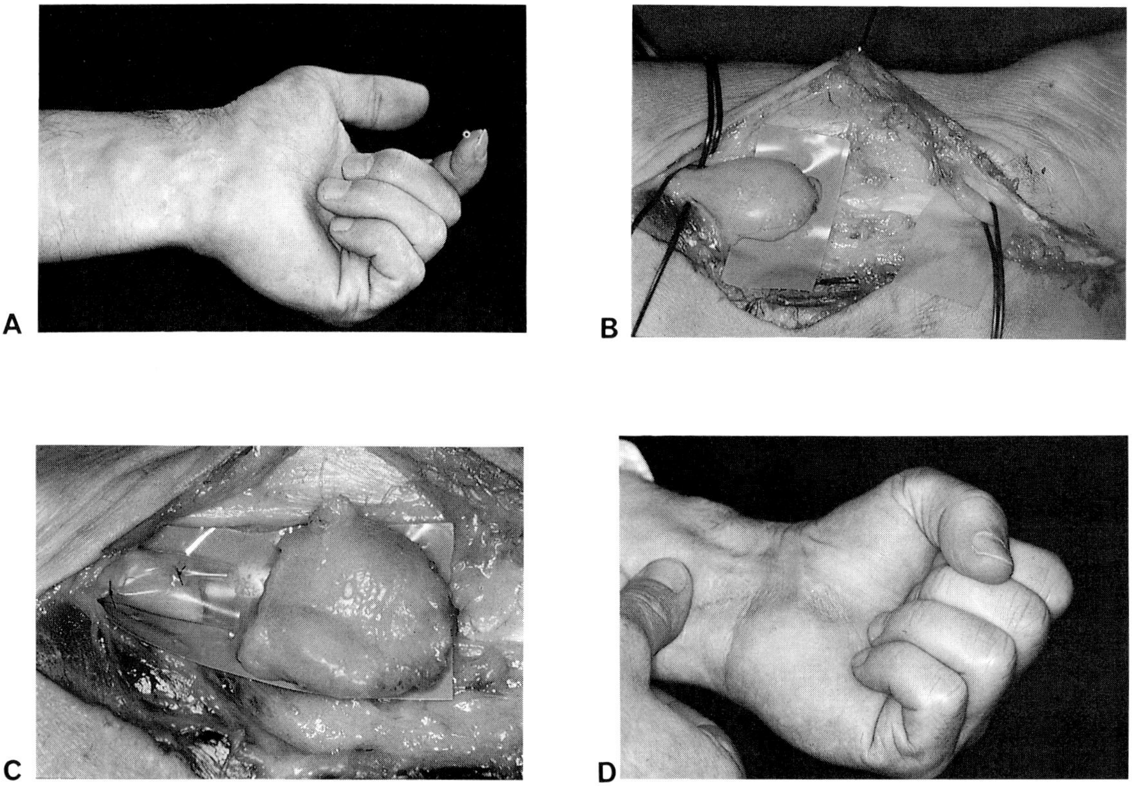

102 MANAGEMENT OF PAIN IN THE HAND AND WRIST

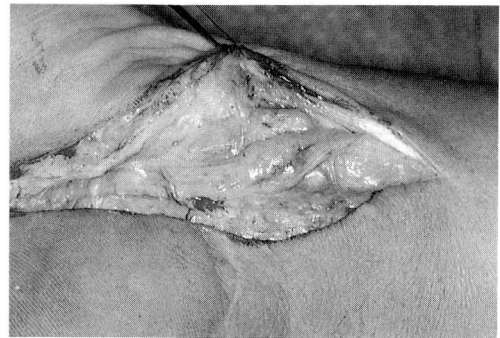

Fig. 7.3 Terminal neuroma of the median nerve. (a) (b) This 45-year-old man sustained laceration at the wrist at the age of 5 years. He had no treatment. 12 months after resection of the neuroma (c) and wrapping of the proximal nerve stump with a silastic sheet he was relatively free of pain. (d) An overlap of function of the ulnar nerve had preserved reasonable hand sensation.

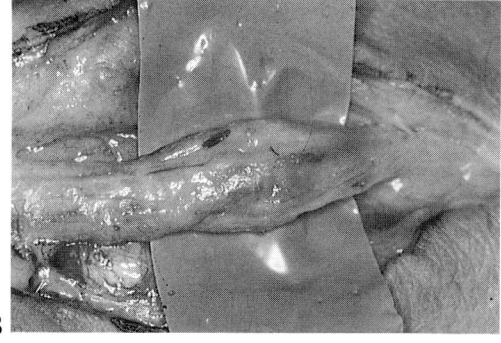

Fig. 7.4a Neuroma in continuity of the median nerve. 9 months after nerve repair there were signs of a median neuroma at the site of repair and no distal median nerve function.

Fig. 7.4b Findings at operation. Neuroma in continuity. 6 months after internal neurolysis this patient had a little less pain at the neuroma site and he had regained some protective feeling in the median nerve distribution of his hand.

b. Terminal neuroma (Fig. 7.3). These occur after complete section of a peripheral nerve trunk or branch or distal ramifications of a branch.
2. After partial nerve division (these are called neuromas in continuity) (Fig. 7.4)
  a. Lateral neuroma. Partial damage to the side of the nerve allows axons to escape. The size of the neuroma will depend on how many axons escape from the gap before proliferating fibroblasts and Schwann cells close the gap.
  b. Neuromas following nerve repair (Fig. 7.4). This is more common where the repair is carried out on cut ends with dissimilar fascicular patterns or where there has been a segment of nerve resected or destroyed.

These neuromas in continuity will be fusiform or nodular enlargements of the intact nerve.

The involved cross sectional area will contain normal axons as well as intertwining regenerating axons and glial tissue.

3. Spindle neuroma
These are not true neuromas but are swellings or enlargements of an intact nerve. Chronic irritation, friction or pressure sufficient to produce fibrous tissue proliferation constricts nerve fibres, causes ischaemia and eventually replaces nerve fibres and vessels. Such a neuroma occurs in a 'bowler's thumb' (Dobyns et al 1972) (ulnar digital nerve of the thumb) and in the posterior interosseous nerve on the extensor aspect of the wrist. In these the perineurium is intact.

Neuromas may also be classified according to:

1. The site – nerve trunk or branch or distal ramifications (Fig. 7.6)
2. The type of nerve, whether it be sensory or motor or mixed.

CLINICAL FEATURES

After any peripheral nerve injury most patients notice an unpleasant feeling of paraesthesiae and an over reaction to normal stimuli. The recovering nerve remains hypersensitive for some time.

In an amputation stump, immediate and early diffuse pain in the stump is more likely to be due to ischaemia, tension in the flaps, low grade infection or traumatic oedema of the stump. With resolution of the wound much or all of this pain sensitivity will subside (Wynn Parry 1981).

After about 3–6 weeks, however, some patients notice a change in the character of the pain, which now becomes burning and more localised. These patients are developing a painful neuroma. Pain is provoked by local pressure or traction on the neuroma.

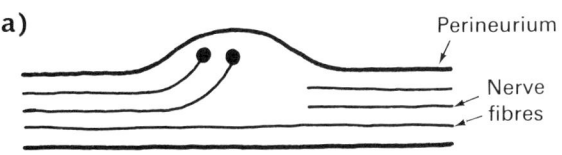
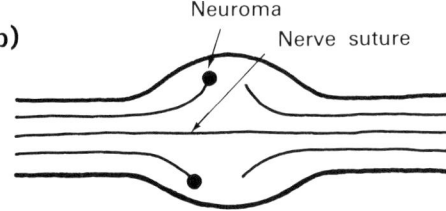
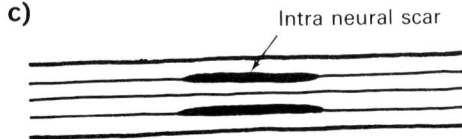
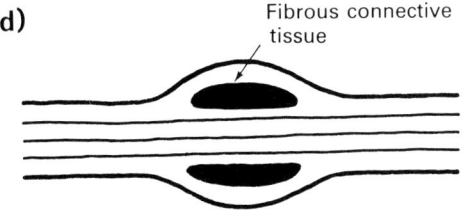

Fig. 7.5 Types of neuroma in continuity. (**a**) Lateral neuroma in continuity. (**b**) Neuroma after nerve repair. (**c**) Neuroma after intraneural injection. (**d**) Spindle neuroma (pseudoneuroma).

CAUSES OF PAIN IN A NEUROMA

Probably about two thirds of neuromas are asymptomatic. There are no distinguishing pathological features between painful and non-painful neuromas.

The vagaries of neuroma formation are such that similar nerve trunks sectioned at the same level in the same patient, will develop neuromas of varying sizes and symptomatology (Eaton 1980). Local tissue factors such as anoxia, foreign material or infected or necrotic tissue at each specific neuroma site play an important role in their formation and symptomatology.

The extrinsic factors include the tight fibrous capsule around the neuroma and the adhesions of the neuroma to adjacent tissue such as bone and soft tissue. Boyes (1956) believed that infection during healing and excessive wound scar were the major causes of painful neuroma.

The intrinsic causes of pain in neuroma include the electrical activity in the sprouting axons.

SYMPTOMS

Patients with painful neuroma complain of burning pain or painful paraesthesiae in the area of supply of the severed nerve. There may also be symptoms of an associated autonomic dystrophy with sweat, colour and temperature changes. There may be associated joint stiffness and weakness. Some patients with a neuroma have such pain and disability that they develop depression.

PHYSICAL SIGNS

A symptomatic neuroma is always tender and there may be a strongly positive Tinel sign. A positive sign distal to the level of injury indicates fine fibres have regenerated to that point. It does not guarantee functional recovery.

The neuroma may be visible and palpable as a nodule (see Fig. 7.3).

There may be signs of disuse of the part, e.g. the amputation stump or the area of innervation of that particular nerve.

There may also be signs of an associated autonomic dystrophy.

DIFFERENTIAL DIAGNOSIS

A tender nodule in an amputation stump may be due to an implantation dermoid cyst.

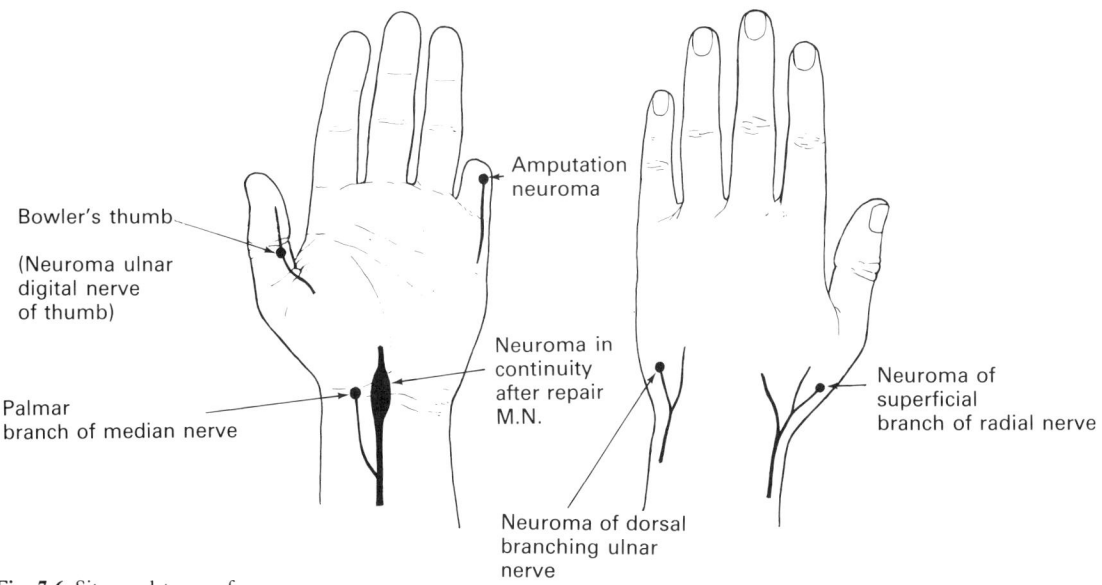

Fig. 7.6 Sites and types of neuroma.

A glomus tumour or an osteoid osteoma can be mistaken for a neuroma.

IMPLICATIONS

A painful neuroma is a relatively common cause of severe hand disability.

A painful neuroma can affect not only the function of a part, e.g. the amputation stump or the wrist in the case of a radial neuroma, but can result in painful stiffness and disuse of the adjacent digits and occasionally the entire hand or upper limb.

After nerve injury the neuroma pain is far more disabling than the numbness and palsy secondary to the injured nerve. A painful neuroma in any part of the hand can render useless an otherwise normal hand.

Persisting pain can lead to secondary and severe psychological sequelae such as depression. Narcotic addiction and severe social and economic problems can follow.

INVESTIGATION AND ASSESSMENT

The clinical features are sufficient to diagnose a neuroma and to assess the residual nerve function in cases of neuroma in continuity.

Electrophysiological tests will indicate the degree of nerve sparing quantitatively and are useful on a serial basis to indicate the degree of any regeneration.

An X-ray and bone scan may be useful to exclude a glomus tumour or osteoid osteoma.

DIAGNOSTIC LOCAL ANAESTHETIC BLOCKS

All patients should be examined after local anaesthetic is injected just proximal to the neuroma. If most pain and tenderness is relieved by this technique it can be assumed that there was a local somatic nerve problem without secondary autonomic overlay. Local surgery is likely to be more effective in these patients. Such a local anaesthetic block also enables the patient and the doctor to assess the potential function in that part of the digit or hand.

STELLATE NERVE BLOCK

If pain and tenderness persist after the local anaesthetic nerve block, a stellate nerve block should be given. This will mostly relieve any residual pain and give an indication that other anti-autonomic measures may be helpful in management.

PREVENTION AND PRIMARY CARE

Any severed nerve will form a neuroma.

No procedure has yet been discovered that completely and consistently is successful in preventing neuroma formation. Only destruction of a cell body can inhibit axonal regeneration. The perineurium presents the only impenetrable barrier to regenerating axonal sprouts. A meticulous microneural end to end apposition by repair or nerve grafting is the best way of preventing axonal escape and neuroma formation.

Although it is not possible to prevent a neuroma one can control the environment in which a neuroma forms and so lessen the likelihood of a neuroma from being symptomatic. Such measures include avoiding infection and providing a satisfactory soft tissue bed for the neuroma away from any point of compression or traction.

Prevention of amputation neuroma

After fashioning of the amputation stump, dissect the digital nerves, apply very gentle traction and section the nerves as sharply and atraumatically as possible, allowing the nerve to retract about 1 cm into clean well vascularised soft tissue (Fig. 7.7). Surgical electrocoagulation of the divided nerve may minimise neuroma formation. Any tension in closing the stump may produce anoxia with increased wound induration and fibrosis.

Prevention of terminal branch neuroma

In any laceration that overlies a known superficial nerve trunk, examine for a sensory deficit before

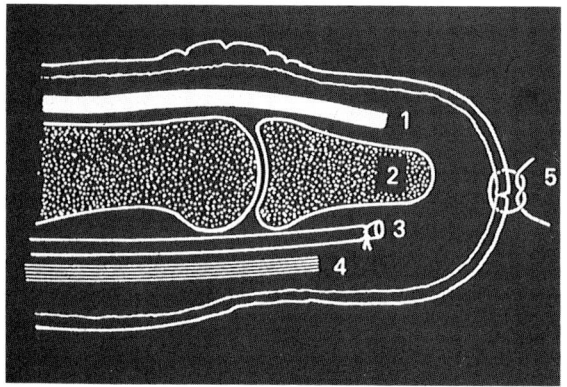

Fig. 7.7 Technique for amputation through a digit to minimise neuroma formation.

administering a local anaesthetic nerve block. Eaton advises primary repair of sharply divided sensory nerve trunks greater than 3 mm in diameter, especially the dorsal branch of the ulnar nerve and the superficial branch of the radial nerve at the wrist. Repair of these nerves is intended to prevent or reduce painful sequelae rather than restore sensibility.

Divided sensory nerves less than 3 mm in diameter may be more difficult to diagnose because of the smaller sensory deficit. They are also more difficult to find at operation because they retract from the wound area. If such a divided nerve is found, draw it distally, resect it sharply and allow it to retract.

The same retraction technique can be used for small sensory branches that are sectioned during surgical exposure. Avoid excessive traction on such a nerve during retraction since intraneural axon ruptures can produce linear microneuromas which are particularly difficult to treat.

The proximal retraction technique is also applicable to intermediate size sensory or mixed nerves that have sustained severe crush lacerations or those that are badly frayed and likewise considered irreparable.

Prevention of neuroma in continuity

Partial lacerations of large and mixed nerves should be readily diagnosed because the acute deficit is usually proportionally greater than that which would be expected for the actual number of axons interrupted. Local anoxia, haemorrhage or compression may contribute to this phenomenon.

In intermediate or smaller trunks the deficit is smaller and may be overlooked. There is no other situation in the management of peripheral nerve injuries in which an accurate anatomic diagnosis is more crucial than in partial nerve division (Eaton 1980).

Such partial lacerations to a nerve should be explored and repaired, preferably at the time of injury or certainly within 3 or 4 days before the architecture and orientation of the axons have become obscured by fibrin, clot or granulation tissue. One should be aware and take precautions to avoid damage to the uninjured nerve fibres.

Subsequent repair is far more difficult and the results far less satisfactory.

Prevention of terminal branch neuroma

Most accidental surgical sections of the superficial branch of the radial nerve or the dorsal branch of the ulnar nerve or the palmar branch of the median or ulnar nerve can be avoided by awareness of the anatomy and variations and by careful incision and exposure.

In operations on the radial or ulnar side of the wrist, e.g. in surgery for de Quervain's conditions, it is safer to incise obliquely or longitudinally rather than transversely to avoid damage to the superficial branch of the radial or the dorsal branch of the ulnar nerve. These nerves usually lie adjacent to the superficial veins in the fat layer superficial to the deep fascia.

In carpal tunnel decompression, incision of the flexor retinaculum and the volar carpal ligament and antebrachial fascia on the ulnar side of the interthenar crease, in the line of the ring finger, should avoid the palmar branch of the median nerve.

In patients prone to postoperative superficial neuroma formation, or those having revision surgery for persistent or recurrent carpal tunnel syndrome, first block that palmar branch of the median nerve. Inject local anaesthetic on the ulnar border of the flexor carpi radialis (FCR) tendon proximal to the wrist. An incision on the ulnar side of the area of innervation should avoid the palmar branch of the median nerve.

SECONDARY CARE – THE MANAGEMENT OF PATIENTS WITH ESTABLISHED PAINFUL NEUROMA

General

The management of patients with established painful neuroma is as difficult and frustrating as any branch of hand surgery. It requires enormous patience, skill and judgment and an understanding of human nature. Although the patient will need to relate and have confidence in one doctor, preferably the surgeon, a team approach may be essential. Specialised hand therapy techniques provided by physio and occupational therapists are vital in management. The social worker, rehabilitation officer, pain consultant, and clinical psychologist may have a role to play.

Early diagnosis and treatment are especially important because untreated painful neuromas can lead to fixed reflex pain patterns. Once established, these reflex patterns can persist even when the neuroma is anaesthetised, resected or otherwise rendered asymptomatic.

Non-operative treatment of painful neuroma

There are measures aimed at relieving pain and those aimed at restoring functional activity in the involved hand (Morrin et al 1985). In Chapter 6 this subject is considered in detail.

1. To relieve pain
   a. Peripheral. Massage and percussion. These are useful hand therapy techniques which can reduce the pain and sensitivity in the tissues around a neuroma.
   Local anaesthetic blocks. These help break the pain cycle and make massage and percussion easier during the phase of anaesthesia.
   Stellate nerve blocks are indicated if there is an autonomic component to the pain.
   Intralesional injections of corticosteroid. Two to 10 mg of triamcinolone acetonide can be injected into localised accessible terminal neuroma at intervals of 2 weeks to 2 months, with some relief in 60–70% of patients (Smith & Gomez 1970). Transcutaneous nerve stimulation (see p. 77).
   b. The central measures include the use of analgesics and tranquilisers, acupuncture and hypnosis.
2. Measures to restore function. Some patients find relief from protective splints and have appliances and tools modified for their games and work. Modification of leisure and work activities may be necessary.

Operative treatment

Over 100 physical or chemical modalities have been proposed for the treatment of painful neuroma (Snyder 1965).

Most of these procedures involve the initial resection of the painful neuroma followed by mechanical or chemical modification of the residual nerve stump to minimise the formation of a painful neuroma.

These methods include the destruction of the nerve end by phenol, alcohol, freezing, crushing, electrocoagulation, steroid injection or CO_2 laser; ligation of the nerve stump with silk or wire; capping of the nerve end with silastic, tantalum, silver or gold; and implantation of the neuroma or nerve stump in a muscle, bone or blood vessel.

These techniques might produce an initial relief of symptoms but a second painful neuroma occurs within 1–3 months in a significant number of patients.

The procedure of choice will depend on whether the function of the affected nerve is dispensable or not. An amputation stump neuroma can be resected. When a neuroma forms on the superficial cutaneous branches of the median, ulnar or radial nerves, these neuromas can also be resected or nerve continuity restored by nerve repair or nerve graft.

Many surgeons favour resection of an established painful neuroma, transferring that nerve stump into an area of uninjured soft tissue and away from points of pressure or contact. Tupper (1976), in a comparison of surgical treatments of painful neuroma from all causes, found only 34%

painless or minimally tender operative sites following the first neurectomy. Those undergoing a second neurectomy achieved only 38% painless or minimally tender operative sites. Those undergoing a second neurectomy with silicon capping following unsatisfactory initial simple neurectomy achieved only 25% painless or minimally tender operative sites (Tupper & Booth 1976).

Herndon et al (1976) have adopted a completely different surgical approach to the painful neuroma. They base their technique on making every effort to keep the primary neuroma intact within its matured encapsulating scar. They atraumatically transpose it enbloc to an adjacent proximal area that is free of scar and less exposed to trauma. By this technique 4 out of 5 painful amputation neuromas and 2 out of 3 terminal branch neuromas were rendered symptom-free. 72% had absent to mild sensitivity at the point of relocation and 28% had no sensitivity.

All surgical measures should be attended by adequate pre- and post-operative hand therapy measures.

THE SURGICAL TREATMENT OF PAINFUL TERMINAL NEUROMA

Amputation stump neuroma

Pre-operative measures

For all patients with painful terminal neuromas, conservative desensitising measures should first be tried. Differentiate the amputation stump which is painful and tender due to a neuroma, from that which is associated with an unsatisfactory stump with tension of the tissues over the stump, a nail fragment or an implantation dermoid. X-ray the stump.

If the neuroma is too tender for adequate examination, use a local anaesthetic digital nerve block. If this does not relieve pain in the stump it may be unwise to plan a local operation. A stellate nerve block should then be given to exclude and then be part of the management of an associated autonomic dystrophy.

Operative technique

Dissect the neuroma and nerve proximally with microneural instruments, avoiding unnecessary damage to that nerve. One then has to decide whether to resect the neuroma or transfer the neuroma itself into a new tissue bed, where compression is unlikely and traction is minimal.

Tupper advises neurectomy and Eaton advises relocation of the neuroma. The author of this chapter relocates moderately painful neuroma but resects those associated with severe pain.

Neurectomy combined with silastic capping was advocated by Frackelton et al (1971), Snyder (1965) and Swanson et al (1977). Frackelton noted that his best results were those in which the transected nerve and its silicone cap were definitively transposed and transfixed to a separate soft tissue site (Frackelton et al 1971). All authors stress the critical nature of the length and fit of the silicone cap. Improper fit may lead to necrosis if the cap is too long or too tight, or proximal and distal axon escape if the cap is short or loose (Biddulph 1972; Frackelton et al 1971; Swanson et al 1977; Tupper and Booth 1976). These potential problems do not occur with relocation of the intact neuroma (Herndon et al 1976).

In those digital amputation stumps which are diffusely dysaesthetic with one predominantly palpable and sensitive neuroma and the other that is not palpable, Herndon (1988) advises relocation of both neuromas. He also emphasises that there must be no tension on the nerve being relocated otherwise the finger movement will cause traction on the neuroma thus producing pain.

Optimal sites for relocation of a palmar neuroma include the dorsal web space, within or deep to the muscle and between the metacarpal shafts. A dorsal site is preferable to a volar one where the neuroma may be subjected to direct trauma or bimanual activity such as gripping tools.

Eaton's technique. Eaton's (1980) technique for relocation of a neuroma is as follows: the neuroma in continuity with its nerve stalk is carefully dissected proximally until the neuroma bulb can be transferred to its optimal relocation site without tension. When a bifurcation is encountered, such as the dorsal sensory branch of the digital nerve, careful teasing of this filament from the main branch under magnification will permit full mobilisation. Care must be taken to leave the adjacent digital vessels undisturbed. A 5/0 or 6/0

TRAUMATIC NEUROMA IN THE HAND 109

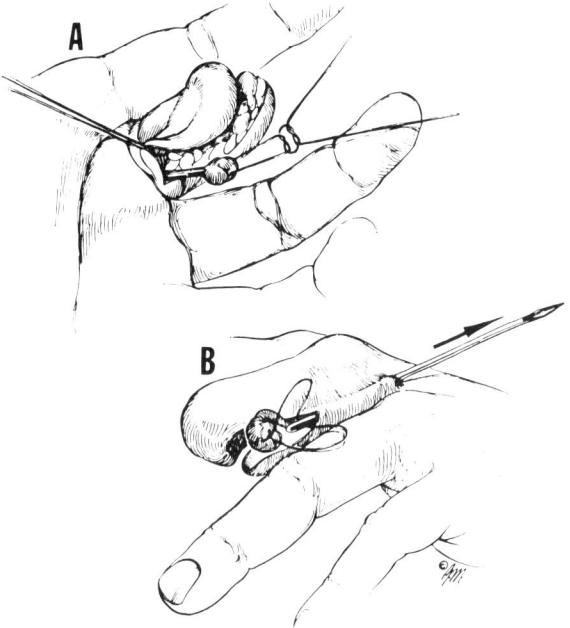

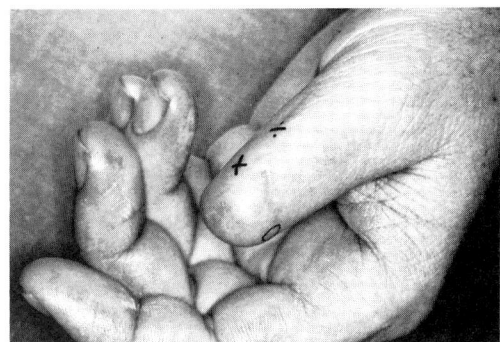

Fig. 7.9a Amputation neuroma recurring one year after neurectomy.

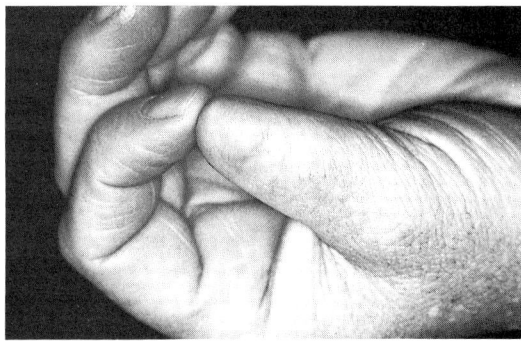

Fig. 7.8 Relocation of an intact neuroma. (a) After the neuroma is dissected free, a suture is placed in its capsule. A second knot is tied about 3–4 mm from the capsule. (b) A tunnel is bluntly dissected in the soft tissues. The neuroma is pulled through the tunnel into an area free of recurrent trauma. The suture is passed through the skin and tied, pulling the second knot up to the dermis. (Reproduced from *Operative Hand Surgery* 2nd ed. by D. P. Green 1988 by kind permission of Churchill Livingstone Inc. © Elizabeth Roselius).

Fig. 7.9b 2 years after revision neurectomy, this 42-year-old teacher was relatively free of pain and had useful thumb stump function.

catgut suture is placed through the capsule and not the neuroma and tied. The free ends of this suture are passed through a subcutaneous tunnel to the relocation site and then out through the skin proximal to the site. The neuroma is then drawn proximally into this location by traction on these sutures. The free end of the suture is tied loosely to the skin leaving subcutaneous tissue between the neuroma capsule and the skin (Fig. 7.8).

Superficial positioning of the neuroma or fixation to the skin are complications that have an unfavourable influence on the final result. Before closure, the nerve trunk is inspected to be certain that it is completely free of tension. The most common cause of failure in this procedure is displacement of the relocated neuroma from rebound due to residual tension in the proximal stalk as the catgut sutures absorb.

Associated surgical measures for the stump may be indicated, e.g. shortening of the bone, removal of associated nail fragments or dermoid cysts, releasing of any tethered tendons and a general fashioning of the healthy loose soft tissue pad.

Recurrent amputation neuroma

If a patient is referred with an amputation neuroma recurring after neurectomy or translocation by an experienced surgeon, one more surgical procedure, translocation or neurectomy, may be worthwhile (Fig. 7.9).

Post-operative care

Protect the wound until healing is established. After the sutures are removed begin massage of the scar with lanolin. Begin percussion and other desensitising measures as soon as the wound is adequately healed. Begin exercising the joints of the finger and hand as early as possible. Explain and encourage the patient to exercise and use that part of the hand and maintain a regular follow up.

NEUROMA OF THE SUPERFICIAL BRANCH OF THE RADIAL AND DORSAL BRANCH OF THE ULNAR NERVE

The surgical technique is basically similar to that used for amputation neuroma. These nerves, however, may not mobilise as well as digital nerves. The superficial branch of the radial nerve, in particular, may be relatively fixed by its multiple terminal branches. The aim is to isolate the neuroma atraumatically and relocate it on a relaxed proximal stalk to a bed free of scar and well protected. Neuroma of the radial sensory nerve may be inserted into the fleshy portion of the flexor pollicis longus (FPL) or FCR muscles and more proximal ones into the brachioradialis muscles.

In Herndon's series 2 out of 3 terminal branch neuromas treated by this technique were relieved, including 5 of 7 superficial radial sensory neuromas (Herndon 1976).

NEUROMA OF THE PALMAR BRANCH OF THE MEDIAN NERVE (Fig. 7.10)

This is best treated by resection of the entire palmar branch at its origin from the trunk of the median nerve in the distal forearm (Carroll & Green 1972).

MANAGEMENT OF PAINFUL NEUROMA IN CONTINUITY (see Fig. 7.11)

These neuromas follow partial division of a peripheral nerve and may be:

1. Lateral neuroma after partial damage to the side of the nerve
2. Neuromas following nerve repair.

Indications for operation

If 3–6 months after injury or operation there is persisting neuroma pain or failure of progression of regeneration of the nerve one should consider surgical exploration.
The timing will depend on:
1. The nature of the injury. If one suspects

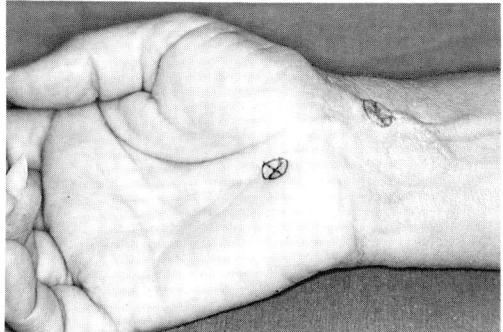

Fig. 7.10a Neuroma of the palmar branch of the median nerve and a very tender scar causing severe local pain 5 months after carpal tunnel decompression.

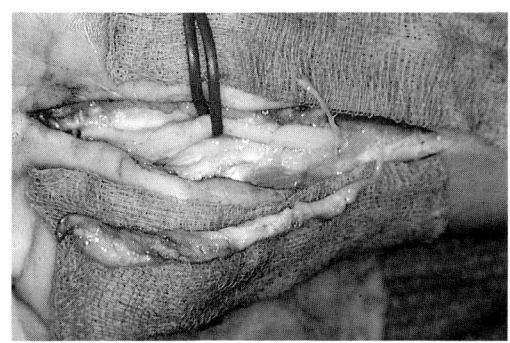

Fig. 7.10b Complete relief following resection of the neuroma. Local anaesthetic blocks gave temporary relief of pain and the inter thenar scar.

neurapraxia following a crush injury one would tend to wait longer, hoping that this was a reversible lesion. Likewise, one would tend to delay operation longer for a gunshot wound and operate earlier for a glass laceration.

2. A severe open injury might suggest a neurotmesis necessitating earlier surgical intervention. Immediate operation is indicated if one suspects partial nerve injury.

3. If the wound is associated with infection or gross scar, one would tend to wait until those complications have subsided.

4. Level of the lesion. The higher the lesion the poorer the prognosis for clinical recovery if there is to be delayed nerve repair or grafting.

5. Type of nerve. Because of the difficulties of distinguishing motor from sensory fibres, delay

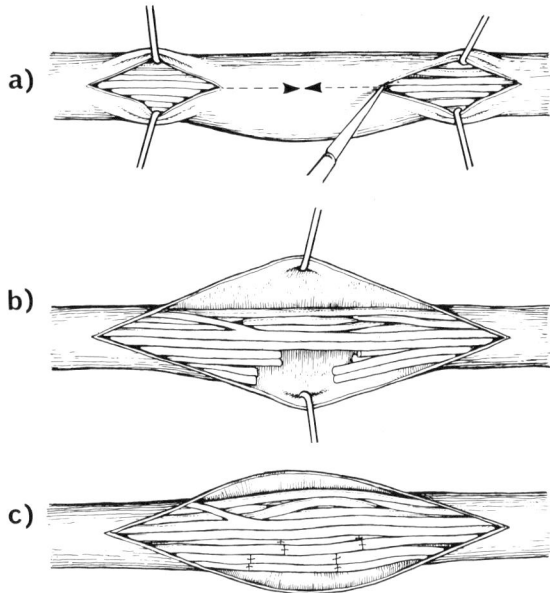

Fig. 7.11 Internal neurolysis for neuroma in continuity. (**a**) Incision through the epineurium exposing proximal and distal to the neuroma and scar. (**b**) Resection of the damaged segment of the nerve preserving those fascicles still in continuity. (**c**) Interfascicular grafting to the defect.

operation in the case of mixed nerves such as the median or ulnar nerve.

Assessment

Inspection and palpation of a neuroma in continuity, although important, can be misleading.

A large bulbous neuroma may comprise excessive epineural scar with a relatively organised intrafascicular pattern of regenerating axons. A smooth neuroma in continuity secondary to injection injury may have severe intrafascicular disorganisation and minimal potential for regeneration. A very firm neuroma suggests dense internal scar and neurotmesis. A lateral neuroma suggests partial transection on the side of the nerve. A very large neuroma, twice the normal diameter, usually indicates neurotmesis.

One should also evaluate the site and type of nerve affected by the neuroma (median, radial or ulnar) and the distal function of that nerve (sensory, motor, autonomic). If distal nerve function is deteriorating despite adequate conservative therapy, one would tend to operate earlier to prevent irreversible changes. Nerves can only be as functional as the residual sensory receptor and muscle tendon motor units.

Types of surgical procedure

These may include:
  external neurolysis
  internal neurolysis
  nerve repair or graft
  nerve transposition.

External neurolysis

Simple freeing of the nerve and the neuroma in continuity from the surrounding scarred tissues may give some temporary relief of pain and, on occasions, temporary improvement in distal nerve function. Omer, however, in his study of 59 nerves, found this procedure unreliable (Omer 1974).

At least there is minimal risk from such external neurolysis. Recurrence of adhesions between the neuroma and the surrounding tissues can be minimised by using thin silicone sheeting.

Internal neurolysis (see Fig. 7.8)

This may be a useful procedure when there is an isolated area of intraneural scarring, such as may occur after crush injuries or accidental intraneural injections. It is essential to use the most delicate microneural technique to avoid damage to uninjured and functional axons. Begin the dissection proximal and distal to the neuroma and leave the nerve as far as possible in its posterior bed, thus maintaining circulation to the neuroma. Make a longitudinal incision in the normal nerve on the proximal side of the neuroma in continuity. Use a 21 scalpel blade and small dissecting microscissors. As the area of the neuroma is approached, the epineurium thickens and becomes lost in the entrapping scar. Single out each fascicle and trace it into the scarred area. An operating microscope is needed to confirm the continuity or disruption of individual groups of fascicles. It is extremely difficult to determine exactly when the intact fascicles have been freed and to avoid unnecessary dissection with damage to intact axons. If there is scar blocking nerve continuity, resect it and close the resulting gap by nerve graft. Internal neurolysis can be followed by reasonable results if one can maintain fascicular continuity through the neuroma.

Williams & Terzis (1976) have described the use of electric stimulation during operation. For this technique the tourniquet should be deflated at least 15 minutes before the recording is attempted and the anaesthetist should avoid using paralysing anaesthetics.

Nerve repair or nerve graft

If after injury or at reoperation after nerve repair there are few intact axons and poor distal function, it is probably wiser to resect the entire neuroma and those few intact axons and perform a definitive reconstruction of the nerve by direct repair or more likely by appropriate nerve grafting. One at least would know then that a definitive procedure under optimal conditions had been carried out and the patient can be reassured accordingly.

Nerve transposition

This is sometimes applicable for neuromas in continuity of the ulnar nerve at the elbow. Transposition of the ulnar nerve relieves tension from the nerve and may make it possible to make a direct suture rather than graft a nerve defect after resection of a neuroma.

Smaller nerves with painful neuroma in continuity may be treated by mobilising the proximal and distal nerve trunks and transposing the neuroma to a less scarred area. The new position of the neuroma in continuity can be maintained by a fascial sling sutured to the dermis to prevent the nerve slipping back into its previous position. Where such mobilising of the nerve is not sufficient to ensure a relaxed repositioning in a satisfactory bed one may section the nerve distal to the neuroma and use the relocation technique as with a terminal neuroma (Eaton 1980). The sensory deficit is really increased whereas the relief of symptoms may be significant.

Spindle neuroma ('Bowler's thumb')

Traumatic perineural swellings can develop in bowlers (Dobyns 1972), tennis players and professional drummers at the site of repeated localised trauma. These thickenings are composed predominantly of hyperplastic perineural elements and rarely contain divided axons.

In bowler's thumb there is a fibrotic nodule of the proper ulnar digital nerve at the base of the thumb. The patient presents with pain and numbness over the ulnar aspect of the thumb.

Conservative treatments include the use of a protective thumb guard or redrilling the bowling ball. Avoiding bowling for 4–6 weeks is always advisable.

Surgical treatment is indicated if conservative measures do not relieve the problem. Neurolysis with excision of the markedly thickened epineurium and rerouting the involved digital nerve into a new soft tissue bed should give satisfactory results. Excision of this nodule would result in loss of sensation in that part of the thumb and the likely formation of a painful terminal neuroma.

Where such fibrotic nodules occur in a dispensable nerve such as the dorsal branch of a digital nerve (in bakers), such a nerve can be sacrificed.

REFERENCES

Badalamente M A 1985 The pathology of human neuromas: an electron microscopic and biochemical study. Journal of Hand Surgery 10B: 49–53

Biddulph S L 1972 The prevention and treatment of painful amputation neuroma. Proceedings of the South African Orthopaedic Association. Journal of Bone & Joint Surgery 54B: 379

Boyes J H 1956 Bunnell's surgery of the hand, 3rd edn. Lippincott, Philadelphia, p 426

Carroll R E, Green D P 1972 The significance of the palmar cutaneous nerve at the wrist. Clinical Orthopaedics 83: 24–28

Dobyns J H 1972 Bowler's thumb: diagnosis and treatment. A review of seventeen cases. Journal of Bone & Joint Surgery 54A: 751–755

Eaton R G 1980 Painful neuromas, management of peripheral nerve problems. Saunders, Philadelphia, pp 195–202

Frackelton W H, Teasley J L, Tauras A 1971 Neuromas in the hand treated by nerve transposition and silicone capping. Proceedings of the American Society for Surgery of the Hand. Journal of Bone & Joint Surgery 53A: 813

Herndon J H, Eaton R G, Littler J W 1976 Management of painful neuromas in the hand. Journal of Bone & Joint Surgery 58A: 369–373

Herndon J H 1988 In: Green D P (ed) Neuromas in operative hand surgery. Churchill Livingstone, Edinburgh

Huber G C, Lewis D 1920 Amputation neuromas. Their development and prevention. Archives of Surgery 1: 85–113

Mitchell S W 1874 Traumatic neuralgia. Section of median nerve. American Journal of Medical Science 67: 2–16

Morrin J, Davey V, Conolly W B 1985 The hand. Fundamentals of therapy. Butterworth, London

Odier L 1811 Manual de médècine pratique. Paschaud, Geneva, p 362

Omer G E Jr 1974 Injuries to nerves of the upper extremity. Journal of Bone & Joint Surgery 56A: 1615–1624

Smith J R, Gomez N H 1970 Local injection therapy of neuromata of the hand with triamcinolone acetonide. A preliminary study of twenty-two patients. Journal of Bone & Joint Surgery 52A: 71–83

Sunderland S 1978 Nerves and nerve injuries, 2nd edn. Churchill Livingstone, Edinburgh

Swanson A B 1977 The prevention and treatment of amputation neuromata by silicone capping. Journal of Hand Surgery 2: 70–78

Snyder C C 1965 Traumatic neuromas (abstract). Journal of Bone & Joint Surgery 47A: 641–642

Tupper J W, 1976 Treatment of painful neuromas of sensory nerves in the hand: a comparison of traditional and newer methods. Journal of Hand Surgery 1: 144–151

Williams H B, Terzis J 1976 Single fascicular recordings: an intraoperative diagnostic tool for the management of peripheral nerve lesions. Plastic & Reconstructive Surgery 57: 562–569

Wood W 1828–1829 Observations on neuromas, with cases and histories of the disease. Transcripts of the Med-Chir Society of Edinburgh 3: 68

Wynn Parry C B 1981 Rehabilitation of the hand, 4th edn. Butterworth, London

E. A. Zancolli and E. R. Zancolli Jr

8 The painful hand, problems and solutions

The hand surgeon is confronted in daily practice with three principal types of complaints: (1) deformities (including tumor formations); (2) functional impairment; and (3) pain (Steindler 1959).

Pain is an unpleasant sensory and emotional experience associated with actual or potential tissue damage, or described in terms of such damage (Mersky 1979). Pain may preceed or accompany objective manifestations, being in many cases the prominent presenting symptom.

From the 'evolution of science' point of view, the efforts expended in our speciality for the study of pain have been little compared with those for investigations on deformity and dysfunction. Several reasons may have been the cause of this delay: (1) the complicated and multiple mechanisms and interrelations of pain; (2) the precise application of the present knowledge to different everyday problems; (3) the absence of an objective and scientific way to measure pain, and (4) the reliance on patients' judgement. The latter is obviously subjective and usually mixed with constitutional and emotional factors, which makes perception of pain different for everyone.

We would like to mention all those colleagues who have helped to unfold the mysteries of pain applied to our speciality, among others Arthur Steindler, George Omer Jr and Wynn Parry, who have put on paper tremendous amounts of study, observations and experience.

From the specialist's point of view we believe that pain should be considered along with other modalities of clinical investigation such as deformity, functional impairment and complementary studies for diagnosis. It is interesting to note that as a specialist increases in experience, pain becomes a more important focus of attention and a special target to attack.

From the patient's point of view, pain in the hand is a real problem that prevents or interferes with daily activities, work and hobbies. Pain is, therefore, an important symptom and unmeasurable condition which needs to be taken into account, sometimes easy to treat and at other times nearly impossible. There are two principal goals in the treatment of pain involving the upper extremity: (1) relief of the subjective pain experience; and (2) restoration of the involved extremity to active function (Omer & Spinner 1975; Omer 1978, 1979).

In this chapter we shall refer to different aspects which have been found useful in our daily practice for the diagnosis and treatment of pain conditions involving the hand, dividing it into four parts:

I. General clinical manifestions
II. Characteristics of pain according to the tissue involved
III. Interrogation and examination
IV. Pain in different pathologies.

I. GENERAL CLINICAL MANIFESTATIONS OF PAIN

Pain speaks its own language which may be crude or inarticulate according to all linguistic standards (Steindler 1959). But pain assumes diagnostic meaning by its accessory characteristics:

1. type
2. intensity

3. presentation
4. mode of production
5. duration
6. quality
7. localisation and distribution
8. functional impairment (Table 8.1).

Table 8.1 Analysis of different pain manifestations

Type	I	– acute	
	II	– chronic	
	III	– chronic syndrome	
Intensity	I	– annoying	1. sleep unaffected
	II	– moderate	2. sleep disturbance
	III	– severe	3. sleep impeded
Presentation	I	– continuous	
	II	– intermittent	
Mode of production	I	– spontaneous	
	II	– provoked	1. by movement without strength
			2. by specific function using strength
			3. by strenuous activity
			4. by external pressure or compression
Duration	I	– remissions	– duration of attacks
	II	– minor remissions	– duration of asymptomatic periods
	III	– no remissions	
Quality	I	– sharp	
	II	– dull	
	III	– burning	
Location and distribution	I	– sharply localised	– trigger points (or areas)
	II	– diffuse	– usually muscles
	III	– irradiated	– referred proximally or distally and with or without metameric or peripheral nerve distribution
	IV	– reflex sympathetic overflow	– burning pain, abnormal vasomotor response and dystrophy – vascular pattern
Functional impairment	I	– none	
	II	– interfered	1. strenuous activity
	III	– prevented	2. usual work
			3. daily life activities

Type

Pain can be *acute or chronic*. Chronic pain is defined as pain that persists or recurs at intervals for months or years (Bonica 1979). We must differentiate chronic pain from *chronic pain syndrome*.

Chronic pain may be present in long-standing pathology, as in osteoarthritis, with a stable emotional personality.

On the other hand, a chronic pain syndrome includes some other characteristics:

1. symptoms longer than 6 months
2. minimal objective physical findings
3. evidence of medication abuse
4. somatic preoccupation, with poor appetite, loss of energy, insomnia, and diminished ability to concentrate
5. attempts to manipulate the surgeon, family and environment (Omer & Thomas 1974).

The pattern for development of a chronic pain syndrome follows a sequence: nociceptive stimulus – sensation of pain – suffering – pain behaviour – which may continue in the absence of tissue damage (Omer & Thomas 1974). The chronic pain syndrome occurs in a patient with an unstable emotional personality, in whom the 'pain state' becomes a permanent 'memory bank', and the total personality may become focused on the pain (Omer & Thomas 1974). This is a pernicious energy that imposes excessive psychological, social and economic stresses on the patient.

Intensity

Pain may be *annoying*, *moderate* or *severe*. In intense pain sleep can be disturbed or even impeded.

Presentation

Pain may present as *continuous* or *intermittent*. Continuous pain can be the expression of expanding inflammation or a growing tumor (usually dull). It is also the ache of muscle strain. If sharp and associated with other nerve symptoms, such as paresthesiae, it suggests a peripheral nerve pathology.

Mode of production

According to the mode of production, pain can be *spontaneous* or *provoked*.

Spontaneous pain usually correlates with direct irritation of peripheral nerves at any level. It is also observed in increasing inflammatory conditions of soft tissues as well as bone in growing tumors. In fact, most of the pain situations which start intermittently and are brought out by continuous eliciting causes can be expected to become spontaneous and continuous as they increase in intensity (Steindler 1959).

Provoked pain may be produced by different situations: (1) by an active or passive (less frequent) movement without using strength; (2) by a specific function using some strength (as with grip action in tennis elbow; (3) in strenuous activities, such as sports; (4) by an external pressure or compression, as in neuromas. Each one of these mechanisms can provoke pain always or occasionally. Special preconditioning factors should be noted.

Duration

Pain may present with *remissions, minor remissions* and *no remissions*. In the first case, associated with intermittent pain, the specialist should investigate the duration of attacks and the duration of asymptomatic periods.

Quality

Pain may be identified as *sharp, dull* or *burning*.

Dull pain is generally the expression of a deep seated lesion, most often bone or muscle.

Burning pain is usually associated with causalgias or minor causalgias with compromise of the sympathetic system.

Localisation and distribution

Location of pain can be: (1) *sharply localised*; (2) *diffuse*; (3) *irradiating* with or without metameric or peripheral nerve distribution; or (4) *with reflex sympathetic overflow*.

Sharply localized pain usually depends on increased peripheral nociceptive stimulus (Omer 1984). The peripheral nociceptive stimulus is often associated with trigger points. A trigger point, or area, is a small hypersensitive region from which impulses bombard the central nervous system and give rise to referred pain (Travell & Rinzler 1952). This condition is generally induced by local trauma but may also be produced by other types of circumscribed lesions in highly sensitive tissues such as periosteum.

Diffuse pain is present when deep tissues are involved. This is frequent in muscular lesions which may respond with a protective muscular spasm. Pain sensation in tendons is often also poorly localised.

Irradiating pain, originating in trigger areas and referred distally and/or proximally, can occur with or without a metameric or peripheral nerve distribution. Usually proximal referred pains do not correlate with peripheral nerve distributions.

Reflex sympathetic overflow (Omer & Thomas 1974) correlates with burning pain, abnormal vasomotor response and dystrophy. It usually affects a whole region, as the hand in Sudeck's atrophy, or the whole upper limb in the shoulder–arm–hand syndrome. The innervated vessels serving nutrition and thermo-regulation of the body are irritated by pain, and convert the corresponding area into a 'target zone'. This syndrome is thought to be a prolongation of the normal sympathetic response to injury (Bonica 1976). The pain impulses to the cortex are greatly amplified, causing intense discomfort, and can result in cross stimulation between sympathetic and sensory fibres (Doupe et al 1944). Signs of 'target zone' irritation are vasomotor changes (abnormal vasoconstriction or dilatation) that show a vascular rather than a segmental pattern, with accompanying pain, oedema and atrophy of subcutaneous tissue, skin, muscle and bone (patchy osteopenia) (Omer & Thomas 1974; Omer 1987).

Functional impairment

Correlating pain with the consequent functional impairment it may: (1) interfere with strenuous activity, usual work and daily activities, or (2) prevent these same activities partially or totally.

In clinical situations anxiety is correlated with acute pain, while depression is associated with chronic pain. The pain threshold is the least stimulus at which a subject perceives pain (Mersky 1979). The pain tolerance level is the greatest stimulus intensity causing pain that a subject is prepared to tolerate (Mersky 1979). Age, sex, race, ethnic groups, religion and other factors influence pain tolerance (Schachtel 1981). A number of traits such as anxiety, expressiveness, depression and hypochondriasis are characteristic facets of personality and can also modify pain tolerance (Lankford 1980). Pain tolerance is negatively correlated with neuritocism and positively correlated with extroversion (Lynn & Eysenck 1961).

We have analysed the different characteristics with which we can evaluate pain with more or less precision, but remaining conscious that the recognition of pain is subjective and depends upon the intensity of the peripheral stimulus, the central summation and the personality of the patient.

II. CHARACTERISTICS OF PAIN ACCORDING TO THE TISSUE INVOLVED
(Steindler 1959)

Each of the different tissues affected has its own way of expressing pain. In general, the farther from the periphery the more scant is the distribution of sensory end organs in the tissues and less precise is, therefore, the allocation of the pain source. There are some exceptions such as the periosteum, which is a highly sensitive structure, and the sensory nerves. The latter are obvious exceptions to the rule since they are themselves conductors of pain.

Joint pain originates from the synovial membrane and fibrous capsule and ligaments. There is also a response of the vasomotor system (sympathetic), in different degrees, which may add to the patient's disability as much or more than does the primary stimulus following irritation of sensory fibres. Articular cartilage seems to be insensitive. No sensory nerve fibres have been found in cartilage and since it carries no blood vessels, there are also no sympathetic fibres penetrating it. In cases of articular cartilage lesions, pain may originate from subchondral bone and synovitis.

The localisations of muscle pain is much less accurate than in the highly sensitive tissues such as skin and periosteum, but more distinctly localised than in viscera. Muscle usually reacts with a protective spasm with the intention of pain suppression. Pain sensation in tendons is generally also poorly localised and is a low sensitive tissue (except when entering compartments).

Fascia has a sensory network of finely beaded terminals, somewhat in between the looser ones in muscles and the dense network of the periosteum.

Bone pain originates from the blood vessels (sympathetic fibres) as well as the sensory fibres from the peripheral nerve which accompany the blood vessels. There is also ample sensory supply in the marrow cavity, making bone probably sensitive to intraosseous pressure. Periosteum is extremely sensitive and in many cases periosteal pain can be the presenting symptom. It has a quite definite trigger point, more superficial (extracortical) and pain can usually be elicited by pressure. Some nearly painless conditions, such as many benign bone tumors, can be explained by an intact periosteum and the absence of an increased intraosseus pressure.

All stimuli of sensory nerves have some effect upon sympathetic nerves in the surrounding territory. Leriche stated that any pain sensation causes reflexly a vasomotor condition (Leriche 1923, 1937). When tissue is injured, the nociceptors are influenced by the sympathetic efferents, chemical environments, vasculature, temperature and high frequency antidromic impulses (Omer 1987).

III. INTERROGATION AND EXAMINATION

To arrive at a correct interpretation of a pain complaint from the patient's own statements often requires a lot of interrogatory skill and experience. As we have already described, the different tissues involved have their own way of expressing pain. However, what makes the analysis of the situation more difficult is that many times they may all 'cry' at once. On the other hand, many patients are very imprecise in their pain description and particularly confused about the sequence of attacks, remissions and circumstances, so important for diagnostic and prognostic purposes. But the physician can usually arrive at a presumptive diagnosis of the different pathologies where pain is the presenting and leading symptom. An important mental attitude for the physician is not to believe that what he cannot explain is non-existent (Steindler 1959).

In this section, dedicated to the clinical record, we have to consider:

1. history and analysis of pain characteristics
2. physical examination
3. complementary studies useful for diagnosis.

History of pain and analysis of clinical characteristics

In the study of pain history there are 3 well defined phases that have a logical sequence (Table 8.2):

Phase I – cause for consultation
Phase II – patient's spontaneous narration of symptoms
Phase III – methodically induced interrogation.

Phase I: cause for consultation

After asking the patient the reason for seeking help, the physician can usually extract the clue for a diagnostic orientation from the first ten words (approximately) of the response. We transcribe those first words in the patient's report.

Phase II: patient's spontaneous narration of symptoms

In the second phase the patient continues with the narration of symptoms, which may be clear or lead to confusion.

Phase III: methodically induced interrogation

In phase III the specialist's skill and method are the clue to the interrogation. It must be clear that at the end of this third phase the physician should arrive at a presumptive diagnosis and the possible differential diagnoses. This will be later confirmed or rechecked by the physical examination and complementary studies.

There can be many ways to perform this interrogation, but we shall describe the sequence which we prefer.

1. Time of beginning of symptoms
2. Circumstance/s and cause/s attributed to origin
   trauma
   idiopathic
   etc.
3. Methodical analysis of pain characteristics (see Table 8.1)
4. Evolution of symptoms
5. Previous treatments (if any)
6. Necessity and response to rest, medication, or other form of treatment
7. Associated symptoms
   crepitation
   clicks
   functional impairment
   loss of strength
8. Subjective evaluation of emotional stability.

Having concluded these 3 phases, based on the history and the analysis of the clinical characteristics of pain, the specialist can have either a clear picture or confusion about the situation. If confusion arises from the patient's lack of precision where pain is the leading and presenting symptom, we tell the patient to return home and come back after a careful new analysis. For example, we can ask him to analyse the distribution, localisation, circumstances or any other obscure point in the

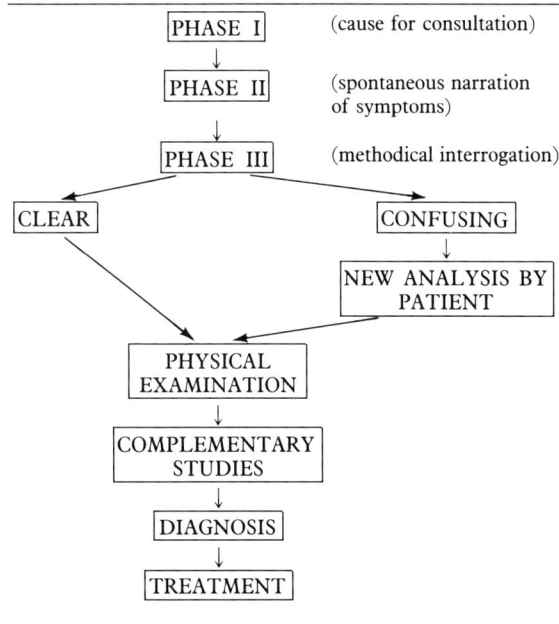

Table 8.2 Sequence for clinical study

first examination. In other cases, where pain manifests only for a short period after a strenuous activity and later disappears, we tell the patient to return next time the pain is present, in order to obtain a precise localisation through physical examination.

During the study of a patient consulting for pain, it is easy for the physician to be confused or misled in different situations: (1) atypical pathology; (2) presentation with wide overlapping into surrounding territories; (3) a diffuse or radiating pain; (4) a difficult personality; (5) a patient's inability to describe pain, with confusion about the different characteristics and factors to be analysed.

Physical examination

When the prominent or unique symptom is pain, it is important that it is present when examining the patient. As we have already explained, if pain appears for short periods only after strenuous activity, usually sporting, the patient is submitted to that specific activity before the specialist's visit. Physical examination may then lead to positive results.

Therefore, conditioned by the presence of pain, or the possibility of reproducing it during the examination, the following steps are taken for a thorough examination:

1. Palpation, searching for trigger points
2. Pain elicited by active or resisted movements
3. Specific tests
4. Anaesthetic blocks.

Palpation searching for trigger points

A trigger point is a circumscribed area in which digital pressure produces a sudden sharp pain. It is by far the most valuable sign for locating the origin of pain and for identifying painful structures. The accuracy of such localisation depends, among other factors, on the anatomical depth of the issue involved and its specific sensitivity. Many times the physician can find more than one trigger point depending on different and contiguous structures. It is convenient to examine first the painless areas and only then search for the trigger point we suspect is the cause of pain. Bilateral investigation of the painful area may give us a lot of information.

In every localisation investigated several questions are useful for orientation:
does this point elicit pain?
is it the same pain you usually feel?
does it radiate to any other part? Where?
if so, is this the same radiation you usually feel?

One should not be satisfied until the patient confirms that the usual pain has been reproduced. Secondary trigger points, probably due to inflammation or overstress of nearby structures, are temporarily dismissed. A profound knowledge of the anatomy is needed for recognition and interpretation through palpation.

Occult silent trigger points can be considered in 3 different situations: (1) in persons without pathology; (2) in a patient with a pathology which has other trigger points interconnected; and (3) interrelation of associated pathologies.

It is interesting to point out that in a person without symptoms, mild silent tender points can be found, elicited by digital pressure, in the dominant upper limb, comparing these same points to the corresponding ones on the non-dominant side. These points are usually found over the anterolateral aspect of the radiohumeral joint and at the glenohumeral joint (approximately 2 cm lateral to the coracoid process). Occasionally the lateral and anterior aspects of the ulnohumeral joint are also silently tender.

When one of the following pathologies is present, the trigger points of the others generally become more tender in the homolateral side (dominant or non-dominant): medial epicondylitis, lateral epicondylitis, de Quervain disease and supraspinatus syndrome.

The 'tender points association' previously described might correlate, in some way, with the clinical observation that even though only one pathology initiates symptoms, other posterior or simultaneous 'predisposed-interrelated pathologies' (in both upper-limbs) may present. Association between the following 'predisposed-interrelated disorders' may occur: de Quervain disease, trigger finger/s, trigger thumb, Dupuytren disease or palmar fasciitis, carpal tunnel syndrome, painful basal joint of the thumb, lateral epicondylitis, medial epicondylitis and painful shoulder.

Pain elicited by movements

Now we ask the patient to reproduce the movement(s) that provoke pain. The same questions should be asked as in investigating trigger points. Also the different active movements with or without resistance are investigated. Dynamometry is useful for evaluating loss of strength caused by pain.

If pain is produced by passive movements, it is almost invariably a sign that the joint or structures in its immediate surroundings are involved. Pain elicited only at the extremes of the arc of motion generally corresponds to a synovial origin, but if present through all the arc of motion, destruction of the articular cartilage must be suspected.

Specific tests

Having localised the site of pain, the examiner has already usually elaborated a diagnostic orientation. This is the time for utilising the specific tests for the different suspected pathologies. The Allen test (Allen 1929) is used to evaluate circulatory problems. Muscle and tendon functions are investigated by tests that isolate their individual function, as for example the Apley test (Apley 1956) for the flexor superficialis tendons. When nerves are compromised, sensibility, muscular and sudomotor functions should be explored. In Table 8.3 we mention some specific tests for the study of joint instability and degeneration. Axial compression usually reproduces pain of cartilage destruction, while different stress manoeuvres are utilised for discovering instabilities. Some tests, such as the Watson's scaphoid shift test (Watson et al 1988), investigate both components. Many of these tests can produce clicking or crepitation. Every one of them should be examined bilaterally in order to compare and evaluate their pathological significance, especially if the contralateral hand is normal.

Anaesthetic blocks

Anaesthetic blocks are very useful for confirming or dismissing the localisation of trigger points. They are a very valuable instrument in the specialist's armamentarium for diagnosis.

Only the point desired is blocked with 2% lignocaine hydrochloride. In order to avoid dispersion to other areas, the smallest possible amount of anaesthetic should be used. Sometimes, in difficult diagnostic cases, several different points have to be blocked in sequence or after the effect of the previous block has disappeared, according to circumstance.

When injecting a steroid (triamcinolone acetonide) as an anti-inflammatory treatment in a localised trigger point, we combine it with lignocaine in order to evaluate post-injection if the painful area has disappeared.

After a few minutes of an anaesthetic block (with or without steroid association), the patient and/or examiner try to reproduce the movement or manoeuvre that provoked pain. If pain has disappeared, one can be sure that the trigger point has been hit and only now we can confirm a diagnostic localisation or evaluate the effect of local steroid injections in the corresponding pathology. Reasons for persistence of pain after the injection can be: (1) the wrong area has injected, or (2) the coexistence of other trigger point(s). In the latter situation, if the main trigger point was hit but other trigger point(s) are present, pain diminishes but does not disappear.

Complementary studies useful for diagnosis

Complementary studies are used to investigate, complete or corroborate the data obtained through history and physical examination. Usually with a meticulous history, a careful physical examination and regular X-ray films, a correct diagnosis can be made. An experienced examiner reduces the need for sophisticated procedures, but in some atypical or difficult cases the specialist can obtain sufficient information for the diagnosis only with the help of specific elective studies.

Routine laboratory studies, such as sedimentation rate, are very useful. In the roentgenographic evaluation, special projections, dynamic studies under an image intensifier and tomograms may be needed. If the data are still insufficient an arthrogram may be indicated, depending on the pathology. Arthroscopy has a real place in some wrist lesions. Other studies such as scintigraphy,

Table 8.3 Some specific tests used for diagnosis of joint instability, painful stability and cartilage degeneration. Bilateral comparison for pathological significance

Joint	test for instability or painful stability	test for cartilage destruction	test for both components
Distal radio-ulnar	piano key-board sign (Backdahl 1963; Jackson et al 1974)	axial compression	
Scapho lunate			Watson's scaphoid shift test (Watson et al 1988)
Piso-triquetral			axial compression and displacement stress
Triquetro lunate			Ballottement test (Reagan et al 1984)
Triquetro hamate	passive ulnar deviation (Lichtman et al 1981)		
Ulnar carpometacarpal (4th and 5th rays)			axial compression with flexion – extension stress
Radial carpometacarpal (2nd and 3rd rays)			axial compression with flexion – extension stress
Trapezio metacarpal	pinch in retroposition	axial compression and twisting	
Thumb metacarpophalangeal	– stress for abnormal hyperextension – lateral stress in flexion and extension	axial compression	
Metacarpophalangeal (4 fingers)	– lateral stress in flexion – stress for abnormal hyperextension	axial compression	
Proximal interphalangeal	– lateral stress in extension – stress for abnormal hyperextension	axial compression	
Distal interphalangeal	lateral stress in extension	axial compression	

computerized axial tomography scans, magnetic resonance imaging, doppler, plethysmography and electrodiagnostic studies may have a relative or absolute indication.

In cases of traumatic or non-traumatic origin with persistent pain and negative X-rays, a technetium radionuclide scan is often the next step towards a correct diagnosis.

IV. PAIN IN DIFFERENT PATHOLOGIES, DIAGNOSIS AND TREATMENT

It is not surprising to encounter many pathological conditions in the region of the hand in which pain plays a prominent role, considering how richly this particular area of the upper limb is endowed by sensory fibres (Steindler 1959). There is another factor which favours pain manifestation, and that is the crowding together of sensory structures in comparatively narrow spaces, which do not allow inflammatory expansion without exerting painful pressure on the surrounding sensitive tissues (Steindler 1959). Nearly every traumatic lesion in the hand is accompanied by some degree of pain. Also, non-traumatic pathologies are also associated with pain in some stage of their course. Therefore it would be impossible to describe them all in a few pages.

In previous sections we have analyzed the different general characteristics and aspects of pain that can be found in different pathologies. In this section we shall only refer to some pathologies associated with pain, which are worthy of special mention. Reasons for these particular choices for analysis are: (1) the belief that a detailed surgical technique (as will be described) is a fundamental factor for the goal of pain relief, or (2) to mention different aspects of diagnosis and/or treatment from the authors' experience, some published here in English for the first time.

The selected pathologies are:

1. de Quervain's disease
2. Lateral epiconylitis
3. Fractures and non-unions of the hook of the hamate
4. Chronic lesions of the second and third carpometacarpal joints
5. Painful disorders of the distal radioulnar joint: a modification of the Darrach procedure
6. Treatment of the different stages of osteoarthritis of the basal joint of the thumb
7. Some indications and techniques for articular denervation of the wrist
8. Chronic first dorsal compartment syndrome
9. Treatment considerations in reflex sympathetic dystrophy.

de Quervain's disease (de Quervain 1895)

We have deliberately chosen this common disorder as a detailed and correct surgical technique is a necessary factor in order to obtain pain relief and avoid multiple complications.

The abductor pollicis longus and the extensor pollicis brevis run through the first dorsal compartment of the wrist beneath the extensor retinaculum. This compartment, located more radial than dorsal, has a great tendency to produce pathology on account of a compartmental tenosynovitis (de Quervain's disease; de Quervain 1895), generally caused by supernumerary tendons.

The presence of supernumerary tendons of the abductor pollicis longus (APL) with distal insertions in different structures – first metacarpal, trapezium, muscles of the thenar eminence and transverse carpal ligament – has been recognised by anatomists and surgeons, but with different incidences: Wood (1867) 68%; Loomis (1951) 89.8%; Lacey et al (1951) 81%; and Bianchi (1978) 56%. These percentages demonstrate the normal presence of 2, 3 or even 4 tendons corresponding to the APL. Wood (1867) in *Variations in human myology*, describes one of the variations of the APL as 'digastric muscle'. This anatomical variation has 2 muscle bellies, one proximal innervated by the radial nerve, and a distal belly in the thenar eminence innervated by the median nerve. This distal belly can easily be separated from the rest of the thenar muscles.

Pain may sometimes be severe with the consequent functional impairment of the thumb and, in some cases, also the wrist. Tenderness over the first dorsal compartment is found. The Finkelstein test (Finkelstein 1930) is performed by asking the patient to place his thumb in the palm, in a flexion – adduction position, and then make a fist over it. In this position, the examiner deviates the wrist in ulnar direction eliciting pain. We usually potentiate this test by making digital pressure over the distal end of the first dorsal compartment. Except in a very early stage and mild cases, we have not obtained effective results with conservative treatment. Differential diagnoses are: synovitis over the radial styloid, osteoarthritis of the basal joint of the thumb or radio-scaphoid joint, and tenosynovitis of the abductor pollicis longus and extensor pollicis brevis just proximal to the first dorsal compartment (usually accompanied by a very distal ending of their muscle bellies).

Surgical treatment is performed under local anaesthesia and pneumatic tourniquet. A subcutaneous injection of 2% lignocaine hydrochloride underneath the programmed incision is usually sufficient. We prefer a transverse incision, placed over the first dorsal compartment 1 cm proximal to the distal end of the radial styloid, for cosmetic reasons and avoiding hypertrophic scars. With this approach, care should be taken not to incise any further than skin with the scalpel. Then dissection of the subcutaneous tissue is achieved with scissors, spreading them in a longitudinal direction. The surgeon must be aware that branches of the radial nerve are located in this anatomical plane. After placing 4 tendon retractors in each cardinal point of the incision, the retinaculum of the first dorsal compartment is incised longitudinally. Resection of this structure should be avoided because of the danger of tendon subluxation. Two or 3 tendons appear inside the compartment. One of them is the abductor pollicis longus and the other(s) depend on the digastric muscle. Identification of each tendon function is accomplished, exerting traction on each one of them. The surgeon must remember that, generally, the extensor pollicis brevis is located in a separate subcompartment within the first dorsal compartment which must also be liberated. The tendon(s) of the digastric muscle are resected (approximately 2 cm of tendon resection). Subcutaneous tissue and skin are closed after a careful haemostasis with a bipolar coagulator. Immobilisation with a volar-radial wrist splint for 10 to 15 days is convenient, leaving the thumb free for immediate active movements in the post-operative period.

Lateral epicondylitis (tennis elbow)

This condition was first described by Bernhard in 1896 as a strain produced by forceful pronation and supination movements, hence given the name of tennis elbow (Steindler 1959).

It usually begins as an acute attack of differing intensity after strenuous activity using the extensors of the wrist and pronation–supination movements. If the condition continues its course, acute attacks become more frequent and intense and may evolve into a chronic inflammatory disorder.

Usual symptoms are: provoked sharp moderate to severe pain, localised tenderness in the lateral epicondyle and anterolateral aspect of the radiohumeral joint, distal radiation over the wrist extensor muscles, usually diurnal pain (sometimes nocturnal exacerbations awaking the patient), diminished grip strength and pain on full extension of the elbow, pain upon resisted extension of the middle finger, painful opposed pronosupination, prolongation of the periods with rest pain with the evolution of the disease (with pain exacerbated by function).

Multiple pathogenesis have been described for this condition. Meherin and Cooper (1951), who studied 200 cases, concluded that there is little that is definite about the pathological background of tennis elbow. Cyriax (1936) in a comprehensive article enumerated no less than 26 pathological conditions among which were mentioned: traumatic periostitis, sprain of collateral ligaments, fibrosis of the extensors, tears or sprains of muscles or ligaments, synovial or ligamentous impingement and inflammatory joint changes. Bosworth (1955) later attributed the main aetiology of pain in tennis elbow to the orbicular ligament, while Osgood (1922) described a bursitis between the 2 extensor carpi radialis tendons.

Nowadays it is accepted by the majority of authors that the most frequent pathogenesis of lateral epicondylitis or tennis elbow is a degenerative change in the insertion of the epicondyle extensor tendons. If the tender point is over the lateral epicondyle it is usually catalogued as a lateral epicondylitis, but if it is located near the neck of the radius with a positive middle finger test and painful resisted supination with the elbow fully extended, it is usually described as a radial tunnel syndrome (Lister et al 1979).

In our daily practice we have found mainly 4 different tender points in the lateral epicondyle region:

1. over the anterior aspect of the lateral epicondyle, probably due to degenerative changes of the common extensor from the epicondyle
2. over the anterolateral aspect of the radiohumeral joint (some 1 cm medial and 1.5 cm distal to the lateral epicondyle with the elbow flexed 80°), which can be precisely localised with pronation and supination movements. This pain is produced by a chronic synovitis (which we have

corroborated with anatomopathology) of a synovial fold ('pseudomeniscus', de Goes 1961) between the radius and humerus, being produced as any other impingement syndromes (see p. 119)
3. over the posterior aspect of the lateral epicondyle caused by a tenosynovitis of the triceps tendon (not frequent)
4. over the wrist extensors (some 3 to 4 cm distal to the lateral epicondyle), presenting as a palpable muscle contracture.

It is interesting to note that points 1 and 2 usually coexist, the radiohumeral point being frequently more tender than that of the lateral epicondyle. In a few cases the localisation of pain can be encountered only in one point (1 or 2), without tenderness in the other point. To differentiate a chronic synovitis of the 'pseudomeniscus' from a radial tunnel syndrome we perform an anaesthetic block. The cc of lignocaine hydrochloride are injected into the joint through a posterolateral approach (palpating the joint between the lateral epicondyle and the olecranon).

If this is not done, and the patient is operated on for a radial tunnel syndrome (RTS), when presenting a chronic synovitis, the relief of pain may be the result of an indirect denervation of the elbow joint (when employing the surgical technique described for RTS). In some of these cases, after this operation, in which pain persists but only in a minor degree, it may be due to the articular nervous fibres entering posterior to the joint over the anconeus muscle as described by Bateman (1948).

Our experience with steroid injections has been very encouraging over many years. We perform this with triamcinolone acetonide (up to 2.5 cc, 15 mg) and 4–5 cc of 2% lignocaine hydrochloride. The elbow is placed in 80° of flexion and the skin point of injection lies over the tender point previously described. From here the needle is directed to the radiohumeral joint and afterwards to the lateral epicondyle. In the latter localisation a wide area is injected through corrections of the needle's direction (Figs 8.1, 8.2). A minute or two later pain is provoked again through forceful movements. If the injection hit the intended target area, pain should be absent. Usually, with one or

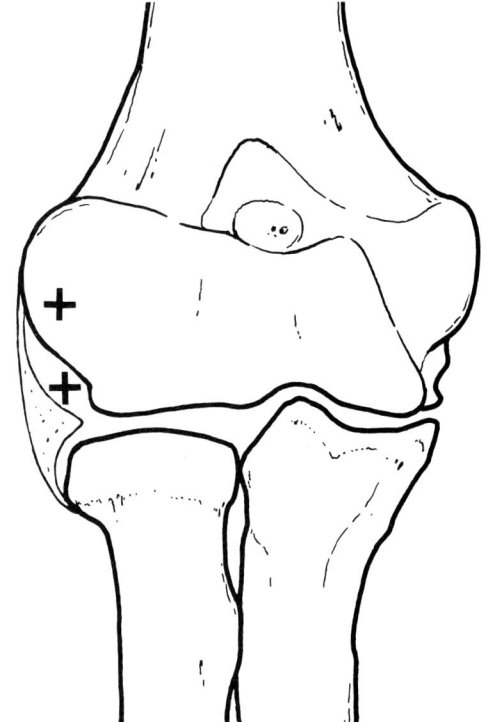

Fig. 8.1 Target points for steroid injections.

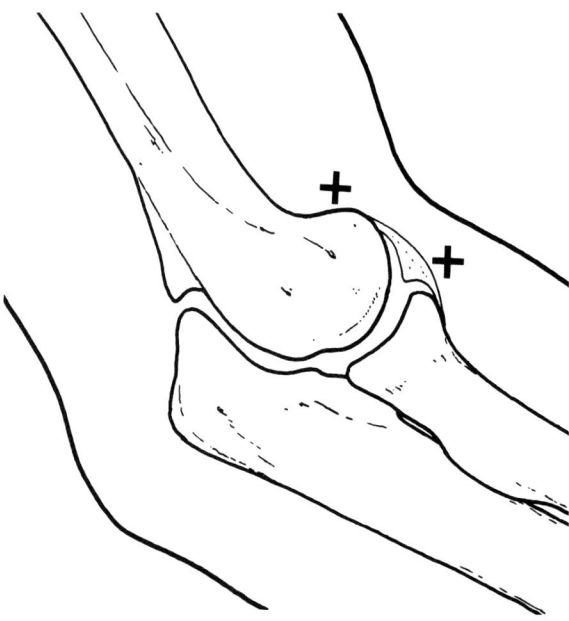

Fig. 8.2 Target points for steroid injections.

two injections, symptoms will completely disappear. The first injection usually relieves about half of the pain. When asymptomatic a strengthening–stretching programme for the extensor muscles is begun.

In those cases where conservative treatment is not effective (approximately 5%), after a reasonable period of time surgery is indicated. Resection of the 'pseudo-meniscus' is accomplished (Fig. 8.3), associated with a small tenotomy of the tendinous origin.

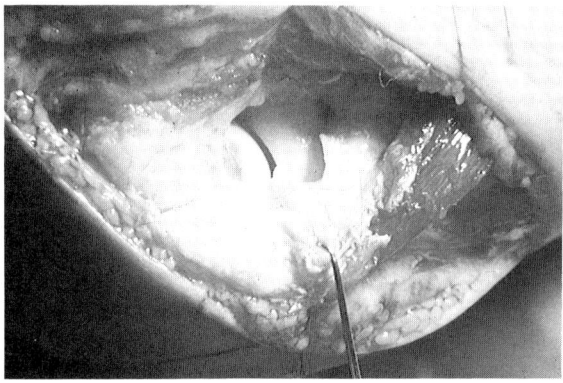

Fig. 8.3 Surgical case – resection of radio-humeral 'pseudo-meniscus'.

Fractures and non-unions of the hook of the hamate

We decided to consider this entity for 2 important reasons: (1) if the treating physician is not aware of this injury, the diagnosis and appropriate treatment will not be accomplished; and (2) the surgical technique must be meticulous because of the vulnerable anatomic structures in the vicinity. Defects of surgical technique are usually the cause of fair or poor results.

The most important clues for diagnosis are: (1) gripping function producing pain and diminished strength; (2) tenderness over the hook of the hamate; and (3) pain elicited by forced abduction against resistance of the little finger. Other diagnostic features can be: pain over the dorsum of the hamate; crepitation, tenosynovitis or rupture of the flexor tendons of the little finger; and ulnar nerve paresthesiae or paresis.

Fractures of the hook of the hamate can be produced by direct trauma or by indirect mechanisms. The most frequent are falling on an outstretched hand and sports activities such as golf, polo, etc. Non-unions are diagnosed usually several months after symptoms have begun, as the initial diagnosis can be difficult.

The presumptive diagnosis must be confirmed by bone imaging. Anteroposterior and lateral X-rays usually do not give the physician any information. Oblique views in supination, carpal tunnel views and other special projections have been described, but all can have false negatives. Our first choice is computed tomography (Egawa & Asai 1983) and the second lateral tomography.

The knowledge of the surgical anatomy is paramount when considering the surgical intervention. The hook of the hamate projects 1 to 2 cm distal and lateral to the pisiform in the hypothenar eminence. At this point it can be palpated beneath the skin, subcutaneous tissue and palmaris brevis. It is important to remember that it is the most important structure for attachment, on the ulnar side, of the flexor retinaculum. It has insertions, also, of the opponens and short flexor muscles of the small finger, as well as the piso-hamate ligament. The superficial branch of the ulnar nerve passes ulnarly in proximity to the tip, while the deep branch is located near the base of the hook and has a turning point at the distal end of the hook in a transverse and radial direction. The flexor tendons of the small finger pass along its radial border in the carpal tunnel and utilise the hook as a point for orientation.

For the excision of the hook of the hamate we use a longitudinal incision of approximately 6 cm, beginning 5 mm distal to the distal volar wrist crease, passing over the hook of the hamate in direction to the ulnar border of the ring finger. The transverse carpal ligament is visualised after some dissection of the subcutaneous tissue. The hook of the hamate is palpated and the ligament incised longitudinally, approximately 2 mm radial to the tip of the hook. The flexor tendons of the little finger are explored and afterwards retracted radially. The motor branch of the ulnar nerve, turning around the base of the hook, must be identified.

Then the ulnar side of the hook is approached, opening the Guyon's canal (Guyon 1861). The sensory branch of the ulnar nerve and the ulnar artery are identified and retracted ulnarly. Only then, the motor branch is dissected proximally and very carefully retracted ulnarly and distally. The flexor retinaculum and periosteum over the tip of the hook are opened longitudinally. A subperiosteal dissection at each side of the hook is performed. The hook is then resected in easy stages and the flexor retinaculum reattached to avoid tendon subluxation.

Immobilisation is obtained with a volar splint for 10 to 15 days, allowing flexion–extension digital movements during that period.

Chronic painful lesions of the second and third carpometacarpal (CMC) joints

Acute injuries to the second and third carpometacarpal joints can result in sprains, fractures (usually small intra-articular fragments), or dislocations (rare). If initial diagnosis and treatment are not adequate, chronic instability and osteophyte formation may develop. As noted by different authors (Joseph et al 1981; Gunther 1984), chronic sprains of the CMC joints can produce pain, tenderness, laxity and crepitus on manipulation. With stress testing for instability (flexion–extension manoeuvres), pain is elicited. It is usually caused by an occupational stress (Carroll & Carlson 1989). With strenuous activities, patients experience weakness and disabling pain. The best imaging study, in our experience, to confirm this pathology is a lateral tomogram.

As noted by different authors, arthrodesis will result in an excellent long-term relief of pain. Twenty years ago we began employing a surgical technique for this pathology which we shall describe in this section. The highest incidence of this pathology presents in post-traumatic cases, especially in professional boxers. While boxing, axial forces are transmitted particularly through the second and third rays, with the consequent possibility of sprains and small intra-articular fractures conducive to a chronic instability and osteoarthritis. Of the 8 professionals boxers we have operated on with this pathology, none of them had any pain after the operation and all returned to their original level of competition. Two of them after the operation fought for their world championship, one of them winning it.

We shall describe some important aspects of the surgical technique. The carpometacarpal joints are palpated and a dorsal transverse incision is made over them. Care should be taken with the sensory branches of the radial nerve. The extensor tendons of the fingers are retracted. The extensor carpi radialis brevis is separated radially, while the extensor radialis longus is sectioned 1 cm proximal to its metacarpal insertion. Sometimes a ganglion emerging from this area can be found. The dorsal capsule is opened and 4 joints are exposed: the 2nd carpometacarpal, 3rd carpometacarpal, intermetacarpal between 2nd and 3rd, and capitate–trapezoid. The articular cartilage of the 4 joints is removed. Subchondral bone is curetted. The joints are stabilised with 3 or 4 K-wires (Figs 8.4, 8.5). Bone graft (spongiosa) of the distal radius is packed inside the 4 joints affected by the arthrodesis. This type of cross shaped arthrodesis is covered by suturing the capsule over it. The

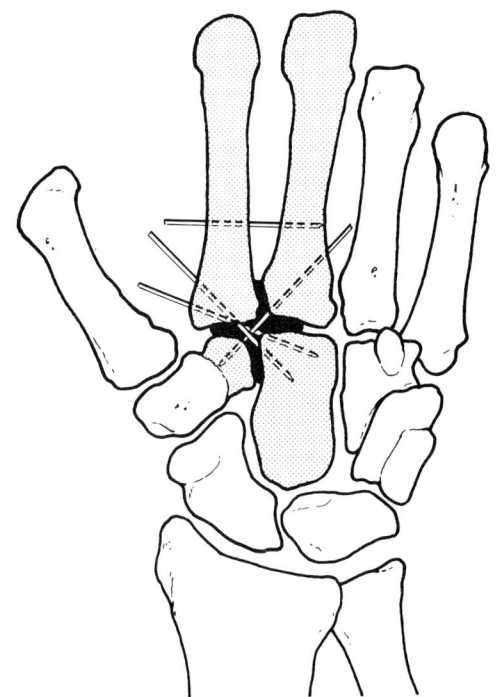

Fig. 8.4 Arthrodesis of the 4 joints.

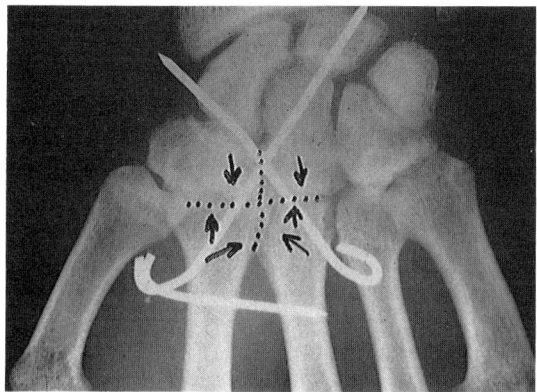

Fig. 8.5 X-ray of a surgical case – arthrodesis of the four joints.

ECRL is sutured to the distal stump. Immobilisation for 1.5–2 months is accomplished by a short cast, leaving the fingers free for motion. The K-wires are removed after confirming the consolidation of the arthrodesis. This confirmation is difficult to visualise in standard X-rays because of the special configuration of the CMC joints. Anteroposterior and lateral tomograms are useful for confirming the healing of the arthrodesis (Fig. 8.6).

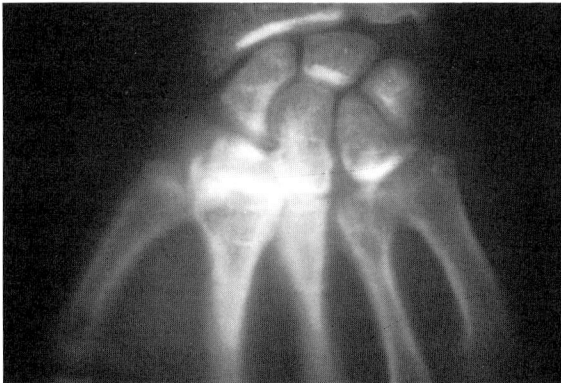

Fig. 8.6 A-P tomogram demonstrating healing of the arthrodesis.

Painful disorders of the distal radio-ulnar joint: a modification of the Darrach procedure

Excision of the distal ulna is usually indicated in conditions that cause derangement of the articular surfaces of the radio-ulnar joint, interfering with function and resulting in limited and/or painful motion. Recent studies have arrived at conclusions which must be considered before deciding on resection of the distal ulna: (1) operations that alter the radio-ulnar length relationship can be expected significantly to change contact pressures at the radiocarpal joint as well as forearm load transmission (Werner et al 1986); (2) the ulna bears an average of 17–18% of the axial load in the neutral position, increasing in wrist extension and ulnar deviation and decreasing with flexion and radial deviation (Werner et al 1986; Trumble et al 1987); (3) anatomical studies have emphasized the importance of the triangular fibrocartilage complex (TFCC) in stabilising the ulnar side of the wrist (Bowers 1985) and the ulnar; (4) one third of the lunate normally articulates with the TFC in neutral position, increasing with radial deviation. Therefore ulnar translocation and ulnocarpal instability can be produced by the Darrach procedure, which destroys the bony support for the TFCC. The classical Darrach procedure has been modified by several authors to avoid the mechanical disadvantages of that method.

Our intention is to describe another modification for the Darrach procedure, which we have been using for the last 2 years with encouraging results, even though the follow up time and the number of cases are not yet sufficient to reach definite conclusions. This modification is particularly indicated in rheumatoid arthritis. The main intention is to prevent progressive ulnar translation of the carpus due to progressive destruction of the lunate fossa of the radius.

The idea for considering this technique was to give bony support to the TFCC and tense the ulnar collateral ligament and periosteum of the ulna by preserving their attachments in the styloid process which is fused to the sigmoid notch of the radius. The distal ulna is approached through the sixth dorsal compartment of the wrist. The distal ulna is dissected subperiosteally, preserving the ligament's and periosteal attachments to the base of the styloid process. An oblique osteotomy of the styloid is made, leaving a remnant 1 by 1 cm. Then a transverse osteotomy of the ulna is performed 2 mm proximal to the upper border of the sigmoid notch of the radius, making an oblique

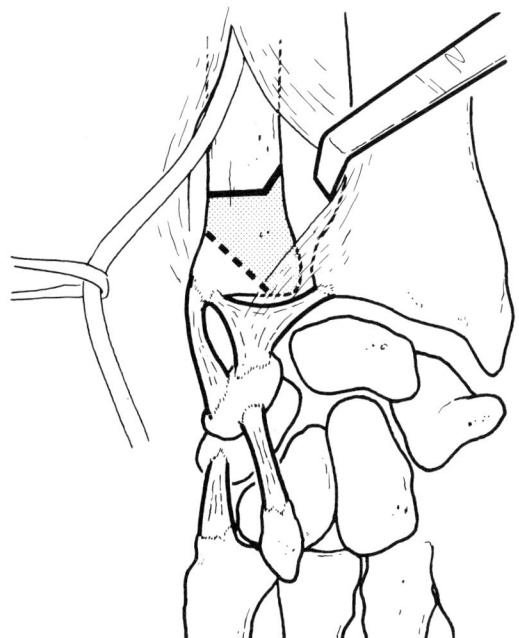

Fig. 8.7 Transverse osteotomy of the ulna.

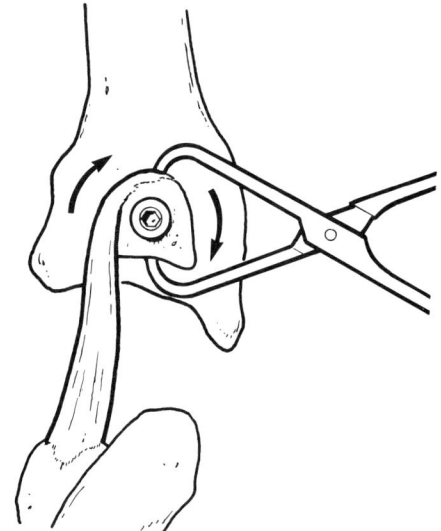

Fig. 8.9 Tightening of styloid process.

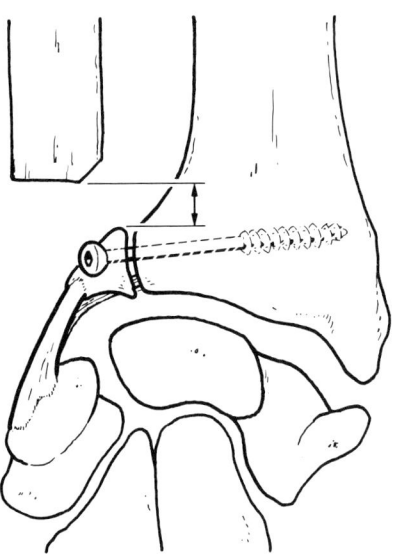

Fig. 8.8 Removal of articular cartilage for fusion with the styloid.

small resection of the radial margin (Fig. 8.7). The articular cartilage is removed from this notch for fusion with the styloid, which is fixed by a 4 mm malleolar screw (Fig. 8.8). If the ulnar collateral ligament (UCL) remains somewhat lax, before completing the screwing, the styloid process is turned until tension is obtained in the UCL and ulnar periosteum (Fig. 8.9). If the extensor carpi ulnaris is unstable it can be introduced in the fifth dorsal compartment.

The intention with this technique is to offer some support to the carpus, as with other procedures, like the ones described by Sauve-Kapandji (1936) or Bowers (1985).

Treatment of the different stages of osteoarthritis of the basal joint of the thumb

In this section we shall discuss our preferred treatment of the different stages of trapeziometacarpal (TMC) osteoarthritis. The TMC joint can oppose, through rotational movements, the tip of the thumb to the tips of the remaining digits, using the areas with the highest sensibility discrimination during prehension (Zancolli et al 1987). Rotation of the first metacarpal during opposition (pronation) and retroposition (supination) depends on three factors: muscular activity, ligament tension and congruence of the spherical portion of the TMC joint.

Absence of pain is fundamental for a normal function of the thumb. The symptoms and signs that can be present in osteoarthritis of the basal

THE PAINFUL HAND, PROBLEMS AND SOLUTIONS 129

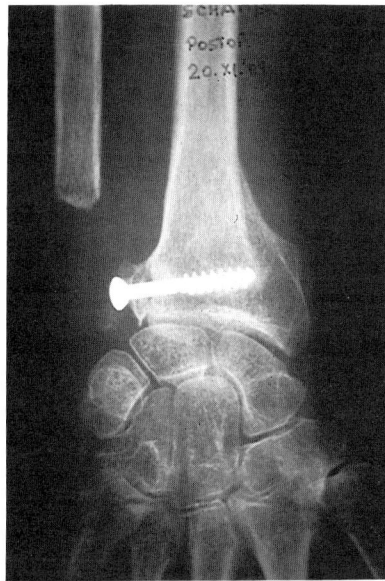

Fig. 8.10 X-ray of a postoperative case.

joint of the thumb are: (1) pain usually present at rest, exacerbated by pinch grip (it may be severe); (2) loss of strength and great functional disability of the thumb; (3) deformity produced by the subluxation of the base of the first metacarpal; (4) inflammation and oedema; (5) crepitation with axial compression; and (6) with time a hyperextension deformity of the MP joint of the thumb.

We utilise Burton's (1973) classification for the different stages of the disease. The most important features of each stage are:

Stage I: ligament laxity, pain with heavy pinch on repeated use, negative X-rays or a small osteophyte, some dorso-radial subluxation, and pain with axial compression

Stage II: very limited activity, pain and crepitation with axial compression, and definite degenerative changes in X-rays

Stage III: pan-trapezial osteoarthritis

Stage IV: associated pain and articular degeneration of the MP joint of the thumb.

In Stage I, as symptoms can be reversible for a period of time, the goal is some type of treatment

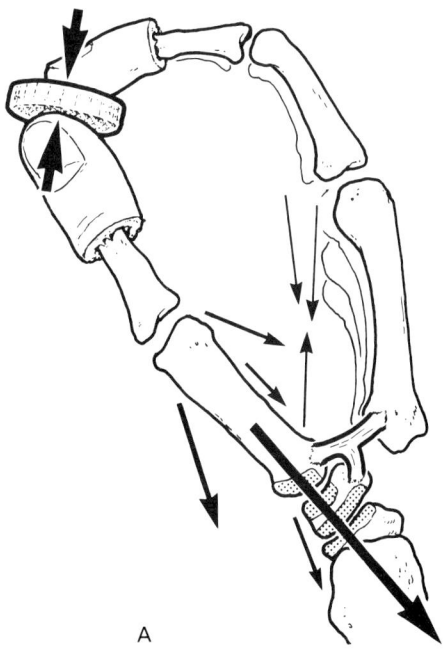
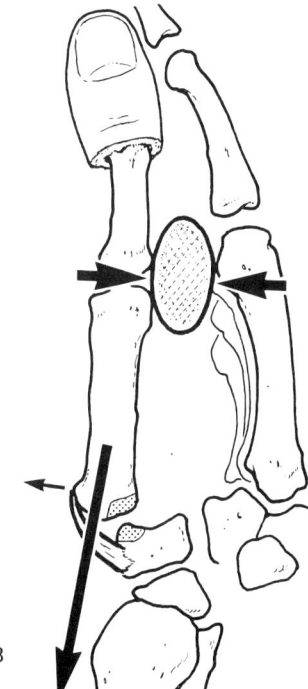

Fig. 8.11 Stages in the treatment of pain in TMC osteoarthritis.

for pain. In our opinion the best method for this purpose has been placing the thumb in a 'resting functional position'. In opposition, the TMC joint is stable and depends on the automatic screwing mechanism produced by the opposition muscles, dorsal ligaments, and ample articular contact (a strong grip is possible) (Zancolli et al 1987) (Fig. 8.11a). During retroposition, however, the articular congruence at the spherical portion of the joint is reduced, and pinching under these conditions might be harmful. The reason for this last situation is that a longitudinally directed force tends to sublux the metacarpal base, to elongate the palmar ligament, and to increase pain and TMC arthritis (Fig. 8.11b) (Zancolli et al 1987). Therefore to place the thumb in a 'resting functional position', an adhesive tape is located with the thumb in maximal palmar abduction, preventing retroposition and abduction, and in this position pulp prehension is allowed (Fig. 8.12). Usually, having the thumb in this position, symptoms disappear in a few days at the beginning of Stage I. If pain persists with this technique and other forms of conservative treatment we sometimes recommend a surgical denervation of the TMC joint.

In Stage II surgery is indicated. We utilise a technique consisting of a trapezium resection with capsular interposition arthroplasty and active stabilisation of the base of the first metacarpal. This procedure was presented in 1979 (Zancolli 1979a) and published in 1981 (Zancolli et al 1981a, b).

A 5 cm transverse incision is made over the lateral and dorsal aspects of the TMC joint (Fig. 8.13a). Only skin is incised with the scalpel. Subcutaneous tissue is liberated with scissors with rome dissection, because of the branches of the superficial radial nerve.

The EPL is retracted towards the ulna. The first dorsal compartment is opened longitudinally and the tendons retracted to the radial side. Beneath the floor of the first dorsal compartment the radial vessels are dissected and separated proximally. A T-shape capsulotomy is made in the metacarpo-trapezial-scaphoid joint (Fig. 8.13b). The trapezium is divided longitudinally in 2 parts, with an osteotome, in order to facilitate the resection and avoid damaging the flexor carpi radialis (FCR) tendon (Fig. 8.13c). Once the trapezium is resected, the tendon of the digastric muscle is cut as proximally as possible (if not present a strip of the ABPL is utilised). Two holes are made in the base of the first metacarpal: one dorsal and the other one in the centre of the articular surface (they must be interconnected). The tendon is passed

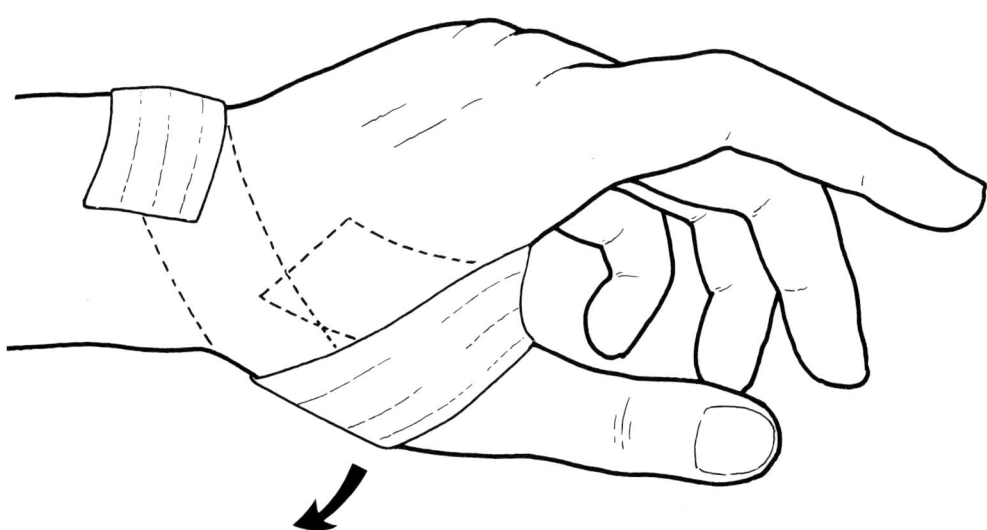

Fig. 8.12 Adhesive tape for 'resting functional position'.

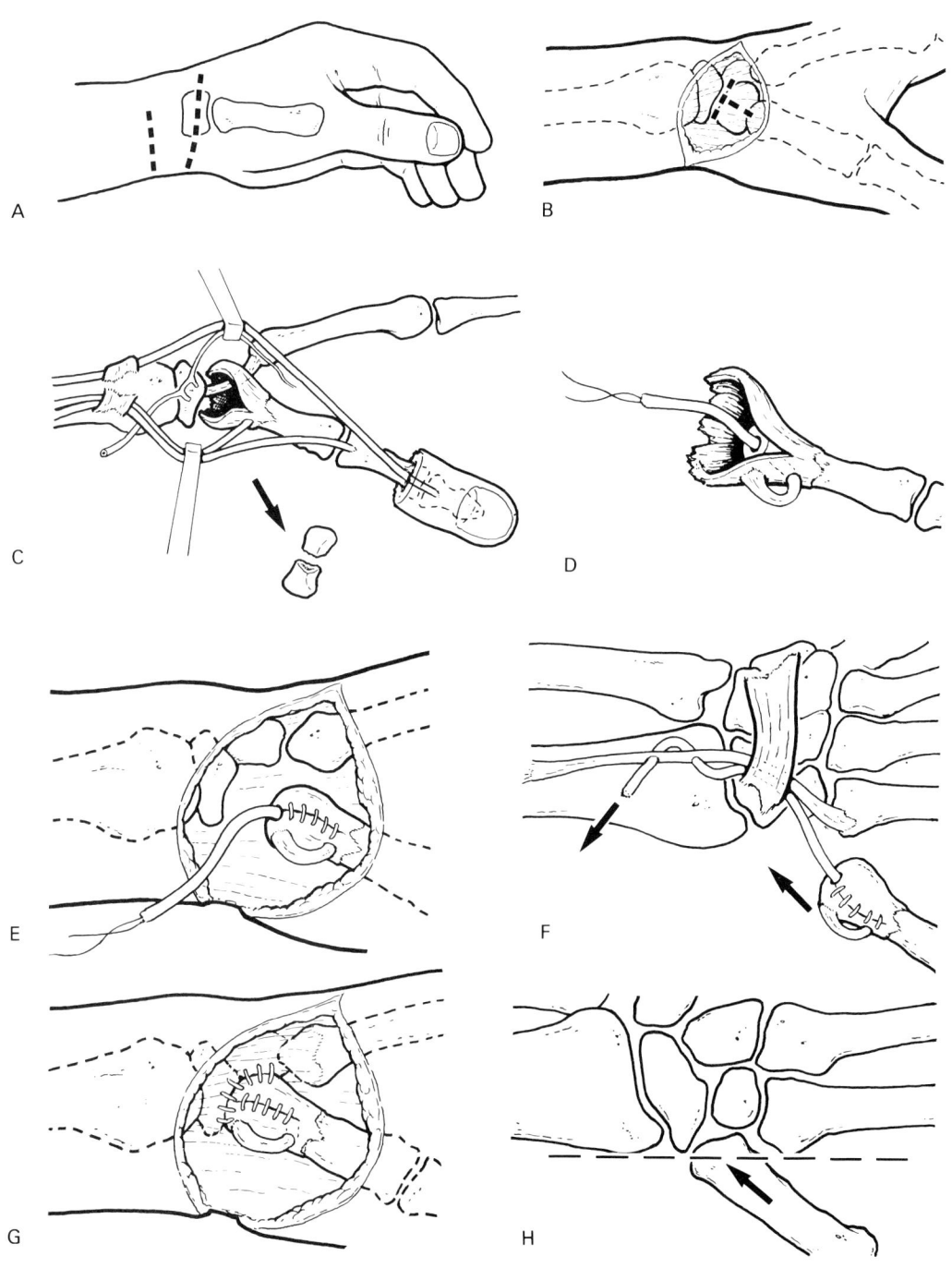

Fig. 8.13 Surgical technique.

from the dorsal hole to the central hole (Fig. 8.13d). The capsule is sutured around the tendon, making a complete covering of the metacarpal base (Fig. 8.13e). Then the tendon is passed around the tendon of the FCR tendon at the bottom of the surgical field. A complementary transverse incision of 2 cm is made 5 mm proximal to the proximal wrist crease over the FCR tendon. The tendon transfer is then passed from the distal incision to the proximal one through the FCR tunnel and sutured to this tendon at the level of the accessory incision (Fig. 8.13f). This suture is performed maintaining the metacarpal base reduced in the original location of the trapezium, with the thumb in moderate radial abduction. Afterwards, 2 or 3 sutures are applied between the metacarpal's capsule and the scaphoid capsule (in the radial side) to strengthen the maintenance of a slight radially abducted position (Fig. 8.13g). Incisions are closed and a cast, including the thumb, is applied for 30 days. If hyperextension of the MP joint is present (Stage IV) a sesamoid–metacarpal arthrodesis should be performed in the same surgical stage.

This technique has proven, with 10 years follow up, to be an effective and durable method for the relief of pain, thumb stability, recovery of strength and normal motion (Zancolli et al 1981a, b). Shortening of the thumb (3–4 mm) was not noted by patients and only an assessment finding. We believe that this technique offers all the advantages of resection–interposition arthroplasties with the aggregate of an active stabilisation of the metacarpal base (the FCR normally contracts in pinch grip).

Denervation of the wrist joint for some painful conditions

Denervation of the wrist joint is an important procedure in the specialist's armamentarium for some well selected painful conditions. It can be performed in conjunction with other techniques or as an isolated procedure. It is our intention to refer to the normal innervation of the wrist, mention some possible indications, and describe the surgical technique.

Different authors have agreed that the main innervation of the radiocarpal joint is the posterior interosseous nerve (PIN). Some describe participation of other nerves: the anterior interosseous nerve (AIN) sending branches to the volar ligaments of the carpus (Cozzi & Nemirosky 1971); and the dorsal cutaneous branch of the ulnar nerve (DCBUN) (Kaplan 1984).

The posterior interosseous nerve supplies 90% of the innervation of the carpus (Cozzi & Nemirosky 1971). After sending branches to the muscles of the dorsal compartment of the forearm it reaches the level of the proximal border of the radio-ulnar ligament dividing, there, into sensory branches for innervation of the radio-ulnar joint, radiocarpal joint and mid-carpus, and ending in small fibres (1 to 2 mm) at the base of the second and third intermetacarpal spaces. Cruveilhier (1852) described this distribution, but Froment (1846) described a more distal one ending at the proximal phalanges.

According to our clinical investigations with anaesthetic blocks in different painful situations of the wrist: (1) the posterior interosseous nerve block relieves most of the pain if not all, in pathologies affecting the distal radio-ulnar radiocarpal and midcarpal joints; (2) the triangular fibrocartilage complex (and sometimes the triquetrum and lunate) can be innervated by the dorsal cutaneous branch of the ulnar nerve; and (3) the radioscaphoid joint can sometimes be supplied by a branch of the superficial radial nerve.

Denervation of the wrist joint can be indicated as an isolated procedure or associated with another one, in some cases of: Kienbock disease, osteotomies for malunions of the distal radius, Darrach (or similar) procedures, lesions of the triangular fibrocartilage complex, carpal instabilities, painful scaphoid, non unions, chronic painful carpometacarpal lesions, reflex sympathetic dystrophy, fracture-dislocations of the carpus, fractures of the distal radius and ganglion excisions.

A denervation procedure should only be performed after determining through anaesthetic blocks (see p. 120) precisely which nerve(s) give innervation to the pathologic area involved.

We shall only describe the surgical techniques we use for denervation of the PIN, AIN and DCBUN.

Technique for the PIN and AIN

A 4 cm longitudinal incision is made on the dorsum of the distal forearm, ending at the radiocarpal joint and located over the centre of the distal radio-ulnar joint. The extensor retinaculum of the fourth dorsal compartment is incised. The tendons are retracted radially. The PIN can be found on the floor of this compartment in an ulnar position. The nerve is freed from the vessels and sectioned. The proximal and distal stumps are the coagulated with a bipolar coagulator. Dellon (Dellon & Seif 1978; Dellon 1985) prefers to divide this nerve proximal to the extensor retinaculum.

If the AIN is also to be divided, the distal part of the interosseous membrane – very thin at this level – is sectioned and the AIN is immediately visualised. The same technique as for the PIN is utilised for this branch.

Technique for the DCBUN

A 4 cm long oblique incision is made just over to the ulnar styloid in a proximal–volar to distal–dorsal direction. The nerve is dissected, thus dividing the twigs going to the joint.

We believe that when different surgical procedures are planned for the solution of painful conditions, denervation of the wrist joint should be considered, if the anaesthetic block results in pain relief.

Chronic compartment syndrome in the first dorsal interosseous muscle (FDIM)

This is a very infrequent pathology with great difficulties for diagnosis. Styf, Forssblad & Lundborg (1987) added 4 cases to the 3 already described in the literature. Patients complain of a heavy sensation, pain, and swelling located in the first intermetacarpal space over the FDIM. These symptoms, together with weakness of grip, are induced by exercise. After some hours the hand returns to normal until the clinical picture repeats, when a new vigorous activity is accomplished. Recordings of intramuscular pressure in the FDIM at rest and during exercise are recommended for confirming the diagnosis (Styf et al 1987).

Among our patients we had only one case, a polo player who complained of swelling and tenderness over the FDIM, associated with fatigue and muscle weakness after an intense game or practice. In the first visit symptoms were absent, so we examined him after an intense polo game corroborating the symptoms and point of tenderness. We operated on him with a presumptive diagnosis of a chronic compartment syndrome of the first dorsal interosseous. The intraoperative finding was a hernia of the FDIM (Fig. 8.14). When completing the fasciotomy the muscle came out, giving the impression that the compartment was not ample enough for that muscle. As in all the other cases described, fasciotomy of the FDIM alone cured the symptoms and allowed him to return to a high level of competition without any handicap.

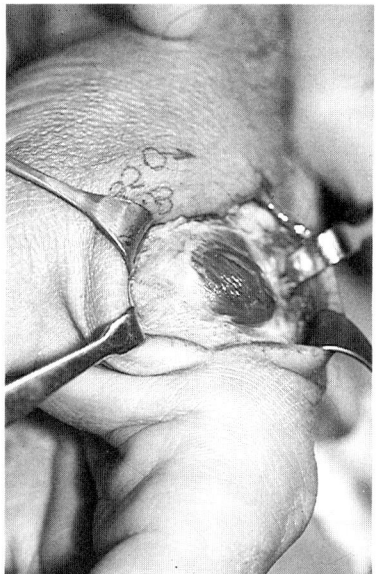

Fig. 8.14 Hernia of the FDIM in a polo player.

Reflex sympathetic dystrophy (RSD) – our method for distal anaesthetic blocks

During the last 2 years, one of us (E.R.Z. Jr) has been using a technique which we have not found described in the literature, for distal *anaesthetic blocks of peripheral nerves and arteries*. As the results with this method of treatment have been surprisingly effective, we shall describe it in this chapter.

Lankford (1988) has given an exhaustive description from personal experience, of reflex sympathetic dystrophy. This disorder is characterised by a devastating amount of pain, swelling, discoloration, and stiffness in an extremity as a result of vasomotor dysfunction of the sympathetic nervous system, which can occur following trauma, surgery or local and systemic disease (Lankford 1988). It is caused by a prolongation and overreaction to the normal response to injury (Bonica 1976).

Diagnosis is made on 4 cardinal signs (Lankford 1988):

pain. Usually burning, continuous (present at rest), exacerbated by passive or active motion
joint stiffness
swelling
discoloration. It can present as cyanosis, redness, paleness or a combination of all 3 and varies according to the stage of RSD).

Secondary signs for diagnosis are osseous demineralisation, sudomotor changes, temperature changes, trophic changes, vasomotor instability and palmar fasciitis. Diathesis, in its 2 types, is another of the components for diagnosis (Lankford 1988).

Many treatments have been described in the literature (quoted by Lankford): stellate ganglion blocks, sympathectomy, guanethidine blocks, reserpine blocks, sympatholytic drugs, alpha blockers, oral reserpine, oral guanethidine, calcium channel blockers, transcutaneous nerve stimulation, acupuncture, systemic steroids, calcitonin, periodic perineural infusion (for continuous blocking of trigger points) and somatic nerve blocks.

Peripheral (somatic) nerve blocks are based on the possibility of blocking the sympathetic efferent fibres (carried by the peripheral nerves). Axillary, median, radial and ulnar nerve blocks have been used. The general impression, according to different authors, is that they are useful for cases of minor causalgia and minor traumatic dystrophy, being quite effective in producing a temporary interruption of the sympathetic nerve reflex, but not lasting as long as a stellate ganglion block (Lankford 1988).

The goal of any treatment in RSD is to block the sympathetic efferent impulses, therefore preventing the continual feedback of pain reflex. For this purpose, we presumed that the more complete the sympathetic block could be, the better and longer the results that could be obtained.

In this decade, this concept has proven to be true for digital vascular insufficiencies. Digital sympathectomies, performing a distal interruption of the sympathetic system at the base of the fingers, have been more effective than proximal preganglionar or postganglionar denervations (Flatt 1980; Wilgis 1985). The reason for this difference in results is the special anatomical distribution of the sympathetic fibres, some of which bypass the sympathetic chains and enter the plexus or vessels. Therefore it is reasonable to assume, as demonstrated with digital sympathectomies, that a distal sympathetic block has more chance of being complete, producing a total sympathetic inhibition with a major clinical effect.

When all the hand is involved in RSD, the most distal point to apply this concept is at the level of the wrist joint. It is a well known fact that at this level sympathetic fibres are localised not only in the peripheral nerves but also in the arteries. Therefore our method blocks all nerves and main arteries at the level of the wrist in order to obtain a complete sympathetic block.

The method we employ is performed as follows:
1. The patient is taken to the operating room and given 10 mg diazepan intravenously.
2. The upper limb is draped as for an usual hand operation.
3. Then the different target structures are blocked at the wrist level with 2% lignocaine hydrochloride. The sequence we follow for sympathetic blocking at the wrist level is (Fig. 8.15):

a. radial superficial nerve and artery
b. musculocutaneous superficial branch
c. palmar cutaneous branch

THE PAINFUL HAND, PROBLEMS AND SOLUTIONS 135

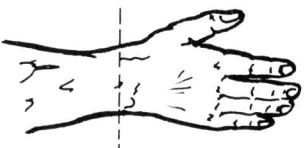

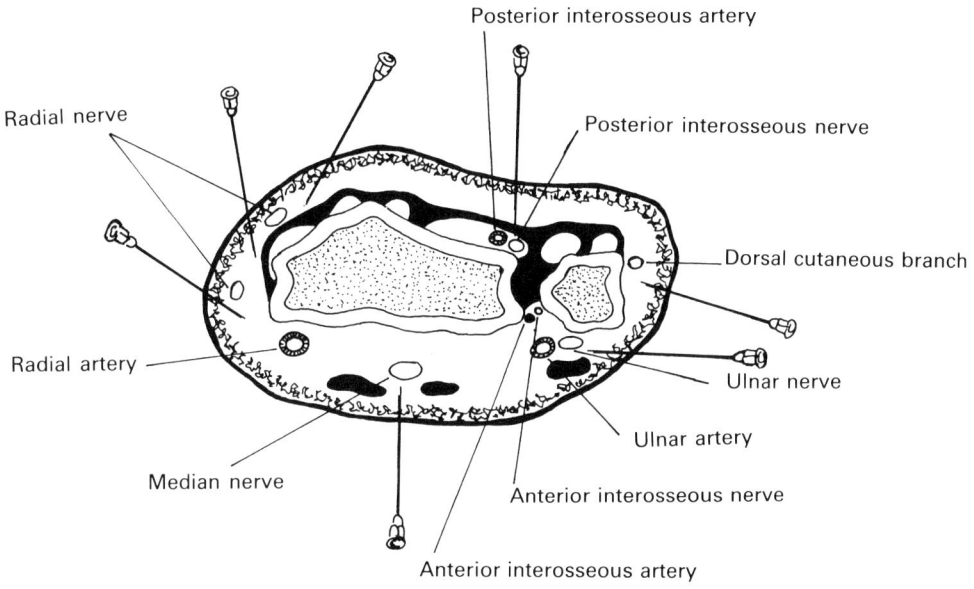

Fig. 8.15 Different target points for anaesthetic blocking.

d. median nerve
e. ulnar nerve and artery
f. dorsal cutaneous branch of the ulnar nerve
g. posterior and anterior interosseous nerves and arteries.

4. After checking with the patient that all the selected structures have been blocked, the surgeon proceeds to passive mobilisation of the stiff joints. We believe that only an experienced surgeon can do this mobilisation, being aware of the harm that can be done to a hand by forced manipulations when the joints present severe stiffness. This phase is accomplished by placing the surgeon's unopposed hand over the dorsum of the patient's affected hand with the wrists in hyperextension. The volar aspect of each of the physician's fingers should be placed over the dorsum of the corresponding digit of the patient. Then gentle and controlled active flexion induces passive flexion in the patient's fingers. This is done in each isolated digit and in all the fingers (the latter making a fist). These manoeuvres, repeated several times, permit differentiation of reducible from unreducible joint stiffness. Unreducible joint stiffness should be forced, but limiting the procedure to those articulations which respond with ease. In reducible stiffness, complete digital passive flexion can usually be obtained. Afterwards, gentle passive extension mobilisation of the MP and PIP joints are performed.

5. The improvement gained in passive motion is shown to the patient who now begins active movements trying to reach the range of motion obtained by passive mobilisation. This point is one of the advantages of the procedure because extrin-

sic flexors and extensors are not paralysed and a painless active motion can be instituted immediately.

6. If pronation and supination were also limited and painful, the same mobilisation concepts are applied. This can be done because the distal radio-ulnar joint has been also blocked.

The patient is then put in an intense rehabilitation programme and asked to maintain the improved range of motion through an intense effort. The work done during the first week after this procedure is one of the clues to a good result.

We have used this procedure in 12 cases of major traumatic dystrophy *in the first half of the second stage*. In all of these patients resting pain disappeared (except in one in whom it diminished about 50% until the second block). Forceful manoeuvres in unreducible stiffness can produce persistence of pain. The active range of motion gained during the procedure (less than the passive motion) could be maintained, and moderate pain, which didn't prevent flexion-extension exercises, was elicited in the extremes of the arc of motion. This pain diminished with time and finally disappeared 1 or 2 months after the block. In some cases we tried a second block only with the intention of improving the last degrees of motion in reducible joint stiffness, because sympathetic pain was not a problem any more. Swelling did not increase with this technique but tended to disappear slowly in a couple of months. The colour of the hand immediately improved, hyperhidrosis disappeared, and the temperature was very close to normal, as stated by the patients. These changes were maintained over time.

The interesting point about this type of block is that the evolution of the disease is immediately stopped, and if reducible joint stiffness is present, motion can be regained. Two or 3 months after the disappearance of pain we can perform surgery, if indicated, without complications. From retrospective analysis, a *posterior interosseous nerve lesion* must have been the trigger for the abnormal sympathetic reflex in the majority of cases. In the first stage of RSD anaesthetic blocks of the posterior interosseous nerve are sufficient for relieving pain and regaining progressive motion. If anaesthetic blocks are effective posterior interosseous neurotomy can be considered.

Therefore, as the main treatment of RSD should be some type of blocking of the sympathetic efferent and sensory afferent impulses that produce the sympathetic abnormal reflex, we believe that this method of distal anaesthetic block of peripheral nerves and arteries is another valid way to break the 'vicious cycle' described by Lankford.

REFERENCES

Allen E V 1929 Thromboangeitis obliterans, methods of diagnosis of chronic occlusive arterial lesions distal to the wrist with illustrative cases. American Journal of Medical Science 178: 237–244

Apley A G 1956 Test for the power of the flexor digitorum sublimis. British Medical Journal 1: 25–26

Backdahl M 1963 The caput ulnae syndrome in rheumatoid arthritis: a study of the morphology, abnormal anatomy and clinical picture. Acta Rheumatologica Scandinavica, Suppl 5: 1–75

Bateman J E 1948 Denervation of the elbow joint for relief of pain. Journal of Bone & Joint Surgery 30B: 635

Bianchi H F 1978 Abductor largo, extensor corto y enfermedad de de Quervain. La semana médica 153: 23: 790–793

Bonica J J 1976 Causalgia and other reflex sympathetic dystrophies. Postgraduate Medical Journal 53: 143–148

Bonica J J 1979 Current status of pain therapy. In: Perry S (chairman) The interagency committee on new therapies for pain and discomfort. Report to the White House. US Dept of Health, Education and Welfare, Public Health Service, Bethesda, MD, National Institute of Health, pp 111–114

Bosworth D M 1955 The role of the orbicular ligament in tennis elbow. Journal of Bone & Joint Surgery 37A: 527

Bowers W H 1985 Distal radioulnar joint arthroplasty: the hemiresection interposition technique. Journal of Hand Surgery 10A: 169–178

Burton R J 1973 Basal joint arthrosis of the thumb. Orthopedic Clinics of North America 4: 331

Carroll R E, Carlson E C 1989 Diagnosis and treatment of injury to the second and third metacarpal. Journal of Hand Surgery 14A: 102–107

Cozzi E, Nemirosky C 1971 Denervación articular de la muñeca y de la mano. Revista de ortopedia y traumatologia latino americana 16: 2

Cruveilhier J 1862 Traite d'anatomie descriptive, 3rd edn. 4 vols Paris Labé

Cyriax J H 1936 The pathology and treatment of tennis elbow. Journal of Bone & Joint Surgery 18: 921

De Goes H 1961 The radio-humeral meniscus and its relation to tennis elbow. Journal of Bone & Joint Surgery 43-1, 2: 302

Dellon A L, Seif S S 1978 Anatomic dissections relating the posterior interosseous nerve to the carpus and the etiology of dorsal wrist ganglion pain. The Journal of Hand Surgery 3, 4: 326–332

Dellon A L 1985 Partial dorsal wrist denervation: resection of the distal posterior interosseous nerve. Journal of Hand Surgery 10A: 527–533

de Quervain F 1895 Veber eine form von chronischer tendovaginitis. Correspondenz-Blatt F. Schweizer Aerzte 25: 389–394

Doupe J, Cullen C H, Chance F Q 1944 Post-traumatic pain and causalgic syndrome. Journal of Neurology, Neurosurgery & Psychiatry 7: 33–48

Egawa M, Asai T 1983 Fracture of the hook of the hamate: report of six cases and the suitability of computerized tomography. Journal of Hand Surgery 8: 393–398

Finkelstein H 1930 Stenosing tenovaginitis at the radial styloid process. Journal of Bone and Joint Surgery 12: 509–540

Flatt A E 1980 Digital artery sympathectomy. Journal of Hand Surgery 5: 550–556

Francois Y 1987 Effect of a splint to maintain opening of the first web in basal osteoarthritis of the thumb. Ann chir main 6: 245–254

Froment 1846 Traite d'anatomie humaine. (2° jol) Mc Quignon-Marvis Fis.

Gunther S F 1984 The carpometacarpal joints. Orthopedic Clinics of North America 15: 259–277

Guyon F 1861 Note sur une disposition anatomique prope a la face anterieure de la region du poignet et non encore descrite. Bulletin of the society of Anatomy (Paris) 36: 184–186

Jackson I T, Milward T M, Lee P, Webb J 1974 Ulnar head resection in rheumatoid arthritis. Hand 6: 172

Joseph R B, Linscheid R L, Dobyns J M, Bryan R S 1981 Chronic sprains of the cmc joints. Journal of Hand Surgery 6: 172–180

Kaplan E B 1984 Functional and surgical anatomy of the hand, 3rd edn. Lippincott, Philadelphia

Lacey Th, Bolstein L A, Tobin Ch 1951 Anatomical and clinical study of the variation in the insertion of the abductor pollicis longus tendon, associated with stenosing. Journal of Bone & Joint Surgery 33A: 2

Lankford L L 1980 Reflex sympathetic dystrophy. In: Omer G E Jr, Spinner M (eds) Management of peripheral nerve problems. Saunders, Philadelphia, pp 216–244

Lankford L L 1988 Reflex sympathetic dystrophy. In: Green D P (ed) Operative hand surgery, 2nd edn. Churchill Livingstone, New York, pp 633–663

Leriche R 1923 Lyon chirurgie 20: 746

Leriche R 1937 La chirurgie de la douleur. Masson, Paris

Lichtman D M, Schneider J R, Swafford A R, Mack G R 1981 Ulnar midcarpal instability. Clinical laboratory analysis. Journal of Hand Surgery 6: 515

Lister G D, Belsole R B, Kleinert H E 1979 The radial tunnel syndrome. Journal of Hand Surgery 4: 52–60

Loomis K L 1951 Variations of stenosing tenosynovitis of the radial styloid process. Journal of Bone Joint Surgery 33A: 2: 340–346

Lynn R, Eysenck H J 1961 Tolerance for pain, extroversion and neuroticism. Perceptive Motor Skills 12: 161–162

Meherin J M, Cooper E E 1951 Tennis elbow. American Journal of Surgery 70: 622

Mersky H 1979 Pain terms: a list with definitions and notes on usage. International association for the study of pain (IASP) subcommittee on taxonomy. Pain 6: 249–252

Omer G E Jr, Thomas S R 1974 The management of chronic pain syndromes in the upper extremity. Clinical Orthopaedics 104: 37–43

Omer G E Jr, Spinner M 1975 Peripheral nerve testing and suture technique, instructional course lecture. American Academy of Orthopedic Surgery 24: 122–143

Omer G E Jr 1978 Management of pain syndromes in the upper extremity. In: Hunter J M, Schneider L H, Mackin E J, Bell J A (eds) Rehabilitation of the hand. Mosby, St Louis, pp 341–349

Omer G E Jr 1979 Management of the painful extremity. In: Amstrom J P Jr (ed) Current practice in orthopaedic surgery, vol 8. Mosby, St Louis, pp 86–98

Omer G E Jr 1984 Present thoughts on the management of pain of the upper extremity. Clinics in Plastic Surgery 11: 85–93

Omer G E Jr 1987 Management techniques for the painful upper extremity. In: Terzis J K (ed) microreconstruction of nerve injuries. Saunders, Philadephia, pp 145–159

Osgood R B 1922 Radiohumeral bursitis. Archives of Surgery 4: 402

Reagan D S, Linscheid R L, Dobyns J H 1984 Lunotriquetral sprains. Journal of Hand Surgery 9: 502–513

Sauve-kapandji 1936 Nouvelle technique traitment chirurgical des luxations recidivantes isolees de l'extremite inferieure du cubitus. Journal de chirurgie 47: 589–594

Schachtel H J 1981 Pain and religion. Cancer bulletin 33: 84–85

Steindler A 1959 Lectures on the interpretation of pain in orthopaedic practice. Thomas, Springfield

Styf J, Forssblad P, Lundborg G 1987 Chronic compartment syndrome in the first dorsal interosseous muscle. Journal of Hand Surgery 12A: 757–762

Travell J, Rinzler S H 1952 The myofascial genesis of pain. Postgraduate Medicine 11 : 425–434

Trumble T, Glisson R R, Seaber A V, Urbaniak J R 1987 Forearm force transmission after surgical treatment of distal radio ulnar joint disorders. Journal of Hand Surgery 12A: 196–202

Watson H K, Ashmead D IV, Makhlouf M V 1988 Examination of the scaphoid. Journal of Hand Surgery 13A-5: 657–660

Werner F W, Glisson R R, Murphy D J, Palmer A K 1986 Force transmission through the distal radio ulnar joint: effect of ulnar lengthening and shortening. Handchir Mikrochir Plastic chir 18: 304–308

Wilgis E F S 1985 Digital sympathectomy for vascular insufficiency. In: Urbaniak Jr (ed) Hand clinics: symposium on microvascular surgery 2: 361–367

Wood L 1967-8 Variations in human myology. Proceedings of the Royal Society of London, vol XVI, pp 510–515

Zancolli E A 1979 Capsuloplastia con estabilización metacarpiana activa. International hand meeting, Australia

Zancolli E A 1979 Structural and dynamic bases of hand surgery, 2nd edn. Lippincott, Philadelphia

Zancolli E A, Aponte Arrazola F, Zancolli E R Jr 1981 Artrosis trapeciometacarpiana. Capsuloplastia con estabilizacion metacarpiana activa. Prensa médica argentina 68, 20: 919–924

Zancolli E A, Aponte Arrazola F, Zancolli E R Jr 1981 Artrosis trapeciometacarpiana. Capsuloplastia con estabilizacion metacarpiana activa. Revista de la Sociedad argentina de cirugia de la mano 1, 1: 13–22

Zancolli E A, Zaidenberg C, Zancolli E R Jr 1987 Biomechanics of the trapeziometacarpal joint. Clinical Orthopaedics: related research 220: 14–26

J. Siegfried

9 Neurostimulation techniques for intractable pain in the hand and wrist

INTRODUCTION

Classification of organic pain into 2 categories has been the decisive factor governing modern pain therapy. It is of greatest importance for a rational approach to treatment, whether medical or neurosurgical. Neurogenic and somatogenic pain are such distinct entities that a subjective description and a clinical examination allow them to be clearly differentiated.

Somatogenic pain is characterised by deep, dull pain varying in intensity at different times and localised in a territory not presenting any sensory disorders. The somatogenic, also called nociceptive pain arises from the interaction of painful stimulation with peripheral nociceptors and then activates an intact central nociceptive system. The major feature of somatogenic pain is that it is medically generally responsive to opiates and neurosurgically to the interruption of pain pathways.

Neurogenic pain, also called deafferentation pain, is characterised by pain, generally of the burning type, and is localised in a territory presenting sensory disturbances. The neurogenic pain can be defined as pain that follows damage to the nervous system. The resultant degeneration of nerve cells and fibres presumably leads to loss of input to central pathways. The site of injury can occur at virtually any level of the peripheral or central nervous system. The major feature of neurogenic pain is that it is medically generally nonresponsive to opiates and neurosurgically nonresponsive to the interruption of pain pathways. Neurogenic pain is the most distressing pain and one of the most difficult to treat. However, since the introduction of electrical stimulation techniques, it has been demonstrated that this method has its best results in the control of pain due to involvement of nervous tissue. Its application in neurogenic pain of different origin in the hand and the wrist will be analysed.

INDICATIONS

Peripheral and central factors can be at the origin of neurogenic pain in the hand and the wrist, and are good indications for neurostimulation therapeutical techniques (Table 9.1).

Table 9.1 Neurogenic pain in the hand and the wrist: aetiological factors

1. Peripheral origin
    Peripheral nerve lesion
        traumatic
        iatrogenic (surgery, injection, irradiation)
        polyneuropathy
    phantom and stump
    causalgia and reflex sympathetic dystrophy

2. Central origin
    postherpetic pain
    brachial plexus avulsion
    cord lesion
    post-stroke pain

Peripheral nerve lesions

These lesions, which may evoke chronic pain, are commonly seen after traumatic or iatrogenic injury of nervous radialis, n. medianus, n. ulnaris and their different terminal branches. The pain area is well delimited. Direct compression of nerve, like compression of the median nerve in the carpal tunnel, will be first treated surgically for decompression. A postganglion brachial plexus lesion (traumatic or postradiation) may cause a polyradicular neurogenic pain. Chronic neurogenic pain can also indicate a polyneuropathy; the pain area is more diffuse. Phantom and stump pain belong to the peripheral origin of neurogenic pain, as well as causalgia and reflex sympathetic dystrophy.

Central origin of the pain

Traumatic plexus avulsion is a central pain since the lesion is preganglionic. This is also true for postherpetic pain. Cord lesions (traumatic or inflammatory) may elicit pain, as well as cerebrovascular lesions, which may cause the so called thalamic pain syndrome; a better term is central post-stroke pain syndrome, since the lesions do not always involve the thalamus.

Neurosurgically, destructive (ablative) procedures like rhizotomies or cordotomies are not helpful. The only exception may be the dorsal root entry zone (DREZ) thermocoagulation at and above the level of the cord lesion. The precise anatomical and physiological basis for the success of this procedure is not known, but is probably due to destruction of pain generating centres within the spinal cord as well as to a readjustment of inhibitory and excitatory inputs and an interruption of ascending and descending local reflex pathways. The DREZ operation has its best results in cases of pain in plexus avulsion injury and will be described elsewhere in this volume. This operation can also be considered in the treatment of postherpetic pain. However, we always advocate a trial of neurostimulation techniques in the treatment of chronic intractable neurogenic pain in the first instance, since this method does not hurt the nervous system and can be discontinued at any time, instead of performing a destructive or ablative procedure, which is irreversible and which can be accompanied by undesirable side-effects.

The neurostimulation techniques are the best procedures to control neurogenic pain. The choice of structure to stimulate depends on the site of the lesion (Table 9.2). In case of postganglionic

Table 9.2 Choice of structure to stimulate according to location of lesion

Location of lesion	Structure to be preferentially stimulated
Postganglionic deafferentation of 1–3 peripheral nerves (e.g. traumatic, iatrogenic)	Dorsal spinal roots (epidurally)
Postganglionic deafferentation of a wider territory (e.g. ionizing radiation)	Dorsal columns of the spinal cord (epidurally) on the side of the pain
Preganglionic deafferentation (e.g. brachial plexus avulsion, postherpetic pain)	Thalamic sensory nucleus, somatotopically, on the opposite side
Pain of central origin (e.g. post-stroke pain)	Thalamic sensory nucleus, somatotopically, on the opposite side

deafferentation pain of 1–3 peripheral nerves, the structures to be preferentially stimulated are the dorsal spinal roots corresponding to the projection of the pain in the epidural space. In case of postganglionic deafferentation pain of a wider territory, the dorsal columns of the spinal cord on the side of the pain will be stimulated. In preganglionic deafferentation and pain of central origin, the target to be stimulated will be a thalamic sensory nucleus, on the opposite side.

TECHNIQUE

Dorsal spinal root and dorsal cord stimulation

Either by puncture of the intervertebral space and introducing a flexible electrode into the dorsal lateral epidural space via the puncture needle, or by making a small opening into this intervertebral space and inserting a multicontact electrode mounted on a plastic plate, the electrical stimulation of the dorsal spinal root, if the electrode is placed laterally, and of the dorsal cord, if the electrode is placed more medially, must be accompanied by tingling (paraesthesia) in the painful area. The electrode is initially connected to an external stimulation, and if a short repetitive stimulation suppresses or attenuates the pain for a brief period, the electrode is then, after 3–4 days or more, connected to a programmable pacemaker implanted into a subcutaneous pocket, generally in the abdomen. The neuropacemaker is then programmed and experience has shown that on average it requires a 30-second stimulation every 2 minutes to obtain satisfactory control of pain. If the pain is not satisfactorily improved during the trial period, the electrode is withdrawn.

Sensory thalamic stimulation

A smooth monopolar electrode with a central stylet is introduced stereotactically in the medial part of the nucleus ventropostero-lateralis for pain in the upper extremity, on the opposite side. A specially designed watertight burr-hole screw is used to fix the electrode in the bone. The method of evaluation is the same as that for dorsal cord and/or dorsal spinal root stimulation, with connection of the electrode to a temporary external cable allowing the effect to be tested. In case of control of pain, a programmable pacemaker is then implanted into an infraclavicular subcutaneous pocket.

RESULTS

Personal experience

Dorsal spinal root and dorsal cord stimulation

From May 1973 to December 1987, dorsal cord and/or dorsal spinal root stimulation in the epidural space has been applied by us in a series of 608 consecutive patients, among them 471 cases of neurogenic pain (Siegfried 1989). Many cases of this series of neurogenic pain also presented somatogenic pain, like cases of back pain (somatogenic pain) with irradiation in the peripheral nerves with objective signs of radicular deafferentation. After trial stimulation of 3–6 days, 280 patients reported significant pain reduction and subsequently underwent implantation of a permanent subcutaneous receiver or, since 1983, a programmable neuropacemaker. This was followed in all patients by quantitative reports of drug use, measurement of pain severity with a visual analogue scale, changes in work capacity or daily activity, and by the use of a pain profile, which takes into consideration a 5-grade rating

Table 9.3 Long-term results of dorsal spinal roots and/or dorsal cord stimulation for neurogenic pain in the hand and the wrist (1973–1987)

	Implanted	Long-term follow up			
		very good	good	fair	poor
Peripheral nerve lesion	49				
traumatic	30	22	5	2	1
iatrogenic	13	9	3	1	0
polyneuropathy	6	2	2	2	0
Postherpetic	1				1
Phantom/stump	6	2	2	1	1
Reflex sympathetic dystrophy	6	1	3	1	1

Table 9.4 Evaluation of success in long-term follow up of neurogenic pain in the hand and the wrist treated by dorsal spinal roots and/or dorsal cord stimulation (good and very good results) (1973–1987)

	Success in %	Comments
Peripheral nerve lesions (all cases together)	87%	Best indication
Postherpetic	0%	Series too small. Lesion in the cord at level of stimulation
Phantom/stump	66%	
Reflex sympathetic dystrophy	66%	Good for hyperpathia. Poor for deep dull pain

score (the duration of pain, the intensity of pain, the level of activity, the influence on mood and behaviour, and the use of drugs).

From this series of 280 patients with long-term follow up, 62 patients were suffering neurogenic pain in the hand and the wrist and are analysed in Tables 9.3 and 9.4. Neurogenic pain from peripheral nerve lesions do best with 43 very satisfactory cases out of 49 (87%). Only one case of postherpetic pain in C8/D1 roots has been treated by epidural dorsal spinal root stimulation; after clear improvement during the test period, the pain was reported later on to be the same as before the operation. This is probably due to the loss of myelin and axons in the dorsal spinal root and dorsal horn of the cord following the acute onset (Watson et al 1988). In cases of causalgia, the effect of neurostimulation is very good on the hyperpathia and poor on the deep dull pain. Until 1978 we tried to control brachial plexus avulsion pain with dorsal spinal cord stimulation; 11 patients were treated and 4 received a definite device. No cases responded at all to the dorsal cord stimulation, as we have already recorded (Hood & Siegfried 1984); this is due to the cord lesion created by the avulsion.

Sensory thalamic stimulation

From March 1977 to December 1987, sensory thalamic stimulation has been applied by us in a series of 128 consecutive patients suffering from chronic intractable neurogenic pain. After trial stimulation of 2–7 days, 108 patients reported significant pain reduction and subsequently underwent implantation of a permanent subcutaneous receiver or since 1983 a programmable neuropacemaker (Siegfried 1989). From this series of 108 patients with long-term follow up, 33 patients were suffering from neurogenic pain in the upper extremities and are analysed in Tables 9.5 and 9.6. In thalamic pain syndrome, the success appears to depend on the location of the lesion (thalamic or parathalamic) on computerised tomography (Demierre & Siegfried 1985). A study of the stimulation parameters long-term, with almost no changes, demonstrates the safety of the method with probably the absence of pathophysiological modifications of the brain tissue over the years (Siegfried 1987).

DISCUSSION

Our 16 years' experience in the treatment of neurogenic pain with implantation of a neurostimulation system shows that pain due to lesion of peripheral nerve is the best indication, with over 80% of very satisfactory pain control on long follow up (Siegfried 1988; Siegfried 1989). This observation has also been made recently by Gybels & Sweet (1989) in a major review of literature. In our series, the failures can be eventually explained in many cases by the possible functionally disturbed area of stimulation in the cord. The majority of these failures were cases with a long history of pain before the implantation of electrodes. This is convincing evidence that peripheral nerve injury does induce alterations in the central nervous system (Wall 1983). Injury to the peripheral branch of a primary afferent neurone results in transganglionic changes in the central branch, including the axonal terminals within the dorsal horn.

Other neurogenic pain in the hand and the wrist may be improved by stimulation of the dorsal spinal root and/or the dorsal cord when the lesion is postganglionic and of the sensory thalamic nucleus when the lesion is preganglionic; however, the results are not so impressive as observed in cases of pain due to lesions of peripheral nerve. *Reflex sympathetic dystrophy* is an extremely difficult and costly syndrome to treat. Evaluation is difficult because of its many different manifestations as well as the difficulty of analysing patients' findings

Table 9.5 Long-term results of sensory thalamic stimulation for neurogenic pain in thalamus and wrist (1973–1987)

	Implanted	Long-term follow up			
		very good	good	fair	poor
Central post-stroke syndrome	15	3	5	4	3
Brachial plexus avulsion	15	4	4	3	4
Cord lesion	3	2	1	0	0

Table 9.6 Evaluation of success in long-term follow up of neurogenic pain in the hand and the wrist treated by sensory thalamic stimulation (good and very good results) (1977–1987)

	Success in %	Comments
Central post-stroke syndrome	53%	Only when sensory nuclei are not involved by infarction
Brachial plexus avulsion	53%	Poor results when long story (thalamic retrograde degeneration?)
Cord lesion	100%	Series too small

accurately (Davidoff et al 1988). Some very satisfactory results can be obtained by dorsal spinal cord stimulation. Broseta et al (1982) report more than 50% of excellent results and 20% of good results in his series of 11 cases. Barolat et al (1987) in a series of 16 cases mention 4 excellent and 3 moderate results and Robaina et al (1989) 16% of excellent and 66% of good results. For this author, in the long run these results are better than those obtained with sympathetic blocks and sympathectomy; I would also emphasise the diminution of oedema. No objective changes of bone decalcification and ankylosis of small joints were observed, but most patients were able later to undergo physiotherapy and rehabilitation because of the amount of pain relief. One of the most interesting observation is the activation of blood circulation. Tallis et al (1983) proposed 4 possible levels of action for the stimulation to explain the changes in peripheral blood flow in reflex sympathetic dystrophy. The first would imply the disappearance of pain by activation of the segmental or suprasegmental inhibitors of nociceptive transmission. The second mechanism would be based on an increase of parasympathetic vasodilatory activity or on a decrease of sympathetic vasoconstrictory activity. The third and fourth mechanisms proposed by that author overlap. They are based on the liberation of substances with a vascular and vasodilatory effect at a local or segmental level: substance P, the intestinal vasoactive neuropeptide, prostaglandins and/or prostacyclins.

Pain due to brachial plexus lesions

These pains may be helped by neurostimulation techniques and Wynn Parry (1983) reported a substantial improvement with transcutaneous nerve stimulation in 50% of the cases of his large series of 122 patients. However, we had poor results of dorsal spinal cord stimulation in this condition in a series of 16 patients, due certainly to the lack of large myelinated afferent fibres from the affected painful region (Hood & Siegfried 1984). The relatively limited success obtained on thalamic stimulation in cases of pain resulting from avulsion of the brachial plexus has been evaluated by Mazars & Choppy in their series (1983); they stated also that patients with more than 2 root avulsions and large areas of anaesthesia have a very low response to thalamic stimulation. They postulated that those patients with multiple avulsions had significant dorsal horn damage with resultant thalamic lesions by ascending degeneration, and thus were less responsive to thalamic stimulation. In C5-Dl dorsal rhizotomized rats, Albe-Fessard & Lombard (1983) demonstrated trains of rhythmic, 10 Hz slow waves accompanied by bursts of spikes in the deafferented animals in the ventroposterior thalamic zone, devoted in the normal animal to the forelimb representation. The abnormal thalamic activity was seen starting 6 months after rhizotomy, followed by the appearance of abnormal activity in the cortex. For these reasons, our policy today is to reserve the use of thalamic stimulation for brachial plexus avulsion patients with severe pain that have failed to respond to all conservative therapies not later than 12 to 18 months after plexus injury. When pain has been present for longer or when the thalamic stimulation does not control the pain satisfactorily, we propose the dorsal root entry zone (DREZ) microthermocoagulations. The success of thalamic stimulation is dependent upon the extent of the central lesion from the periphery up to the thalamic regions (Siegfried 1987).

Phantom pain may benefit from spinal cord stimulation in more than 60% of cases. This method should have a high priority, since it is least destructive (Siegfried & Cetinalp 1981).

There are two theoretical reasons why the use of spinal dorsal cord stimulation may be proposed for the treatment of intractable neurogenic pain. First the gate control theory of pain perception, proposed by Melzack & Wall (1965), argues that a rise in pain threshold should occur after stimulation of large low-threshold fibres, whose central action is accompanied by an inhibition of cells that transmit injury signals. Second, advances in electronics permit the design of small implantable programmable neuropacemakers. Since activation of A-fibres, which are concentrated in the posterior columns of the medulla, inhibits spinal input from nociceptive fibres, the epidural placement of electrodes along the dorsal part of the cord seems reasonable. It must be stressed, however, that the neural mechanism responsible for pain relief by dorsal cord stimulation is still controversial: activation of the posterior columns can influence the higher centres of the brain by orthodromic conduction and can influence neural activity on a medullary level by antidromic invasion. Sensory thalamic stimulation has many characteristics in common with dorsal cord stimulation, suggesting essentially the same physiological background. Thus, paraesthesia in the painful area occurring concomitantly with the stimulation is a prerequisite for pain relief. Like dorsal cord stimulation, the effect cannot be reversed by naloxone, and the concentration of B-endorphin in cerebrospinal fluid is not influenced. It is generally assumed that the analgesic effect resulting from the activation of the specific supraspinal sensory system is an inhibitory influence on nociceptive functions.

It should be stressed that these stimulation techniques should only be considered after a full regime of drugs and rehabilitation has been applied. However, the use of such techniques in relieving pain from peripheral nerve lesions has been so successful that the author recommends implementing them fairly soon after injury has taken place, in view of the danger of dorsal horn and dorsal root ganglion alterations occurring.

SUMMARY

Pathogenesis of pain in the hand and the wrist after traumatic or iatrogenic lesions to peripheral nerves and after central lesions in the spinal roots, in the cord or in the brain is briefly reviewed. If the pain, which is of neurogenic and not somatogenic nature, persists, or in the case of relapse with establishment of a chronic pain-state, a very attractive method of treatment is the implanting of a programmable neurostimulator. The electrodes are placed near the dorsal sensory roots in the cervical epidural space for pain of postganglionic origin or in the sensory thalamic nucleus in case of pain of preganglionic origin. The technique is described, and the long-term results with success rates of 50% to 80%, according to the type of neurogenic pain, are presented. A tentative reason for the failures is suggested as well as the mechanism of electrical stimulation of the nervous system as a means of alleviating pain.

REFERENCES

Albe-Fessard D, Lombard M C 1983 Use of animal model to evaluate the origin of and protection against deafferentation pain. In: Advances in pain research and therapy, vol 5. Raven, New York, p 691

Barolat G, Schwartzmann R, Woo R 1987 Epidural spinal cord stimulation in the management of reflex sympathetic dystrophy. Applied Neurophysiology 50: 442

Broseta J, Roldan P, Gonzales-Darder J et al 1982 Chronic epidural dorsal column stimulation in the treatment of causalgic pain. Applied Neurophysiology 45: 190

Davidoff G, Morey K, Amann M, Stampe J 1988 Pain measurement in reflex sympathetic dystrophy syndrome. Pain 32: 27

Demierre B, Siegfried J 1985 Le syndrome douloureux thalamique. Corrélations anatomo-cliniques et traitement par la stimulation intermittente des noyaux sensitifs du thalamus. Neurochirurgie 31: 281

Gybels J M, Sweet W H 1989 Neurosurgical treatment of persistent pain. Karger, Basel

Hood T W, Siegfried J 1984 Epidural versus thalamic stimulation for the management of brachial plexus lesion pain. Acta Neurochirurgica, Suppl 33: 451

Mazars G J, Choppy J M 1983 Reevaluation of the deafferentation pain syndrome. In: Advances in pain research and therapy, vol 5. Raven, New York, p 769

Melzack R, Wall P D 1965 Pain mechanisms: a new theory. Science 150: 971

Robaina F J, Rodriguez J L, de Vera J A, Martin M A 1989 Transcutaneous electrical nerve stimulation and spinal cord stimulation for pain relief in reflex sympathetic dystrophy. Stereotactical Functional Neurosurgery 52: 53

Siegfried J, Cetinalp E 1981 Neurosurgical treatments of phantom limb pain: a survey of methods. In: Siegfried J, Zimmermann M (eds) Phantom and stump pain. Springer Verlag, Berlin, p 148

Siegfried J 1987 Sensory thalamic neurostimulation for chronic pain. Pace 10: 209

Siegfried J 1988 Neurostimulation zur Behandlung von chronischen Schmerzen durch Schädigung peripherer Nerven. In: Lücking C H, Thoden U, Zimmermann M (eds) Nervenschmerz. Gustav Fischer Verlag, Stuttgart, p 292

Siegfried J 1989 Neurosurgical treatment of neurogenic pain. In: Advances in pain research. Raven, New York (in press)

Tallis R C, Illis L S, Sedgwick E M, Hardwidge C, Garfield J S 1983 Spinal cord stimulation in peripheral vascular disease. Journal of Neurology Neurosurgery Psychiatry 46: 478

Wall P D 1983 Alterations in the central nervous system after deafferentation: connectivity control. In: Advances in pain research and therapy, vol 5. Raven, New York, p 677

Watson C P N, Morshead C, Van der Kooy D et al 1988 Postherpetic neuralgia: post-mortem analysis of a case. Pain 34: 129

Wynn Parry C B 1983 Management of pain in avulsion lesions of the brachial plexus. In: Advances in pain research and therapy, vol 5. Raven, New York, p 751

B. S. Nashold Jr and C. Shieff

10 Phantom and avulsion pain

The illusion that a body part still exists following its physical loss is well recognised. The phenomenon has been recorded frequently in medical, military and popular literature (Whitaker 1979). Ambroise Paré observed as long ago as 1551 that amputees might complain of pain in the missing part long after its amputation (Jensen & Rasmussen 1984) and Nelson himself wrote after the loss of his arm that he could still sense its presence (Wall 1981). Others, including Herman Melville and Hans Christian Andersen, describe the phenomenon in works of fiction while it was Weir-Mitchell's professional observations in the American Civil War (Mitchell 1872) which led him to coin the term 'phantom limb'. So detailed were his descriptions of the symptoms experienced after traumatic amputation and peripheral nerve injury, even in his lay publications (Mitchell 1905), that the American public sent charitable donations to the non-existent hero of his essay 'The case of George Dedlow' when it was first published anonymously in *Atlantic Monthly* in 1866.

WHAT IS A PHANTOM LIMB?

Despite such extensive documentation, phantom limb cannot be defined in simple terms. It may, perhaps, best be described in the words of Walton (1985) as 'an illusion of the persistence of a part of the body lost by amputation or an illusory awareness of a part from which sensation has been lost through interruption of afferent pathways'. The symptoms (if, indeed, phantom limb is a symptom as this word implies underlying pathology) differ from patient to patient and an individual's experiences of his phantom may vary, appearing as anything from a precise and discrete replica of its antecedent to fleeting and frequently almost imperceptible paraesthesiae (Frederiks 1963). Detailed questioning is often necessary to elicit these protean manifestations of phantom limbs as their owners do not usually volunteer specific details. Once this has been recognised it becomes possible to distinguish between the simple existence of a phantom limb alone and the variety of sensations that may arise within it. These may be of apparent movement, abnormal posture or of seemingly externally generated sensations. Although all of these phenomena are natural sequelae of amputation, it is unusual for any of them to prompt a request for help, probably because, as intrusions on consciousness, they are not particularly unpleasant. Most individuals seeking medical attention with phantom related complaints do so with pain.

INCIDENCE

The number of individuals undergoing amputation is unknown and hence there can be no truly accurate estimate of those experiencing phantom limb pain or sensation in upper or lower limbs. Recent figures from the United Kingdom Disablement Services Centres (formerly Artificial Limb and Appliance Centres) indicate that approximately 1 in 10 000 of the population of England, Wales and Northern Ireland are referred for limb prostheses annually. While the total has fallen slightly (5892 patients in 1981, 5606 in 1985), there has been an even greater reduction proportionately in the number of upper limb amputees seen in the same period (203 in 1981, 145 in 1985) (Ham et al 1989).

Arteriosclerosis and diabetes are the commonest conditions leading to amputation (together accounting for 80% of cases), whilst a greater proportion of amputations in the young follow injury. Neither group is truly representative but as large numbers of amputations occur as a result of warfare and these previously healthy young men become available for study, scientific articles relating to the problems of phantom limb pain inevitably follow military conflict. The socio-economic sequelae of amputation are more significant in this latter group, especially for upper limb amputees, and it may be that this results in bias both in sampling and any in subsequent reporting.

SYMPTOMS

From those that are questioned soon after their amputation it is apparent that most amputees experience some kind of phantom immediately although most do not volunteer such information. Jensen & Rasmussen (1984) reviewed the results from 13 series published between 1872 and 1980 with a combined total of 4112 amputees. 84% reported that they had experienced a phantom sensation at some time after their amputation and 100% experienced it in one series (Carlen et al 1978). This is in contrast to those whose limbs have been lost in utero or early childhood when only individual cases are reported with phantom limbs (Simmel 1962) and when such phantoms do occur it appears that phantom limb pain does not follow. It is popular belief that sudden loss of a limb is necessary for a phantom to develop but Price (1976) has produced evidence that progressive loss (in leprosy) may also result in phantom limb sensations. With the passage of time phantoms usually shorten, become less obtrusive and can disappear completely (Riddoch 1941). A phantom limb may never be complete or, if intact initially, it may foreshorten. The parts most commonly retained are those located distally, especially the digits (in particular the thumb and index finger or the great toe and the heel), while the proximal parts of the upper arm or the thigh may never intrude into consciousness. The relative sizes of those parts remaining are disproportionate, again with a bias to the periphery. The greater the area of cortical representation, the larger the phantom appears and the more likely it is to persist. The process of shortening may progress until the phantom digits approach and seemingly merge with the amputation stump itself – a characteristic called 'telescoping'. The position that the phantom adopts has been said occasionally to mimic that which the limb occupied immediately before its amputation or injury (Berger & Gerstenbrand 1981) but despite individual reports of bizarre posture there appears little in reality to support this hypothesis and even less to explain it neurophysiologically.

The time scale over which these events may take place is fairly predictable. Phantoms usually undergo their most dramatic involutional changes in the first weeks or months after amputation and tend to be unchanging by the time a year has elapsed. Infrequently they remain virtually unchanged for many years. Various factors (see Table 10.1), especially physical or emotional distress may prompt the return or regrowth of the phantom. Some individuals ultimately become aware that such episodes, for them, are henceforth to be associated also with phantom limb pain.

Table 10.1 Potential aggravating factors

Emotion
Stump contact
Weather
Autonomic changes
Distant cutaneous stimulation
Other pain
Prosthesis

PAIN IN THE PHANTOM LIMB

The presence of a phantom limb does not invariably lead to pain. Few amputees have phantom pain either at the time of amputation or later (Bromage & Melzack 1974). The majority of patients developing pain are aware of it within the first week. Many authors (Riddoch 1941; Ewalt et al 1947; Parkes 1973) suggest that it is most common in those who have had pain in the limb for some time before amputation. These are most likely to be elderly patients with pre-existing disease while younger post-traumatic amputees less commonly have phantom limb pain. The characteristics of the pain vary – it does not usually resemble the preceding symptoms (Cronholm 1951) although it is often described in the same terms as an unhealed wound. Jensen and Rasmussen (1984) quote the results of 18 separate reviews of phantom pain, including one series of almost 29 000 amputees (Sherman et al 1980), all of which show that neither pain nor other phantom sensations are an inevitable consequence of amputation. The numbers of patients reported in these series to experience painful phantoms vary widely (2%–90%) but when its severity was graded, severe pain occurred in 10% (0–19.6%). The natural sequence of events is, as for painless phantoms, of gradual resolution; infrequently recurrence of pain may be associated with a temporary return of the phantom.

It must be remembered that these patients may have other causes of pain. Although similar in nature and arising from the same traumatic episode, phantom limb pain differs in its pathophysiology from that which follows nerve root avulsion or exists in the stump itself. This is not always differentiated by physicians (Danke 1981) and sometimes results in misdiagnosis and inappropriate treatment. Stump pain is a purely local phenomenon, arising from neuromata and other peripheral causes. Like most disease, it is better (and more easily) prevented than cured. Poorly planned flaps may not heal satisfactorily. If the deep facia has not been repaired, muscle retraction may result in adhesions between skin and deeper structures (bone and nerve), increasing the likelihood of stump pain. Troublesome amputation stump neuromata are probably more common if attempts have been made to locate the major nerve trunks to shorten them. While the symptoms may be similar, simple questioning and examination should suffice to distinguish the 2 problems, therapy then being directed appropriately. Stump related problems may induce phantom re-expansion or frank phantom pain which usually resolves when the local trigger has been removed. Individuals who are unfortunate enough to sustain brachial plexus injury together with nerve root avulsion will have similar, but seldom identical, symptoms to those of a 'pure' phantom limb. In these cases pain arises from trauma in that region of the spinal cord known as the dorsal root entry zone.

Despite the insistence of some authorities on a strict distinction between the pain of phantom limb, nerve root avulsion, partial lesions of peripheral nerves and stump pathology, any combination of these may exist. Whilst the expected result is to alleviate the painful symptoms, this potentially complex relationship can frustrate even the best planned therapy. In those unfortunate individuals who are physically or psychologically predisposed there may even be other painful conditions. It must constantly be borne in mind that diseases such as intervertebral disc degeneration or arterial occlusive disease can also produce pain 'in' amputated limbs, erroneous labelling resulting in inappropriate surgery and denying the patient speedy relief of his symptoms.

PATHOPHYSIOLOGY

Phantom limb should not be regarded as an inexplicable and purely subjective phenomenon, characterised by an illogical persistence of that part. Together with the various painful experiences and non-painful sensations emanating from the phantom it derives from the residual anamnestic effects of a permanently imprinted image within the central nervous system.

Sherrington, the father of neurophysiology, described the neural system as a superstructure resting upon the two spinal roots, wherein 'the afferent root cell is the alpha of every functional unit in the system . . . (Sherrington 1900); without its sensory input the nervous system cannot prompt any reaction to the environment. Organisation of the nervous system has evolved with specific central and peripheral connections. Neurones persist irrespective of external influences unless they are physically damaged but the interneural connections are fluid and subject to continuous modification both by higher (cerebral) and peripheral (sensory) input. A permanently imprinted body image develops passively when young. This persists within the sensorium even when its peripheral input disappears. Cessation of peripheral neural impulses does not result in total electrical silence within the central nervous system but releases spontaneous and previously damped signals arising from complex networks within the grey matter of the spinal cord and deep cerebral nuclei. The cells that initiate these messages retain their cell signature. Following peripheral injury, dendritic connections within Lissauer's tract and the dorsal horn of the spinal cord can be re-established following new patterns of peripheral innervation or stimulation. The signals arising in this fashion follow conventional pathways to be received, modified and interpreted in the higher centres. As they mimic the messages from an intact body, they are interpreted as such – pain under these circumstances is an individual's interpretation of these signals superimposed on a cellular neurochemical memory. The absence of a specific pain memory is demonstrated simply by the relief of long-suffered pain by a successful hip arthroplasty. Failure of direct stimulation of exposed cortex to provoke pain despite inducing other sensations confirms that the cerebral cortex is not responsible for phantom pain while the fact that the referred pain of myocardial ischaemia radiates into a phantom arm excludes the peripheral nerves as a cause. Adequate regional anaesthesia has been observed to abolish both the phantom and its pain during its action (Carlen et al 1978) while, conversely, phantom limb sensations, infrequently with pain, have been reported during regional or spinal anaesthesia (Melzack 1974) establishing the spinal cord as the source of the phantom.

That pain itself can be regarded as an indicator of tissue damage is well established, the currently accepted definition of pain itself being 'an unpleasant sensory and emotional experience associated with actual or potential tissue damage, or described in terms of such damage' (Merksey 1979). Phantom limb pain might, simplistically, be interpreted as the memory of such damage. The modern concept of pain acknowledges 2 distinct kinds with separate aetiologies:

1. nociceptive pain due to conventionally recognised peripheral painful stimuli, typified by the pain of fracture, tumour infiltration or inflammation
2. central or neurogenic pain arising from changes within the central nervous system, including the deafferentation pain following cerebrovascular accidents.

As individuals we readily recognise the former pain from our earliest experiences but often find it difficult to appreciate that similar symptoms may exist in the apparent absence of physical disease.

TREATMENT

That no universally effective treatment has been found for phantom limb pain is well demonstrated by the number and variety of therapeutic options (see Tables 10.2–10.4) currently used (Sherman et al 1980). The preliminary stages in any therapy involve formal and full assessment of the patient psychologically, medically and socially. Previous therapies must be recorded as patient cooperation and compliance is based on trust – the recommendation of a previously failed treatment can be disastrous! Any additional or related problems must be defined accurately and corrected. Although staunch advocates of specific therapies will often proceed directly to their own forté, most clinicians involved routinely in the control of pain adopt a cautious and logical progression through the various options available. Starting with the simpler physical measures and non-aggressive psychological manipulations, proceeding next to medications, surgical manoeuvres should be reserved for those patients that do not benefit from simpler techniques.

'Non-medical' treatment

The physical and psychological treatment options shown in Table 10.2 are merely representative of those in regular use. Some have proven efficacy and a physiologically sound basis while others are of dubious benefit. Those therapies that improve the stump, making prosthesis wearing more com-

Table 10.2 Physical and psychological treatment for phantom limb pain

Physical	Psychological
Acupuncture	Explanation
Biofeedback	Relaxation therapy
Heat	Hypnotherapy
Ultrasound	Psychotherapy
Physiotherapy	Phantom exercises
Stump manipulation	
Prosthesis fitting and utilisation	

fortable, are likely also to lessen any secondary recurrence of pain precipitated by local problems. Similarly, improvement in the patient's mood or mobility, by whatever means, will lessen the problems experienced and hence the complaints of pain.

Despite irrefutable evidence for its organic basis, there are still physicians who insist that sufferers of phantom limbs are psychologically disturbed. There can be no doubt that there are psychological sequelae of amputation and the existence of a phantom, or worse of phantom limb pain, can only serve to exacerbate pre-existing psychiatric problems but attempts to treat the pain as a purely mental problem are doomed to failure.

Medical treatment

The accompanying list (Table 10.3) of pharmacological agents used in the treatment of phantom pain is not exhaustive.

The use of analgesics is self evident but irrespective of their potency they are of little use in most cases despite inducing narcosis or dependence. Anticonvulsants (particularly carbamazepine) have a specific action in preventing either the generation or the transmission of abnormal neural signals and hence can be useful in the management of neurogenic pain (Elliott et al 1976) but they should be used with some caution, especially in the elderly and those on multiple medications, as they can easily reach toxic levels. Antidepressants also have a specific pharmacological action but are only of infrequent help, possibly providing more benefit in the treatment of the secondary depression that accompanies the pain. Other centrally acting agents, particularly phenothiazines and benzodiazepines, appear most beneficial when used as sedatives. Local anaesthetics have been mentioned previously; when administered intrathecally they permeate the region of the dorsal horn of the spinal cord and can prevent the genesis of abnormal electrical activity. Their action is short lived and may be associated with more extensive and intolerable side effects. Steroids ('membrane stabilisers') do not appear to have any great benefit either administered systemically or locally. Various other medications (like vitamins) have been advocated by some therapists but are used simply for a placebo-like action.

Surgical treatment

When conservative therapy or peripheral intervention fails to produce relief, the neurosurgeon is consulted (Siegfried & Cetinalp 1981). The list of surgical procedures (Table 10.4) used for phantom

Table 10.3 Pharmacological treatment for phantom limb pain

Non-narcotic analgesics
Narcotic analgesics
Anticonvulsants
Antidepressants
Local anaesthetics
Steroids
Phenothiazines
Benzodiazepines

Table 10.4 Surgical treatment for phantom limb pain

Ablative	Stimulation
Peripheral nerve section	Transcutaneous
Dorsal root section	Peripheral nerve
Sympathectomy	Dorsal column
Dorsal root entry root zone lesion	Deep brain
Spinothalamic cordotomy	
Mesencephalotomy	
Thalamotomy	
Cingulotomy	
Gyrectomy	

limb pain is, effectively, a summary of neurosurgical pain relieving procedures.

It must be stressed that, apart from stimulation techniques, all surgical procedures are destructive and should be withheld until alternative therapies have been proven ineffective. It has already been observed that most phantom limb phenomena, including pain, become less obtrusive with the passage of time. When surgical measures are necessary they should be chosen in the light of the individual patient's requirements and with due consideration of any possible secondary effects of an ablative procedure. Whilst pain arising from peripheral causes can be relieved by peripheral procedures, central procedures are necessary for the relief of neurogenic pain.

Peripheral surgery

Peripheral nerve and dorsal root section or ganglionectomy prevent messages passing into the spinal cord. These, and even anterior root section if one supports the belief that occasional aberrant sensory fibres traverse the motor root, will alleviate pain arising from the stump and reduce secondary exacerbations of phantom limb sensation and pain resulting from this, but they have no effect on simple phantom limb pain itself. The various procedures recommended for stump neuromata should, therefore, be considered for those patients with stump problems but should not be regarded as a panacea.

Sympathectomy

Some of the associated autonomic changes accompanying phantom limb pain, like all centrally arising pain, can be likened to the effects of excessive or aberrant sympathetic activity. Occasional temporary relief of the symptoms has been observed to follow sympathetic blockade (Livingston 1976) and because of this chemical, radiofrequency and surgical sympathectomy have all been used but provide little long-term relief (Kallio 1950).

Cordotomy

The mainstay of neurosurgical intervention for pain relief for many years, anterolateral spinothalamic cordotomy, has been used frequently with generally favourable but occasionally varying reports of its success (Falconer 1953; White & Sweet 1969). In this procedure (either performed via a laminectomy or percutaneously) the anterolateral portion of the spinothalamic tract is divided, interrupting second and third order neurones within the pain carrying pathways as they pass rostrally up the spinal cord. The procedure results in reasonable levels of pain relief – 20 out of 52 patients (38%) obtained better than 50% pain relief and 23 patients (44%) lesser degrees of relief in the combined series reported by Siegfried & Cetinalp (1981). It can, however, produce unacceptable and distressing dysaesthesiae within the area of anaesthesia that results (anaesthesia dolorosa), negating its benefits. In addition long term results suggest that the procedure fails after a year or two – a feature seen also when it is used for chronic pain resulting from other non-malignant conditions.

Stereotactic ablation

With the advent of stereotaxy, electrodes can be placed accurately deep within the brain stem or the cerebral hemispheres and small lesions created within specific pathways or nuclear structures to control chronic pain. The chosen targets fall naturally into two groups: the mesencephalon and the thalamic nuclei. Although initial reports of stereotactic mesencephalotomy (Nashold et al 1969) included cases of phantom limb pain whose pains were relieved, the procedure is not widely performed and is generally reserved for patients with nociceptive or thalamic pain. Many targets within the thalamus or adjacent structures are advocated by functional neurosurgeons but these produce only about 50% success and a high subsequent failure rate (Siegfried & Cetinalp 1981). All ablative procedures are destructive and, despite precision and patient cooperation during thalamotomy, anaesthesia dolorosa is again an unwanted but not infrequent result.

Stereotaxy also allows the alternative procedures of psychosurgery, including dorso-medial thalamotomy and cingulotomy, which can be beneficial in relieving the emotional disturbances associated with chronic pain syndromes but at the expense of altering affect and with the moral implications thereof.

Cortical excision

Following clinical observation that cerebral lesions may be followed by the disappearance of phantom limb pain (Head & Holmes 1911) cortical excision or gyrectomy was attempted with occasional success (Erickson et al 1952) but this procedure has fallen into disrepute.

Dorsal root entry zone lesions

Considering the evidence to support the hypothesis that the phantom limb 'exists' within the grey matter overlying the dorsal horn of the spinal cord and that surgery in this area relieves the pain of plexus avulsion (Nashold & Ostdahl 1979), it is logical that thermocoagulation of the substantia gelatinosa (in which multiple small radiofrequency lesions in the dorsal root entry zone are created) should be utilised for the relief of phantom limb pain. A recent survey of the results from this, the 'DREZ' procedure, confirms its efficacy (Saris et al 1985), reporting good pain relief in 67% of the patients treated with phantom limb pain alone and in 83% of those who also had nerve root avulsion; although surgical amputation can be regarded as 'clean', traumatic amputation is not infrequently associated also with some degree of nerve root avulsion. Those with stump pain alone obtained no benefit and only 29% of those with phantom together with stump pain had any pain relief.

Electrical stimulation techniques

Transcutaneous stimulation. Pain perception is modulated following electrical stimulation of the peripheral nervous system. Whether this follows triggering of a gate mechanism in the dorsal horn or activation of descending inhibitory pathways is not fully proven (Melzack & Loeser 1978) but there are a number of published series testifying to the efficacy of transcutaneous nerve stimulation (Cauthen & Renner 1975; Krainick & Thoden 1981). Krainick and Thoden comment, however, that although there is good control of the continuous background pain, severe pain attacks are only slightly diminished. The technique has a major advantage in being completely non-invasive and it can be modified either in respect of the stimulation parameters or the site of stimulation until the optimum effects are obtained.

Dorsal column stimulation. Working on the same theoretical principle, intermittent stimulation of the spinal cord by implanted extradural or subdural monopolar or bipolar electrodes also provides relief in approximately 50% of cases (Siegfried & Cetinalp 1981). Originally this was undertaken as a staged procedure with an initial laminectomy required for electrode placement followed, after a satisfactory period of trial stimulation with the electrode exteriorised, by definitive implantation of the whole electrode and the receiver coil or stimulator. The development of percutaneous access to the epidural space now allows simpler placement of the electrode. Late failures occur; when these are due to local problems like electrode breakage and displacement they can be rectified but pathological changes such as fibrosis around the electrode tip itself are less easily resolved and some permanent failures result from progressive physiological changes and the contrary nature of pain itself.

Deep brain stimulation. This has been shown to be particularly beneficial in deafferentation pain and preliminary reports in 'pure' phantom limb pain suggest that it may help around 80% of patients (Siegfried & Cetinalp 1981). The procedure is performed stereotactically and, like dorsal column stimulation, requires a period of evaluation before its final acceptance. The ideal target is subject to debate but consensus supports structures within the sensory thalamus rather than those within the periventricular and mesencephalic periaqueductal grey matter. These latter sites appear to control a descending pain inhibition pathway which ends in the dorsal horn but this relieves only pain arising from nociceptive causes.

CONCLUSIONS

Phantom limb pain is not an inevitable sequel to amputation. When it occurs, this is usually early and in conjunction with other phantom limb phenomena. Other painful sequelae of amputation may coexist. The natural course is of gradual remission of all phantom related events but a painful stump or other distress can precipitate recurrence of the phantom and its pain. Those patients who attend the surgeon seeking relief of their phantom limb pain have usually been treated with many drugs and a variety of physical remedies on the recommendations of physicians or others. They must be dealt with sympathetically and logically. Frank appraisal of the individual's associated problems may indicate that simple surgical measures to the stump might suffice or that nonsurgical supportive treatment is necessary. Under no circumstances should the patient be allowed to embark on a regime wherein one destructive procedure follows another.

A logical protocol to offer is progression from transcutaneous stimulation to the DREZ operation with the intermediate option (where and when possible) of chronic electrical stimulation of the sensory thalamus.

Transcutaneous nerve stimulation is safe and may control continuous background pain sufficiently to alleviate most of the patient's symptoms. Dorsal column or, preferably, deep brain stimulation provide excellent pain control in at least half of the patients receiving such treatment but the implants are expensive and can fail mechanically; although they are implanted surgically, no lesion is created in any part of the nervous system. The only surgically destructive procedure to be commended is the DREZ operation: the results are good, the incidence of unacceptable side effects low and it is a specific therapy directed at the anatomical locus from which the pain originates.

Although all caring for patients with phantom limb pain will echo the poet Shelley's sentiments in *Prometheus Unbound*, 'I wish no living thing to suffer pain', the physician may ultimately have to accept the inevitable if all sensible remedies have failed and persuade his patient that no more can be done.

BRACHIAL PLEXUS AVULSION

Aetiology

The first verified case of root avulsion was reported by Flaubert in 1827 and later Frazier & Skillern (1911), carrying out a rhizotomy, verified the pathology of brachial plexus avulsion. Over the next few years occasional cases were reported, but brachial plexus avulsion was considered a rare condition. Today hundreds of patients with brachial plexus avulsion have been treated. One reason for the marked increase in the number of brachial plexus avulsions is the increasing speed of vehicular traffic, especially the motorcycle. In the USA motorcycles killed over 4000 cyclists in 1985 and for each one killed 90 others who lived required intensive medical treatment for their injuries. Although wearing a helmet has reduced head injuries, serious injuries to the chest, abdomen and limbs still take a high toll. The medical costs for such a patient injured in a motorcycle accident is $25 000, or more than $2.7 million for 105 motorcyclists followed for injuries up to 20 months. It is obvious that these injuries are significant both from the personal and financial point of view. In the days of the industrial revolution, workers suffered from brachial plexus avulsion injuries after falls from high places, usually striking their neck and shoulder and forcibly depressing the shoulder, avulsing the cervical roots. Today the leading cause of injury is the motorcycle, followed by car, plane, high speed boat and snowmobile.

Mechanism of injury

Forceful depression of the shoulder and lateral extension of the neck are mainly responsible for brachial plexus avulsion (Fig. 10.1). We have seen

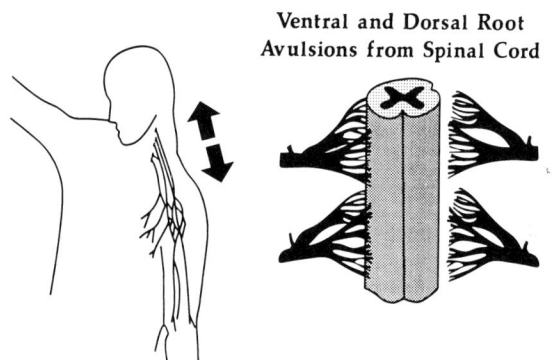

Fig. 10.1 Mechanism of traumatic brachial avulsion injury.

several patients with through-and-through trauma to the upper chest that suffered avulsion of the cervical roots. Immediately after the injury, if no other serious trauma has occurred (cranial or thoracic), the patient exhibits a paralysed arm with loss of sensation in the entire arm. A Horner's syndrome on the side of the avulsion occurs in a high percentage of cases. Initially the paralysis of the arm may go undetected in the face of other serious injuries. A few patients suffer from a partial avulsion and one or two roots may be involved, usually the lower cervical or upper thoracic dorsal roots. A typical brachial plexus avulsion will involve all the dorsal roots from C5–T1 with both the motor and sensory roots damaged (Fig. 10.2).

Pain begins almost immediately after the injury and about 10% of patients develop intractable pain that is not responsive to conservative therapy; they will eventually require a DREZ operation (Nashold & Ostahl 1979). In our experience it is rare that the pain appears years after the avulsion injury. The pain is characterised as burning and crushing, often exacerbated by electrical shocks radiating into the paralysed limb, particularly along the radial aspect of the arm into the thumb and index finger of the hand. A second type of pain usually described as deep, dull aching may also be experienced in the involved arm. The electrical shooting pains usually occur spontaneously. Passive manipulation of the paralysed arm does not usually activate the pain, but there are trigger spots on the intact skin, usually over the neck, suboccipital region or upper chest, which, when touched either by the patient or an examiner may activate the shooting electrical pains into the paralysed arm. One patient had a trigger zone on his forehead on the side of the avulsion. These trigger zones disappear after the DREZ operation, emphasising the extent of the spinal cord connections linking distant segments of the cord that may be activated by pathological lesions.

Diagnostic evaluation

The neurologic findings are straightforward; a history of trauma at high speed, with a flail arm that is senseless and burning pain in the hand. The most useful diagnostic test is a myelogram with a CT or MRI study (Fig. 10.3). The picture seen is one of traumatic myeloceles in the cervical region plus varying degrees of distortion of the dural sac and/or subarachnoid space (Fig. 10.4). The spinal cord may be atrophic on the side of the trauma. The degree of the radiographic or MRI defects does not always indicate the severity of the avulsion. It is not uncommon for at least 4 or 5 dorsal

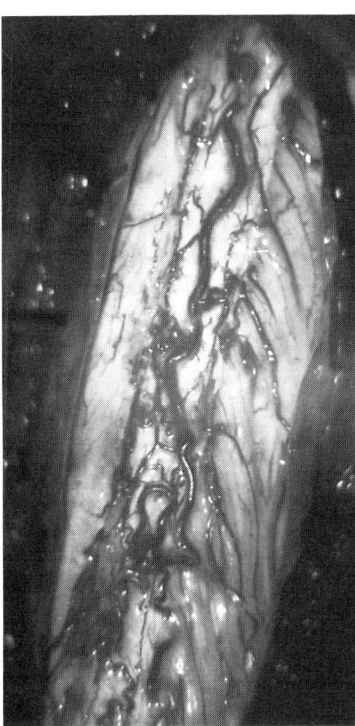

Fig. 10.2 Intraoperative photograph showing area of avulsion on the left (cervical spinal cord).

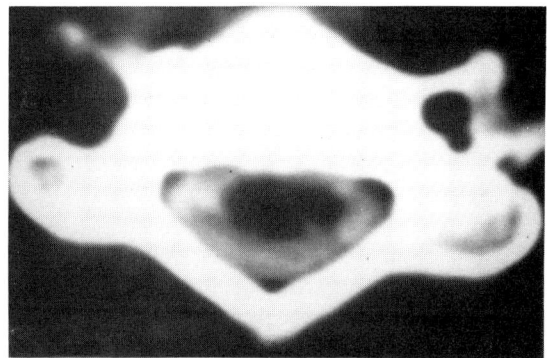

Fig. 10.3 Cross section of cervical spinal cord. Delayed CT scan showing wedge-shaped area of avulsion in spinal cord.

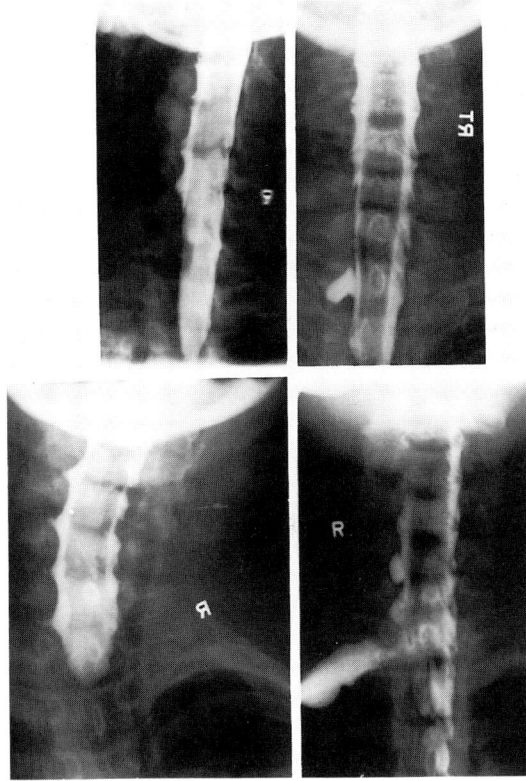

Fig. 10.4 Cervical myelogram in brachial plexus avulsion. Note variety of traumatic myeloceles. Cervical roots C5-T1 avulsed.

and/or ventral roots to be avulsed. However, the radiographic picture may show only 1 or 2 traumatic myeloceles. It is important for the neurosurgeon to recognise this difference and to expose the cervical cord surgically from C5 through T1. We have seen a few patients with only 1 or 2 cervical roots avulsed, but this can be detected on the neurological examination which will reveal only a partial motor and/or sensory deficit; in this case only the 1 or 2 roots avulsed require the DREZ treatment.

Selection of patient for DREZ operation

Initially all patients with brachial plexus avulsion and pain should be treated conservatively with drugs and physical therapy. Eventually 10% of the patients will be candidates for the DREZ operation. The time to consider surgery is about 6 months after injury if there has been no response to intensive conservative therapy. The first patients we operated on in the 1970s had suffered their pain for many years. In fact, our first patient with avulsion had been injured 10 years before. He was successfully relieved, but the subsequent earlier patients had long histories of drug abuse and addiction and did poorly. Two committed suicide after the DREZ failed to relieve their pain. This convinced us not to withhold the operation for too long or to allow the patient to deteriorate. Pain which is burning in character occurring in paroxysms is relieved, while aching pain alone is less successfully relieved.

The DREZ operation

The neurosurgeon must explain the nature of the operation with its risks and benefits. Lawsuits have occurred following the DREZ operation when complicated by weakness of the ipsilateral leg. Weakness occurs in 5% of the operations, and this must be explained carefully to the patient and family. The operation can be divided into two parts – cervical laminectomy and exposure of the cervical spinal cord and the production of the DREZ lesion (Nashold 1988).

All patients receive pre- and postoperative as well as intraoperative steroids. The operation is carried out under general anaesthesia with the patient in the prone position. A complete cervical laminectomy is carried out from C4 through T1 in extensive avulsions. When the dura is exposed, it is possible to see the traumatic myeloceles along the lateral extent of the dural sac with their extensions into the intervertebral foramen. When the dura is opened, the openings of the myeloceles are seen devoid of nerve roots either dorsal or ventral. These sacs may extend for some distance into the neck or even below the clavicle. We make no effort to close the openings. There may be extensive arachnoiditis and scar which must be carefully dissected under the microscope to expose the region of the avulsion. It is important to visualise the entire dorsal extent of the cervical cord so that the avulsed side of the spinal cord can be compared with the normal side (see Fig. 10.2). The area of the dorsal root avulsions can be easily identified under the microscope. As a rule both the dorsal

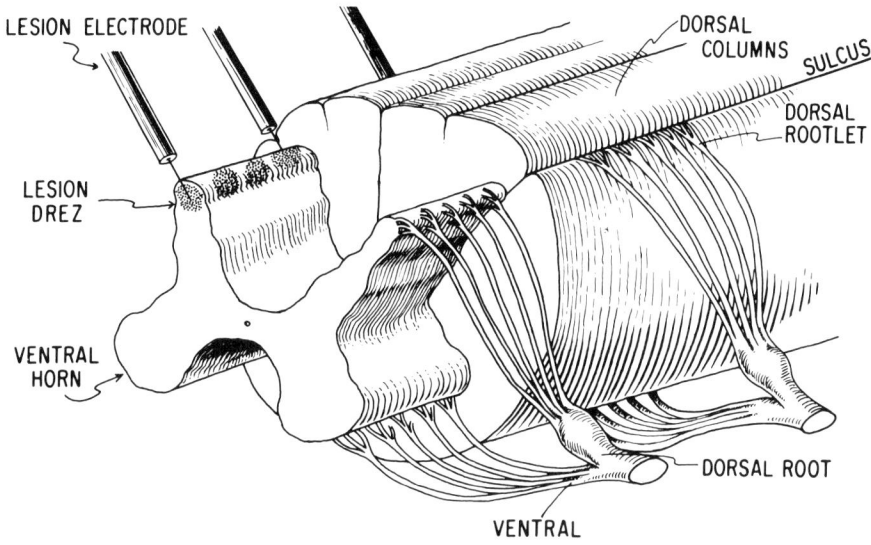

Fig. 10.5 Schematic drawing of spinal cord illustrating the DREZ lesions.

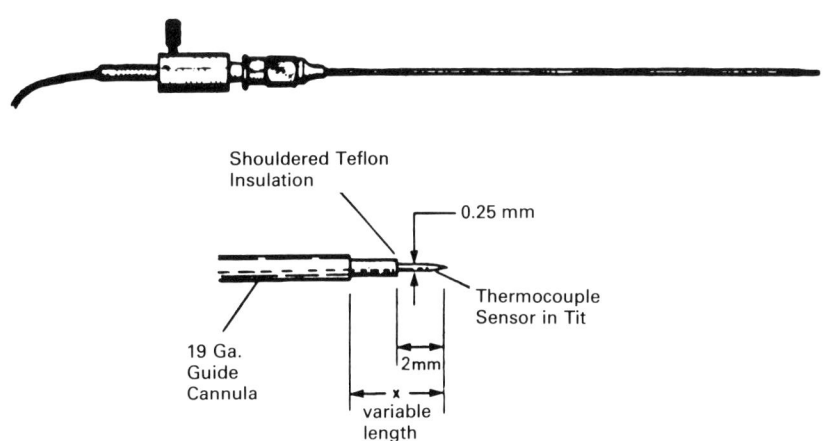

Fig. 10.6 DREZ electrode.

and ventral roots are missing. The important landmark on the dorsal surface of the spinal cord is the intermediolateral sulcus which separates the dorsal roots from the lateral edge of the dorsal columns (Fig. 10.5). The spinal cord may be distorted in this region of the avulsed nerves, so a comparison with the intact normal side is helpful. The DREZ thermal electrode has been used to make the lesions in our group of patients. The DREZ electrode was designed by Dr Eric Cosman of the Radionics Corporation (Fig. 10.6). The electrode is 0.25 mm in diameter, with an exposed lesion tip of 3.0 mm (Cosman et al 1988). There is a cuff just above the lesion tip which prevents penetration of the electrode beyond the 3 mm depth. The Radionics lesion generator produces an RF lesion and the lesions are made at 75°C for 15 s. This results in a lesion approximately 2 mm × 4 mm which is sufficient to destroy the first 5 Rexed layers of the dorsal horn (Fig. 10.7). It is

156 MANAGEMENT OF PAIN IN THE HAND AND WRIST

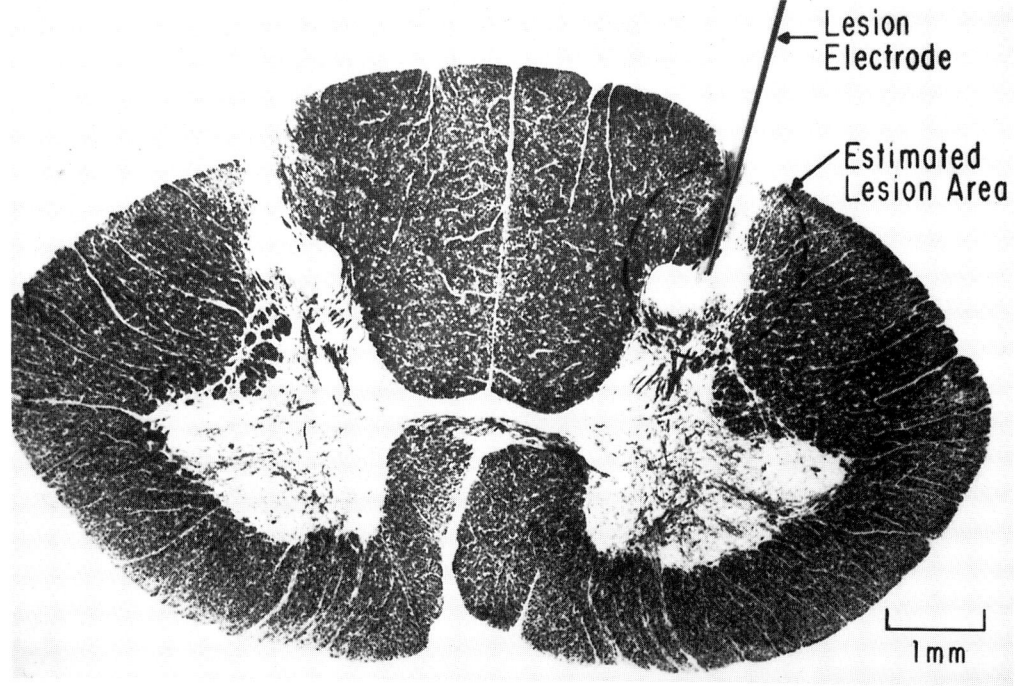

Fig. 10.7 Cross section of normal human spinal cord showing area of DREZ lesions.

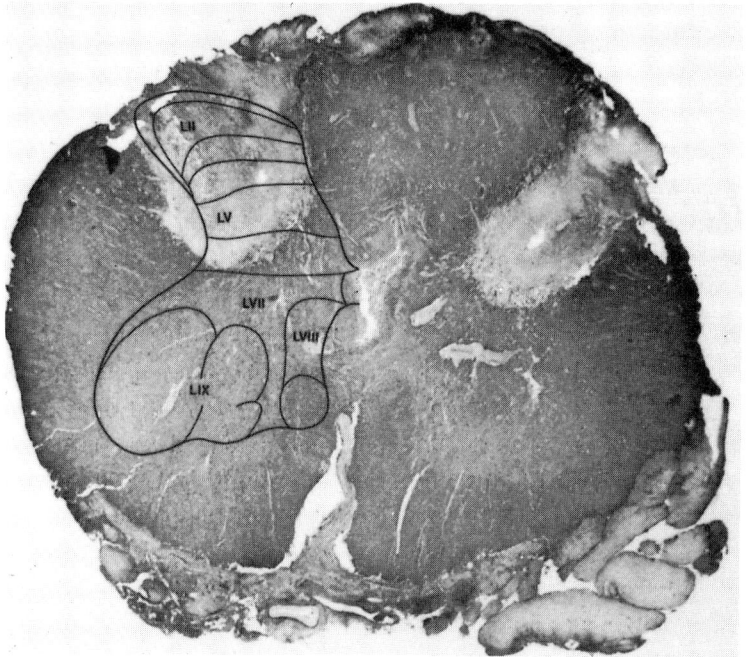

Fig. 10.8 Cross section of spinal cord at lumbar 2 segment.

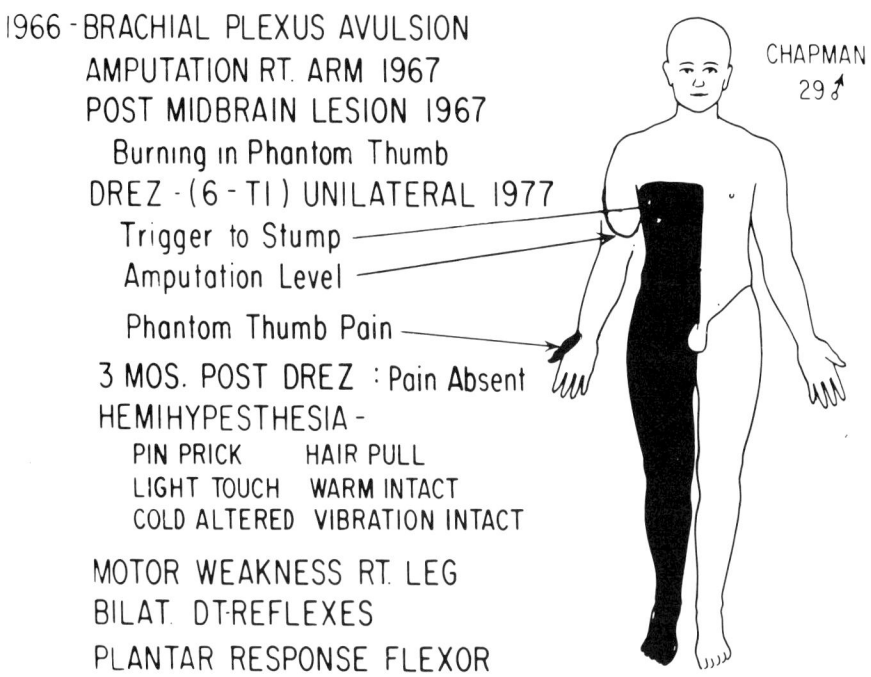

Fig. 10.9 Schematic drawing of postoperative findings in patient with cervical avulsion after DREZ operation. Typical complications in early DREZ operations prior to RF controlled thermal lesions using the Cosman DREZ electrode.

the destruction of the deafferented secondary neurons in these layers which results in the relief of pain (Fig. 10.8). The number of lesions over the involved area of the avulsion is important to the success of the DREZ operation. The region of the cervical avulsion may extend over a distance of 4–5 cm and it is important to space the lesions every millimeter. In the earlier DREZ operations, 10 to 20 lesions might be made over a distance of 4 cm or more and our poorest results in this group of patients may be explained on this basis. At the present time we measure the length of the avulsed region of the spinal cord and if it is 5 cm a total of 50 lesions should be made. This same principle is applied to all DREZ operations in other segments of the spinal cord. The electrode is directed at an angle of about 25° in the cervical region; however, the angle may vary somewhat in other spinal cord regions. The guide of electrode angulation should be about at the angle of exit of the dorsal root in these areas. The lesions always extend from the intact rostral roots, usually C4 in brachial avulsion cases to the lowest intact root T1 or T2.

Results

Complications. To date over 500 DREZ operations have been done with no deaths in the avulsions. The major spinal cord structures at risk in the cervical DREZ are the dorsal columns, the foraminal tract and the crossing fibres of the spinothalamic tract, and an as yet unidentified ipsilateral sensory tract. The major complications are ipsilateral leg weakness (5%) and a variety of transient ipsilateral sensory changes.

One recent patient experienced a contralateral reduction of pain and temperature appreciation (see p. 158). The complications of the DREZ were related to the use of 2 different types of lesion electrodes. In the earliest DREZ operations (1976–1982), a cordotomy type electrode was employed and the lesion size was controlled by the amount of current in milliamperes. These early lesions were not of uniform size and over 60% of the patients showed some initial neurologic deficit, mainly sensory. The sensory changes were always ipsilateral, usually involved the upper thoracic dermatomes just below the level of the lesion and could extend over other large areas of the thorax and upper abdomen (Fig. 10.9). There was reduction of light touch and pinprick with variable changes in appreciation of thermal sensation. These sensory defects all cleared within days, the motor defects were more persistent, but none of the patients were physically disabled. This is in contrast to the thoracic DREZ (post-herpetic pain) which may result in more serious motor disabilities that are permanent. After the DREZ the patient would often complain of an insecure feeling of the involved leg rather than weakness. They would say that they were uncertain as to whether the leg was being placed firmly on the floor. This feeling was not related as far as we could tell to a specific sensory deficit. At first we thought the patient's complaint could be due to involvement of the dorsal column with proprioceptive dysfunction, but on examination it would appear that there was a slight increase in the tendon reflexes on that side with some incoordination or cerebellar deficit. The so called motor weakness, therefore, seemed to be related to changes in the pyramidal and cerebellar dysfunction. About 1982 we began to use the RF thermal electrode (Radionics) and the motor and sensory changes have been minimal and transient since then. One recent patient, however, is worth mentioning because he exhibited evidence of spinothalamic tract involvement on the side opposite the cervical DREZ operation. Post DREZ the patient noted unpleasant sensation over the contralateral abdomen and leg. The skin in this region was hyperalgesic and examination revealed reduction of pain and thermal sensation. Light touch and touching the hairs was also reduced. It was obvious that some portion of the lateral spinothalamic tract was involved: it seemed unlikely to us that this was direct involvement of the lateral spinothalamic tract but that the sensory deficit was due perhaps to involvement of crossing spinothalamic fibres in the central area of the cord. Our reasoning for this explanation was due to the abnormal changes in the spinal cord seen at the time of surgery. The spinal cord was thinned and atrophic on the side of the avulsion distorting the normal anatomy and we reckoned that the 3 mm electrode must have penetrated near to the central grey area of the cord, resulting in the post DREZ sensory change. Fortunately, the unpleasant sensations subsided after 6 months although there is still some mild contralateral sensory change and the patient has experienced good pain relief.

One of the major technical problems in producing small discrete lesions in the spinal cord is illustrated by the above case report, where the abnormal pathology and distortion of the spinal cord structures may have contributed to the complication. We routinely measure the impedance of the spinal cord tissue prior to the lesion making and in the traumatised spinal cord (avulsion or paraplegia) the impedance measurements are always lower than normal, in the range of about 1000 ohms or less (Vieira et al 1988). The normal spinal cord impedance ranges from 1000 ohms to 1200 ohms. The lower spinal cord impedances we believe are associated with extensive scarring in the spinal cord due to the trauma. It is this scarring that makes it difficult to make uniform lesions in the traumatised spinal cord (Fig. 10.10). Some neurosurgeons use the laser to produce the DREZ

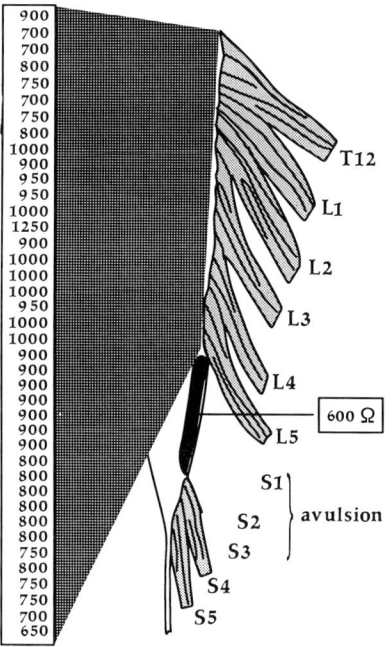

Fig. 10.10 Schematic drawing of the conus medullaris in patient with traumatic avulsion of S1-S2 dorsal roots. Impedance measurements in the dorsal horn region indicated areas of tissue abnormality due to the trauma (normal value 1000 to 1200 Ω) (photograph courtesy of Drs Vieira and Shieff).

lesions and in pain relief the results seem to be similar to the thermal electrode lesion (Ovelmen-Levitt 1988). There has not been a large clinical report as yet using the laser and comparing the complication rate with the thermal electrode. We are concerned that the ability to control the laser lesion size may not be as good as in the thermal lesion. Further data gathered either from laboratory animal experiments or from post mortem examination after the DREZ operation are needed (Iacono et al 1988). The perfect therapeutic lesion that would result in no complications is as yet to be devised. But it is important we continue the search for improved lesion methods, both in the laboratory and in the operating room.

Pain relief. The results of pain relief in patients with brachial plexus avulsion injuries after the DREZ operation range from 82–86% (Rawlings et al 1990). The criteria to judge relief of pain used at Duke Medical Center and reported by my colleagues Friedman and Bullitt are as follows:

good result – no analgesics and no limitation of physical activity due to pain

fair result – patient on analgesics, no narcotics and no physical limitations

poor result — still requiring narcotics and limited physical activity.

Of the 39 patients in our series followed from 1 to 10 years (average 5), 67% experienced good to fair pain relief using the cordotomy type of electrode (1976–1982) (Nashold et al 1989). This group also experienced more postoperative complications. In those patients using the thermally controlled lesion electrode, 82% experienced good to fair pain relief. The recurrence of the pain after the DREZ occurred within the first 6 months and was more common after the use of the cordotomy electrode. The occurrence of a post DREZ dysaesthesia has been rare. Friedman, reviewing our patients in 1988, noted only one patient with mild burning pain 6 months postoperatively. The recurrence of the original pain after DREZ has also been minimal. It occurred more often in the earlier DREZ operations (1978–1982) with the 'cordotomy type electrode' (Fig. 10.11). The recurrence occurs during the initial 6 months after the DREZ operation. The relief of pain after the DREZ operation is directly related to the number of lesions, greater pain relief occurring in patients with multiple lesions placed 1 mm apart (Fried-

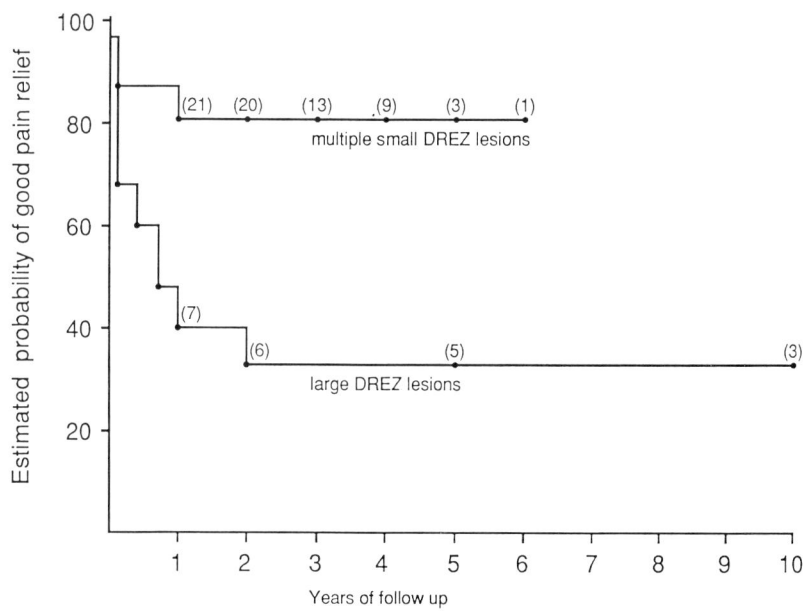

Fig. 10.11 Kaplan-Meier curves depicting probability of pain relief after DREZ lesions. The upper curve charts those patients operated upon using our present protocol. The lower curve notes those patients operated upon using a small number of large DREZ lesions. The two curves are different: $p \leq 0.003$.

man et al 1988). A third of the patients are not relieved by this operation. Campbell reported 85% good and fair results from his series at Johns Hopkins Hospital (Campbell 1988). In the UK, Thomas at the National Hospital for Nervous Diseases reported 86% good and fair results (Thomas & Jones 1984). Using the laser, Powers noted good pain relief in his 6 patients. He also reported fewer complications: proprioceptive abnormality (1) ipsilateral monoparesis (2) (Powers et al 1988).

Conclusions

Painful brachial plexus avulsion represents a pure example of the deafferentation pain syndrome. Since not all patients suffering this injury experience long-term pain, we are still in the dark as to the aetiologic factors responsible for the chronic generation of the pain. In animal experiments after experimental avulsion injuries the experimental results suggest both neurophysiological and neuropharmacological abnormalities occurring in the injured dorsal horn (Ovelmen-Levitt 1988).

Among these some of the changes are the appearance of abnormal electrical activity (epileptiform) in the secondary sensory neurons (as yet not identified) in the deeper layers of the dorsal horn. These secondary neurons begin to fire within 5 hours of the experimental injury and continue for many months. In addition there are behavioural changes (autotomy) noted early on in the animals, which we believe from our laboratory observation are the result of specific responses by the animal (rat) to noxious afferent events, probably originating from the deafferented secondary neurons in the deeper layers of the injured dorsal horn. Initially B-endorphin and substance P are altered after experimental avulsion as well as other neuropeptides. The interactions of these substances may affect the stability of the secondary neurons which begin to fire epileptically. Whether or not these events occur in the injured dorsal horn of man and are responsible for the onset of the pain is still a moot point. In the meantime, the DREZ operation in properly selected patients with deafferentation pain of brachial plexus avulsion can give long-term satisfactory results.

REFERENCES

Berger M, Gerstenbrand F 1981 Phantom illusions in spinal cord lesions. In: Siegfried J, Zimmermann M (eds) Phantom and stump pain. Springer-Verlag, Berlin, pp 66–73
Bromage P R, Melzack R 1974 Phantom limbs and the body schema. Canadian Anaesthetic Society Journal 21: 267–274
Campbell J N 1988 The Hopkins's experience with lesions of the dorsal horn (Nashold's operation) for pain from avulsion of the brachial plexus. Applied Neurophysiology 51: 170–174
Carlen P L, Wall P D, Nadvorna H, Steinbach T 1978 Phantom limbs and related phenomena in recent traumatic amputations. Neurology 28: 211–217
Cauthen J C, Renner E 1975 Transcutaneous and peripheral nerve stimulation for chronic pain states, Surgical Neurology 4: 102–104
Cosman E R, Pittman W J, Nashold B S, Makachinas T T 1988 Radiofrequency lesion generation and its effects on tissue impedance. Applied Neurophysiology 51: 230–242
Cronholm B 1951 Phantom limb in amputees. Acta Psychiatrica et Neurologica Scandinavica (suppl) 72
Danke F 1981 Phantom sensations after amputation: the importance of localization and prognosis. In: Siegfried J, Zimmermann M (eds) Phantom and stump pain. Springer-Verlag, Berlin, pp 56–61
Elliott F, Little A, Millbrandt W 1976 Carbamazepine for phantom limb phenomena. New England Journal of Medicine 295: 678
Erickson T C, Bleckwenn W J, Woolsey C N 1952 Observations on the post-central gyrus in relation to pain. Transactions of the American Neurological Association 77: 57–58
Ewalt J R, Randall G C, Morris H 1947 The phantom limb. Psychosomatic Medicine 9: 118–123
Falconer M A 1953 Surgical treatment of intractable phantom limb pain. British Medical Journal 1: 299–304
Flaubert M 1827 Memoire sur plusiers cas de luxation. Repertoire General de Anatomie et de Physiologie Pathologiques et des Cliniques Chirurgicales 3: 55–69
Frazier G H, Skillern P G Jr 1911 Supraclavicular subcutaneous lesions of the brachial plexus not associated with skeletal injuries. Journal of American Medical Association 57: 1957–1963
Frederiks J A M 1963 Occurrence and nature of phantom limb phenomena following amputation of body parts and following lesions of the central and peripheral nervous system. Psychiatrica Neurologica Neurochirurgica 66: 73–97
Friedman A H, Nashold B S Jr, Bronec P R 1988 Dorsal root entry zone lesions for the treatment of brachial plexus avulsion injuries. A follow-up study. Neurosurgery 22: 369–373

Ham R O, Roberts V C, Luff R 1989 A five year review of referrals for prosthetic treatment in England, Wales and Northern Ireland, 1981–85. Health Trends 21(1): 3–6

Head H, Holmes G 1911 Sensory disturbances from cerebral lesions. Brain 34: 102–254

Iacono R P, Aquire M L, Nashold B S Jr 1988 Anatomic examination of human dorsal root entry zone lesions. Applied Neurophysiology 51: 225–229

Jensen T S, Rasmussen P 1984 Amputation. In: Wall P D, Melzack R (eds) Textbook of pain. Churchill Livingstone, Edinburgh, pp 402–412

Kallio K E 1950 Permanency of results obtained by sympathetic surgery in the treatment of phantom pain. Acta Orthopaedica Scandinavica 19: 391–397

Krainick J U, Thoden U 1981 Transcutaneous electrical nerve stimulation in postamputation pain. In: Siegfried J, Zimmermann M (eds) Phantom and stump pain. Springer-Verlag, Berlin, pp 99–102

Livingston W K 1976 Infiltration of sympathetic ganglia with novocain solution for phantom limb pain. In: Pain mechanisms. Plenum, New York, pp 150–168

Melzack R 1974 Central neural mechanisms in phantom limb pain. Advances in Neurology 4: 319–326

Melzack R, Loeser J D 1978 Phantom body pain in paraplegics: evidence for a central "pattern generating mechanism" for pain. Pain 4: 195–210

Merksey H 1979 Pain terms: a list with definitions and notes on usage. Pain 6: 249–252

Mitchell S W 1872 Injuries of the nerves and their consequences. Lippincott, Philadelphia

Mitchell S W 1905 The case of George Dedlow. In: The autobiography of a quack and other stories. Century, New York, pp 83–109

Nashold B S Jr 1988 Neurosurgical technique of the dorsal root entry zone operation. Applied Neurophysiology 51: 136–145

Nashold B S Jr, Ostdahl R H 1979 Dorsal root entry zone lesions for pain relief. Journal of Neurosurgery 51: 59–69

Nashold B S Jr, Friedman A, Bullitt E 1989 The status of dorsal root entry zone lesions in 1987. Clinical Neurosurgery 35: 422–428

Nashold B S, Wilson W P, Slaughter D G 1969 Stereotaxic midbrain lesions for central dysaesthesia and phantom pain. Journal of Neurosurgery 30: 116–126

Ovelmen-Levitt J 1988 Abnormal physiology of the dorsal horn as related to the deafferentation syndrome. Applied Neurophysiology 51: 104–116

Parkes C M 1973 Factors determining the persistence of phantom pain in the amputee. Journal of Psychosomatic Research 17: 97–108

Powers S K, Barbaro N M, Levy R M 1988 Pain control with laser produced dorsal root entry zone lesions. Applied Neurophysiology 51: 243–254

Price D B 1976 Phantom limb phenomenon in patients with leprosy. Journal of Nervous and Mental Disease 163: 108–116

Rawlings C E III, El-Naggar A O, Nashold B S Jr The DREZ procedure: An update on technique. In press

Riddoch G 1941 Phantom limbs and body shape. Brain 64: 197–222

Saris S C, Iacono R P, Nashold B S 1985 Dorsal root entry zone lesions for post-amputation pain. Journal of Neurosurgery 62: 72–76

Sherman R A, Sherman C J, Gall N J 1980 A survey of current phantom limb pain treatment in the United States. Pain 8: 85–99

Sherrington C S 1900 The spinal cord. In: Schafer E A (ed) Textbook of physiology. Pentland, Edinburgh, vol 2, p 784

Siegfried J, Cetinalp E 1981 Neurosurgical treatment of phantom limb pain: a survey of methods. In: Siegfried J, Zimmermann M (eds) Phantom and stump pain. Springer-Verlag, Berlin, pp 148–155

Simmel M L 1962 Phantom experiences following amputation in childhood. Journal of Neurology, Neurosurgery and Psychiatry 25: 69–78

Thomas D G, Jones S J 1984 Dorsal root entry zone lesions (Nashold's procedure) in brachial plexus avulsion. Neurosurgery 15: 966–968

Vieira J F S, Shieff C, Nashold B S Jr, Bullard D E, Cosman E 1988 Impedance measurements of the spinal cord of man and animals. Applied Neurophysiology 51: 154–163

Wall P D 1981 On the origin of pain associated with amputation. In: Siegfried J, Zimmermann M (eds) Phantom and stump pain. Springer-Verlag, Berlin, p 2

Walton J 1985 Brain's diseases of the nervous system, 9th edn. Oxford University Press, Oxford, pp 63–64

Whitaker H A 1979 An historical note on the phantom limb. Neurology 29: 273

White J C, Sweet W H 1969 Pain and the neurosurgeon: a forty year experience. Thomas, Springfield, pp 50–86

M. Powell

11 The management of malignant hand pain

AETIOLOGY

Cancer virtually never involves the hand directly, but unfortunately malignant hand pain occurs relatively frequently from 2 common and also 2 relatively uncommon sources (Fig. 11.1).

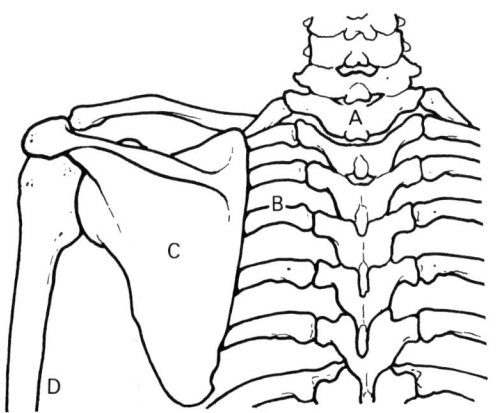

Fig. 11.1 Sites of origin of malignant hand pain. (A) Vertebral body involvement. (B) Apex of lung. (C) Apex of axilla. (D) Shaft of humerus.

Both common sources are in effect direct invasion of the brachial plexus from a tumour mass, the first being direct from the apex of the lung, the pancoast tumour; the second from invasion of the plexus from involved nodes, usually the axilliary nodes from carcinoma of the breast. In both cases, particularly in the axilla, there may also be the side effects of therapy from radiation damage to the plexus itself, although it is uncommon to see this in the UK.

The 2 less common sources are, firstly, hand pain which may derive from malignant involvement of the vertebrae supplying the hand divisions of the plexus, that is C6, 7 and 8 and T1. Although metastatic spread to the vertebrae is common, the cervical spine and upper thoracic are involved only infrequently. Secondly and very rarely, pain may derive from massive involvement of the shaft of the humerus from either primary or secondary malignancy with direct involvement of the nerves as they pass through the upper arm on their way to the hand. Here too, radiation may damage the nerves and cause pain.

CLINICAL FEATURES AND DIFFERENTIAL DIAGNOSIS

The cause of malignant hand pain seldom causes diagnostic difficulties. At the stage of the development of intense hand pain, the tumour origin is usually known.

In *plexus invasion* the pain usually involves the lower brachial plexus divisions, that is C8 and T1, in a patient with a known primary cancer. Progression of the disease will lead to extension of the loss into higher segments. The patient suffers excruciating pain of an unremitting neurogenic type, burning with occasional spasms in the ulnar border of the hand, spreading up to the elbow and in bad cases into the radial parts of the hand. Hand function is frequently lost with C8 and T1 sensory loss and weakness affecting primarily the small hand muscles, and the skin may show disuse and trophic changes similar to Sudek's atrophy. The patient may spend much of the initial interview cradling the arm protectively, as there may be hyperaesthesia in the less severely involved roots. The pain seldom spreads to the chest except in extensive apical lung tumours.

Associated with the lower brachial plexus motor and sensory signs are possibly an absent or diminished triceps reflex and in pancoast tumours a positive Horners sign. A tumour mass may be palpable at the base of the neck or axilla. It is always worth carefully mapping the sensory loss to all modalities as subsequent treatment may alter the clinical picture significantly.

The only clinical condition with a similar anatomical picture is cervical rib compression which is almost never as severe as in malignant pain. Cervical root brachialgia from either spondylitic root canal involvement or simple prolapsed disc pain may be as severe, but usually involves the C6 and C7 dermatomes. The C8 and T1 dermatomes are involved only rarely as spondylitis does not usually affect the C7/T1 or T1/2 spaces.

In *vertebral body* pain involving the hand segments, the pain will also occur locally in the neck itself, usually before the nerve root is involved. The pain is often worse at night, an important diagnostic warning sign often found in spinal canal tumours of all types, which can help to differentiate the condition from cervical spondylitic brachialgia, although the diagnosis will usually be made radiologically. *Malignancy in the humerus* itself will cause intense local pain long before the adjacent nerves are involved.

INVESTIGATIONS

Generally there will be no specific investigations required in pain management, as the diagnosis is clinical. In those cases where the diagnosis is unclear, plain X-rays of the cervical spine, thoracic inlet and apical lung should differentiate the source of the pain. If the cervical vertebrae are involved, computer scanning (CT) or CT myelography will be indicated if surgery is contemplated, otherwise plain X-rays will suffice. Magnetic resonance imaging (MRI) is not so informative as CT in planning surgery for metastatic bone disease because the bone details are lost in the imaging process. Nerve conduction studies and electromyography may occasionally help to clarify the nerve roots involved.

TREATMENT OPTIONS

The treatment of hand pain will be carried out with the close cooperation of radiotherapy and oncology services. Direct treatment of the primary malignancy with deep X-rays or chemotherapy will have been tried or will be continuing during pain management. This can be directed in three ways:

1. Analgesia, systemic and direct
2. Direct surgery
3. Central CNS blocks.

Analgesia

Malignant pain may be brought under control by quite simple drugs in the early stages, when the introduction of nonsteroidal anti-inflammatories such as naproxen may prove very effective, especially when backed up by simple analgesics and nocturnal tricyclics for their analgesia enhancing effect.

When these fail, there is an extensive range of more powerful analgesics for use in intractable malignant pain, morphine sulphate tartarate (MST) starting at 30mg twice daily being the drug of choice. Various other opiates including diamorphine elixir and newer opiate analogues may also be tried.

Dysaesthesias may respond to anti-epileptics such as clonazepam, although carbamazepine (used frequently in benign neuralgias) is often disappointing.

Support groups and pain teams have their own preferences for pain regimes, and are well practised in this part of pain management.

Apart from drugs, other forms of mechanical pain relief may be successful in pain relief, such as TENS and acupuncture. Physiotherapy, using gentle manipulation of the Maitland's type, backed up with heat and ultrasound as appropriate, may be beneficial.

More invasive methods of delivery are available. Support groups regularly use subcutaneous infusions of morphine for long-term pain relief, and a number of slow release infusion pumps are now available, the more recent being of the patient controlled 'demand' type. If effective cordotomy procedures were more widely available nationally, the use of the subcutaneous morphine pump would be restricted to short-term control whilst awaiting a definitive procedure, and, too, in the patient whose prognosis is measured in hours or a few days. In the author's opinion the use of cordotomy is much more effective, and frees the patient from troublesome and expensive gadgetry which requires frequent topping up as well as the inconvenience of being carried about. Epidural morphine administered by indwelling catheter does not have a major part to play in hand pain.

An attractive idea finding favour in the USA is the implanted, programmable continuous slow release pump, holding a month's supply of a chosen analgesia in a built in reservoir. Morphine is the most effective opiate in this role, and is usually given via the lumbar CSF space for pain control. In the UK it may yet have a place in malignant pain management but at present the cost (£3000) effectively prohibits its use.

Direct surgery

Surgery for direct invasion of the plexus from pancoast tumours and axilliary node involvement is not very effective. When attempted, the aim of surgery by brachial plexus exploration is to free the various parts of the plexus from enveloping tumour. Between 40–60% may gain some benefit, but the surgery is technically difficult and the pain relief gained temporary; furthermore the risk of damage to the nerves is high in inexperienced hands.

Surgery for the management of malignant vertebral body disease has undergone a revolution in the last few years and collapse of the cervical spine is not looked on with the same hopelessness as was reported in neurosurgical series until comparatively recently. Most spinal surgeons have abandoned the classical approach of the decompression laminectomy except in the rare case of the unilaterally involved lateral mass and lamina. In the majority of cases, the vertebral body is involved, and often collapsed. Posterior decompression is not only ineffective but also destabilises the vertebral column. In the neck this is particularly disastrous.

The anterior approach to the neck is by contrast very effective. The approach is straightforward, as is the vertebral body resection. Both parts of the procedure are in frequent use for the management of cervical spondylosis by anterior cervical decompression. The incision and approach are along tissue plains, which as a result heal quickly and painlessly, and the bone work is carried out with safety under X-ray control. In fact, tumour involved softened bone usually curettes away more easily than the sclerotic bone of osteoarthritic spondylitis. The missing bone can be replaced with autologous bone from the hip, with bone cement or even purpose built vertebral prostheses in the thoracic spine. At the same time, the collapsed space can be 'jacked open', relieving compressed nerve roots. Patients are usually mobilised in the early postoperative days. If ambulant prior to surgery there are seldom difficulties, particularly if the pain has been relieved.

The posterior elements of the vertebra, which are equally important in the strength of the vertebral column, consist of the spines, laminae and pedicles. If the stability of the spine is in question, following loss of the vertebral body, they can be supported by instrumentation using interlamina wiring onto stabilising rods such as the Hartsill rectangle (a heavy gauge wire loop) or Luque rods (Fig. 11.2). These techniques, though time consuming, are not high risk procedures and are well tolerated.

Central nervous system blocks

It will be appreciated from the preceding paragraphs that surgery, whilst having a useful specific role, has only a limited part to play in the majority of cases of malignant hand pain. When pharmacological analgesia fails, a few patients will respond favourably to sympathetic blockade at the stellate ganglion. Its use is, on the whole, shortlived, although it has the merits of the low risk procedure. Therefore the pain process may have to be blocked by interruption of the spinothalamic tract somewhere within the CNS.

The anterior spinothalamic (ST) tract transmits

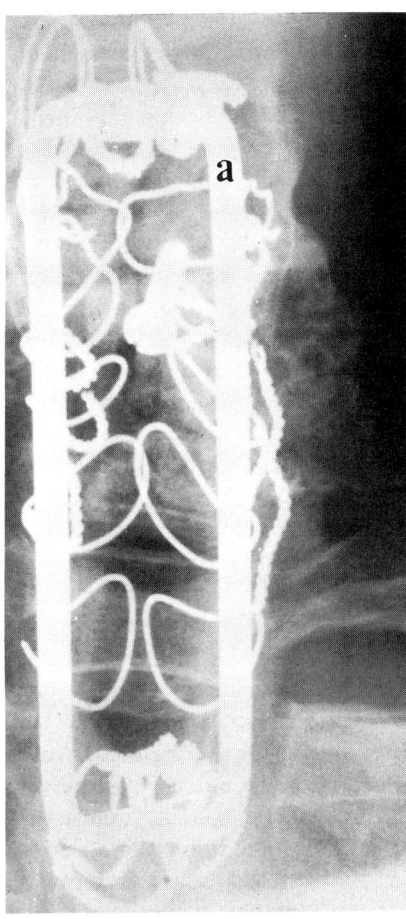

Fig. 11.2a AP view of a cervical spine with malignant involvement of C5 vertebral body from Ca breast. A Hartshill rectangle (**a**) held by interlamina wires stabilises the collapse. A screw locating a cement graft may also be seen.

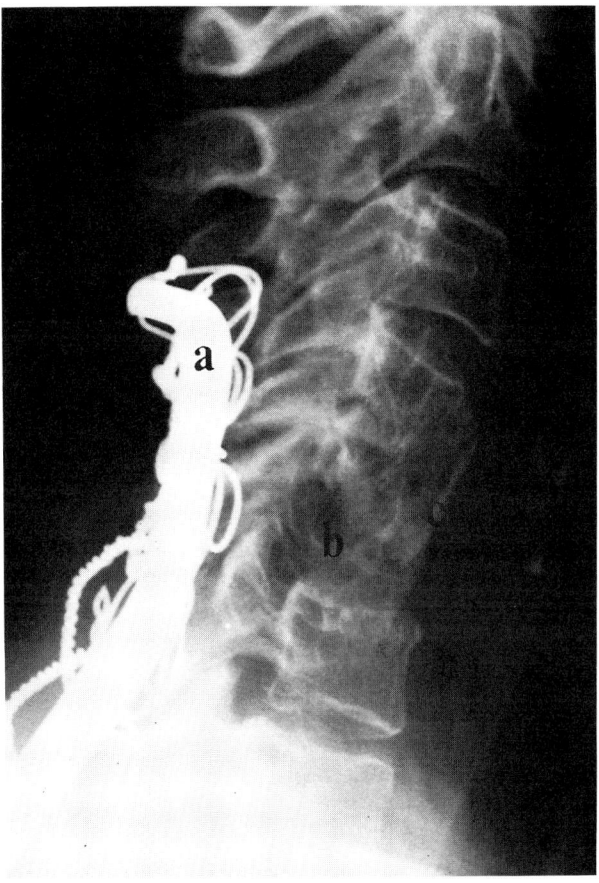

Fig. 11.2b Lateral view of a cervical spine with Hartshill rectangle (**a**) in place. Osteolytic destruction of C5 (**b**) can be seen, as well as a bone graft (**c**) between C6 and C4 anteriorly.

the majority of noxious stimuli to the brain. 70% of the fibres project to the brain stem and only a minority to the thalamus. The tract which is crossed in the cord also transmits temperature but is well separated from the other sensory modalities of light touch, vibration and joint position sense which are transmitted in the uncrossed dorsal columns. Anatomically the closest tracts are the uncrossed corticospinal (motor) tract posteriorly and the bilateral represented spinocerebellar tract laterally. Medially is the grey matter of the ventral horn.

By far the simplest and most effective of ST blocks, as well as being the best tolerated, is the percutaneous cordotomy (PCC), more correctly termed the percutaneous radiofrequency spinothalamic tractotomy. Other techniques exist, including open ST tractotomy and various other blocks made more centrally in the CNS. These have mostly been abandoned as too risky and too short-term in their results. Central stimulating procedures, involving stereotactic placement of thalamic wires, may have a place, but there are only a handful of centres in the world performing these procedures and there remains discussion on the best location for stimulation.

As the technique of PCC is only available from a few centres in the UK, despite its efficacy, the

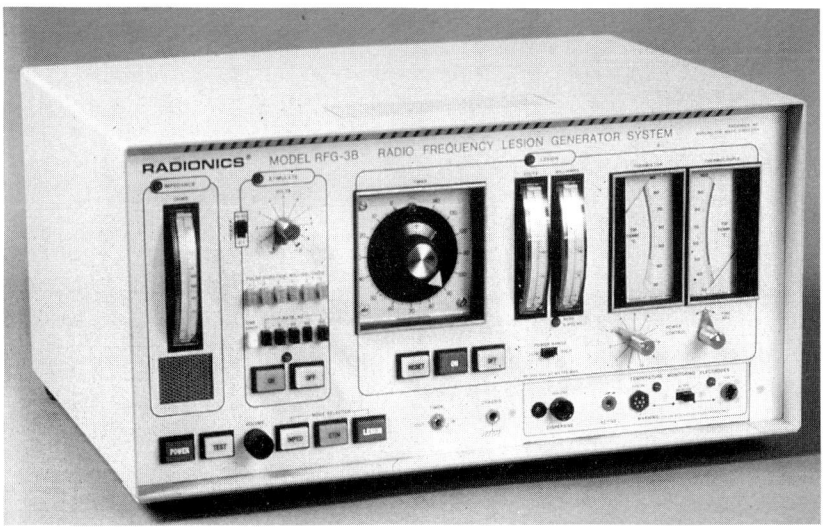

Fig. 11.3 A standard multipurpose radiofrequency generator with impedance gauge, stimulus controls, timer, lesion generator controls (volts or amps), and tip temperature monitors (lesion systems use either thermistor or thermo couples for temperature measurement requiring 2 monitoring controls).

remainder of the chapter will be devoted to its description, in order to stimulate interest in this valuable technique. It involves the placing of a fine needle into the spinal cord at the C1/2 interspace while the patient is awake and localising its position by stimulation prior to creating a heat lesion by passing a radiofrequency current. Originally described in the 50s, the various minor modifications of the technique have made the procedure safe, effective and predictable, even in relatively inexperienced hands.

The radiofrequency generator Fig. 11.3 is in general use in most pain units, and the cordotomy needles, which are Teflon® coated 0.5 mm wires with a 2–2.5 mm exposed tip, may also be used in other pain relief procedures. The needles are introduced using a standard 19 gauge spinal needle as a guide.

The patient lies supine with his head in a special holder (Fig. 11.4) under intravenous anaesthesia such as with propofol, which allows a very quick waking time. The LP needle is introduced into the spinal canal by localising the position on lateral fluoroscopy, usually just below and behind the mastoid. The ideal position in the canal lies immediately in front of the dentate ligament, which should be checked with contrast as seen in Figure 11.5.

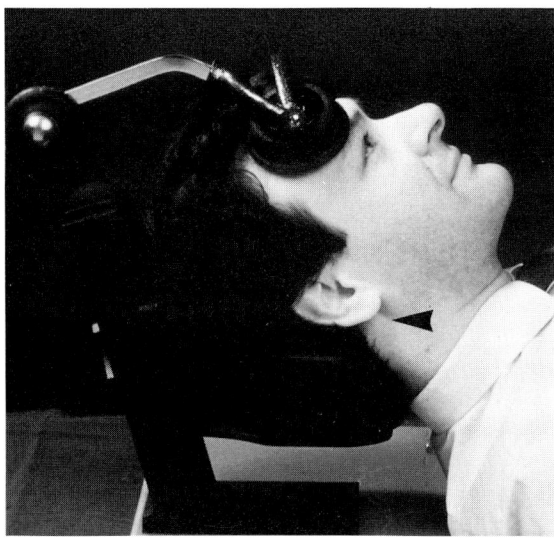

Fig. 11.4 Head holder demonstrated by a volunteer. The arrow marks the approximate entry point.

The patient is then allowed to wake and the cordotomy needle carefully introduced into the cord. This entry is followed by an increase in impedance as the exposed needle tip moves from the CSF into the white matter. The needle's position is then checked by stimulation at 50 Hz. Stimulus in the ST tract is felt as a hot, occasionally unpleasant feeling in either the contralateral hand,

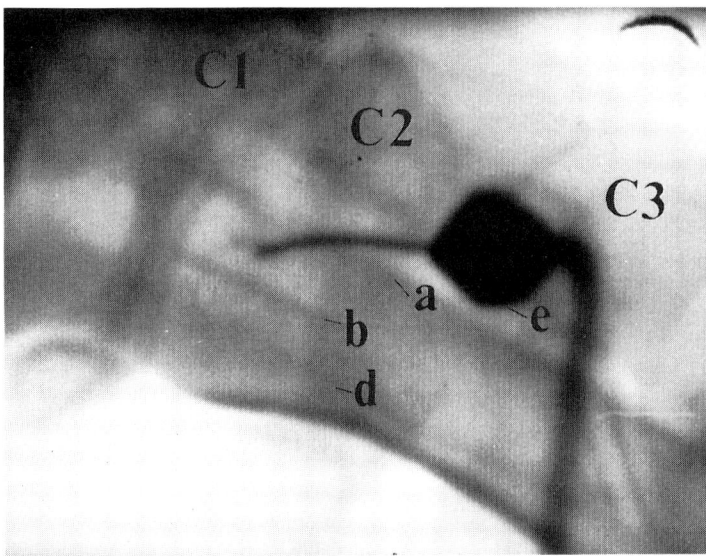

Fig. 11.5 Lateral cervical X-ray taken during a cordotomy. The C1, 2 and 3 vertebral bodies are shown. The front (**a**) and the back (**d**) of the cord are marked as is the dentate ligament (**b**) demonstrated by injection of Iohexol 300 contrast medium from the guide needle (**e**) in perfect position for an arm reference on stimulus.

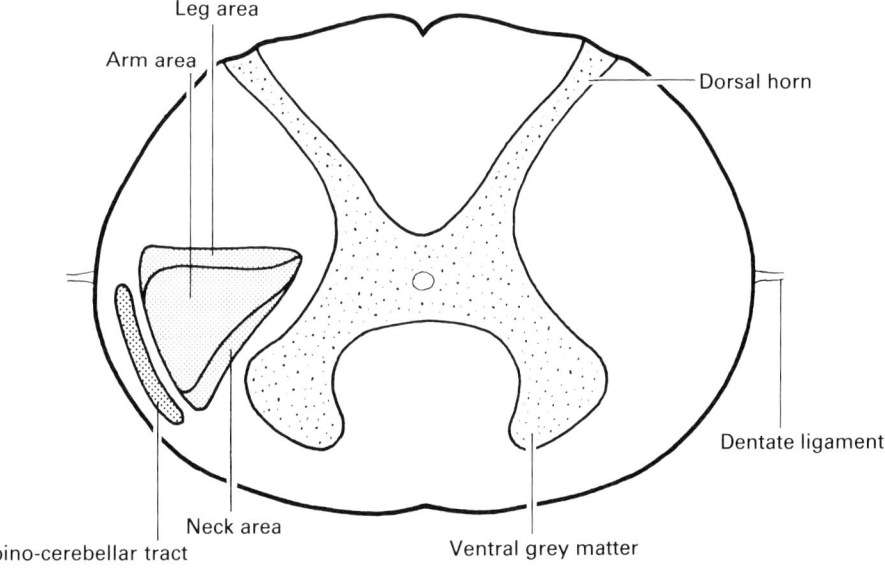

Fig. 11.6 Diagrammatic representation of the cervical cord in cross section at C2. The somatotopic representation of the spinothalamic tract is shown as well as its proximity to the spinocerebellar tract and its relation to the dentate ligament and the grey matter of the cord.

trunk or leg. The needle can be moved anteriorly into the hand area if the stimulus is sensed too low, as the ST tract is organised somatotopically (Fig. 11.6). If the needle lies too posteriorly the stimulus will cause an ipsilateral sensation of buzzing, usually in the hand. This should be checked at 2 Hz when the hand will twitch from corticospinal stimulation. The needle should then be removed. If the needle is too anterior the only stimulus will be to ipsilateral C2 roots.

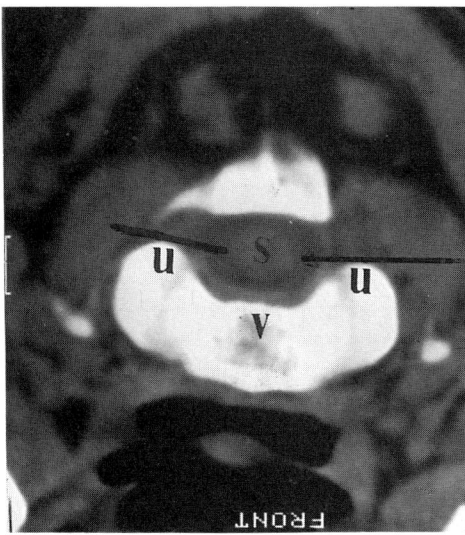

Fig. 11.7a CT scan without contrast of the cord at C2 showing the cord (**s**), the body of C2 (**v**), and the prominent uncinate processes (**u**) which made access to the cord along the lines demonstrated difficult.

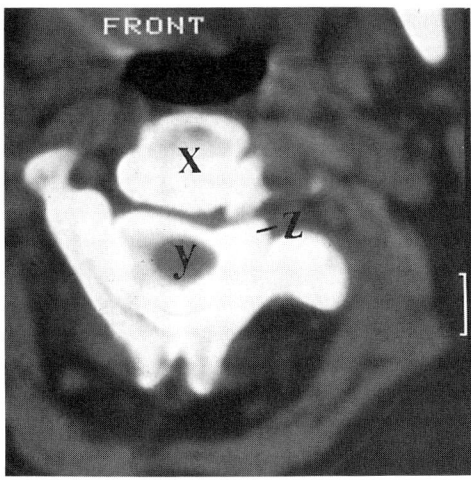

Fig. 11.7b CT scan with contrast in the canal showing an unusually wide AP canal diameter. The cord (**y**) takes an anterior position in the canal, but it may move posteriorly during the procedure. The body of C2 is marked **x**, and the entry root for the needle marked **z**.

Once the correct position has been found, a 2 minute lesion at 75°C is made. Whilst the lesion is in progress the patient must move the ipsilateral hand and toes, as weakening will give warning that the lesion is straying out of the target zone and thus can be safely aborted. The skin sensation is then tested to pinprick. A successful block causes loss over the hand and inner arm, although 3 or 4 such lesions usually have to be made for adequate hand analgesia.

Postoperatively, the patient should be observed for 12–24 hours for pulse BP and respiration, which may be depressed through the loss of afferent stimuli from the chest wall in deep blocks (not seen in the author's series). He is nursed flat as a significant quantity of CSF is usually lost, although it is made up overnight.

The procedure is successful in 85% of cases at the first attempt, but occasionally a second procedure is necessary to extend the block. Occasionally local anatomical abnormalities can make the procedure difficult at the first attempt, but a CT scan of the C1/2 interspace will show unusual bone or the cord position in the canal (Fig. 11.7).

The complications of the procedure are, firstly, weakness of the contralateral side to the pain, but rigorous technique should virtually prevent this, being approximately 2% in the author's series. The second is the development of mild and temporary ataxia from spinocerebellar tract damage, which occurs in 15% of cases, but has usually resolved in a few days. Bladder difficulties are not seen in PCC for arm pain (indeed when they do occur following procedures for leg pain, it usually reflects occult bilateral sacral plexus invasion).

When successful the patient can be slowly weaned off all opiates, although he has often developed some dependancy. Occasionally with the waning of pain the patient seems, perhaps with the withdrawal of the opiates, to become more introspective and very depressed. Finally the loss of pain in a major area sometimes allows a lesser pain elsewhere, such as from other metastases, to become more prominent.

REFERENCES

Lipton S 1984 Percutaneous cordotomy. In: Wall P D, Melzack R (eds) Textbook of pain. Churchill Livingstone, Edinburgh, pp 632–638

Rosomoff H L, Carroll F, Brown J et al 1965 Percutaneous radiofrequency cervical cordotomy. Technique. Journal of Neurosurgery 23: 639–644

Tasker R R 1988 Percutaneous cordotomy: the lateral high cervical technique. In: Schmidek H H, Sweet W H (eds) Operative neurosurgical techniques, vol 2. Grune & Stratton, Orlando, pp 1191–1206

Index

Chapter headings and page references to illustrations are in *italics*.

A fibres, 10, 31
acupuncture, 75, 89, 163
adrenalin, sensitivity to, 5, 6
Adson's test, 73
afferents, 7
  and nerve damage, 4–5
  and tissue damage, 3–4
  unmyelinated, 10–11
Allen test, 120
allodynia
  and causalgia, 83, 84
  and RSD, 20, 85, 86
  and shoulder-hand syndrome, 94
  and TENS, 88
amputation stump, 4
  and neurogenic pain, 140
  neuroma, 100, 101, 103, 104, *105*, 107, 108–9, 147
  see also phantom limb pain
amyloid deposits, 64
anaesthesia dolorosa, 75, 150
anaesthetic, weal, 120
  and central change, 9
  for causalgia and RSD, 86, 87–8
  for cervical spondylosis, 75
  for de Quervain's disease, 122
  for malignant hand pain, 164–8
  for neuroma, 105, 106, 107, 108, 110
  for phantom pain, 148, 149
  for RSD, 134–6
  for tennis elbow, 124
  for wrist joint denervation, 133
analgesics
  for malignant hand pain, 163–4
  ineffectiveness of, 95, 149
angina, 43
angiography, 74
anterior interosseous nerve, denervation of, 133
anticonvulsant drugs, 42, 44, 95, 149
antidepressants
  for central pain 77–8, 94–5
  for M.S., 40
  for phantom limb pain, 149
anti-inflammatory drugs, 3, 94, 163
anxiety and acute pain, 117
Apley test, 120
arteriosclerosis and amputation, 146
arthritis, vii, 3, 19
  osteo — *see* osteoarthritis
  perilunar, 56
  rheumatoid *see* rheumatoid arthritis
arthrodesis, 62, 126–7
arthroplasty, 60, 72
arthroscopy for wrist lesions, 120
aspirin, 3, 64
avulsion pain *see* brachial plexus avulsion
axillary compression syndrome, 57
axons, effects on cut, 4–6

Baldwin's operation, 51, *53*
Barton's fracture-dislocation, *51*, 54
behavioural methods of treating pain, 96–7
Bennett's fracture-dislocation, 62
benzodiazepines, 95, 149
beta blockers, 5
blood circulation, 143
bone
  cysts and tumours of wrist, 63–4
  grafts, 127
  pain, 117
botulinum toxin, 93
bowler's thumb, 112
brachial plexus avulsion injury, 152–4, 160
brachial plexus avulsion pain, 23, 35, 40
  and functional paralysis, 95
  and phantom limb pain, 147
  and RSD, 86
  case histories, 81–3
  DREZ operation for *see* DREZ
  neurostimulation technique for, 143–4
  treatment of vii, 75–81, 140, 142
brachial plexus malignancy, 40, 162
breast, carcinoma of
  and carpal tunnel syndrome, 70
  and hand pain, 162
Brodie's abscess, *61*, 64
burns, 91
Burton's classification, 129–32

calcification around wrist, 64
cancer *see* malignancy
capsaicin, 10, 32

carbamazepine, 77, 88, 95, 149, 163
cardiac patients and causalgia, 88
carpal tunnel syndrome, 35, 37, 43, 57–8, 69–72, 119
  and thoracic outlet syndrome, 74
  and ulnar nerve compression, 73
  recurrent, 106
carpus
  bony swellings around, 58–9
  fracture, 54–5
  instability, 50–1, 133
  osteomyelitis, 61
case histories
  neuropathic pain, 28–31
  painful and injured peripheral nerves, 81–3, 84–5, 90
causalgia vii, 3, 5, 14, 16, 17, 41, 83–5
  and brachial plexus injury, 75
  and neurogenic pain, 140
  and neuroma hypothesis, 18, 19
  and osteoporosis, 86
  and shoulder-hand syndrome, 41, 42
  and ulnar nerve operation, 72
  management of, 86–8
  neurostimulation for, 142
  summary of treatment for, 97–8
  sympathetic mechanisms in, 20
central nervous system
  and cut axons, 5–6
  and pain in hand, 34–45
  and peripheral nerve injury, 8–12, 142, 147–8
  blocks for malignant hand pain, 164–8
cerebrovascular disease, 35–6
cervical disc lesion, 57
cervical rib, 73, 74, 163
cervical spinal cord
  avulsion, *153*, *157*
  disease, 37–40
  DREZ lesions, *155*, *156*
cervical spondylosis, 37–8, 69, 74–5
  fibres, 7, 9, 10, *et seq*
cheiro-oral syndrome, 36
chemical changes and nerve lesions, 11–12
chronic compartment syndrome in first dorsal interosseous muscle, 133

chronic pain syndrome, 115
clonazepam, 163
codeine, 95
Colles' fracture, 51, 54–5, 58, 66
   and carpal tunnel syndrome, 71
computed tomography (CT) scanning, 35, 40, 49
   and brachial plexus avulsion, 153
   and cervical spondylosis, 38
   and hook of hamate fracture, 125
   and malignant hand pain, 163, *168*
   and thalamic pain syndrome, 142
cordotomy vii, 8
   electrode, 159
   for malignant hand pain, 164, 165–8
   for phantom limb pain, 140, 150
cortical excision for phantom limb pain, 151
corticosteroids, 3, 62, 107
   hydrocortisone, 57, 62, 70
costo-clavicular manoeuvre, 73
cramps, 36
crush injuries causing painful, stiff hand, 91
CT scanning *see* computed tomography
cysts
   dermoid and neuromas, 104, 108
   wrist, 62–4

Darrach's operation, 51
   modification of, 122, 127–9, 133
deafferentation pain syndrome, 160
deep brain stimulation for phantom limb pain, 151, 152
degenerative and inflammatory diseases, 59–62
depression
   after percutaneous cordotomy, 168
   and chronic pain, 84, 117
   and neuroma pain, 105
de Quervain's disease, 58, 61–2, 65, 106, 119, 122–3
diabetes and amputation, 146
dislocations
   and RSD, 86
   wrist, 51, 54–5
dorsal column stimulation vii, 7
   for phantom limb pain, 151, 152
   to control neurogenic pain, 140–2
dorsal cutaneous branch of the ulnar nerve, denervation of, 133
dorsal root entry zone operation *see* DREZ operation
dorsal root ganglia, 6, 7
dorsal spinal root stimulation, 140–2
'drawer' sign, 50
DREZ operation vii, ix, 44, 140, 143
   electrode for, *155*
   for brachial plexus avulsion pain, 76, 77, 78–9, 153, 154–9, 160
   for phantom limb pain, 151, 152
drugs
   for brachial plexus pain, 77, 78
   for central pain, 44, 77–8
   for dystonia, 37

   for gout, 61
   for malignant hand pain, 163–4
   for phantom limb pain, 149
   for rheumatoid arthritis, 59, 60
   summary, 94–5
   used in neuroma experiments, 19
Dupuytren's contracture, 93, 119
dystonia, 36–7, 93

ectopic impulses, 31
electromyography, 70, 74 *et seq*
entrapment neuropathies vii, 69–83
epicondylitis, lateral, 119, 122, 123–5
epilepsy, 36, 42

family, role of in pain management programme, 96, 97
Finkelstein test, 122
first dorsal interosseous muscle
   chronic compartment syndrome in, 133
   hernia of, 133, *134*
fitness programme
   for brachial plexus pain, 78, 79
   for functional paralysis, 95–6, 97
fractures
   and carpal tunnel syndrome, 71
   and ulnar nerve compression, 73
   hook of hamate, 122, 125–6
   wrist, 51, 54–5
frozen shoulder, 36, 94
functional block *see* paralysis, functional
functional disorders and painful wrists, 65–7

ganglion, 126
   palmar, 61
   wrist, 62, 63, 72
   gout, 61, 64
guanethedine viii, 5, 87–8, 89, 94

hamate, fractures of hook, 122, 125–6
Hartsill rectangle, 164, *165*
hemiplegia, 42
hernia of FDIM, 133
herpes zoster, 15, 40, 41
   and phantom pain, 43
   and shoulder-hand syndrome, 42
   sympathetic mechanisms in, 22–3
Horner's syndrome, 153, 163
humerus malignancy, 163
hyperalgesia in neuropathy, 31–2
hyperpathia and causalgia, 84
hypnosis for pain relief, 81
hypotension
   and causalgia and RSD, 88
hysterical paralysis *see* paralysis, functional

indomethicin for gout, 61
infective diseases of wrist, 61
inflammation, 3–4

joints
   denervation of wrist, 132–3
   distal radioulnar disorders, 122, 127–9
   lesions of carpometacarpal joints, 122, 126–7
   pain in, 117
   tests for instability, 120, *121*

Kienbock's disease, 51, *52*, 55–6, 133
Klippel-Feil syndrome, 37

laceration of wrist, 58

Madelung's deformity, 51
magnetic resonance imaging (MRI) scanning, 35, 39, 40, 153, 163
Maitland's techniques, 75, 163
malignancy
   brachial plexus, 40
   hand, 162–8
   wrist, 64
management of pain in hand and wrists: central causes of peripheral pain, 34–5
   brachial plexus injuries and malignancy, 40
   cerebrovascular disease, 35–6
   cervical spondylosis, 37–8
   dystonia, 36
   epilepsy, 36
   mechanisms, 43–4
   migraine, 36
   multiple sclerosis, 39–40
   Parkinson's disease, 36
   phantom and referred pains, 42–3
   postherpetic neuralgia, 40–1
   references, 45–7
   shoulder-hand syndrome, 41–2
   spinal trauma, 39
   spinal tumour, 38
   spyringomyelia, 39
   treatment, 44–5
management of traumatic neuroma in hand, 100–1
   classification, 101–3
   clinical features, 103
   investigation, 105
   management, 107
   prevention, 105–7
   recurrent, 109
   references, 112–13
   spindle neuroma, 112
   surgery, 107–12
   symptoms, 104–5
Martin Grueber anastomosis, 72
mechanisms of pain in relation to hand
   axonal injury effect, 5–7
   classical approach, 1
   inner and outer sensory worlds, 1
   nerve damage and afferent barrage, 4–5
   peripheral injury effect on spinal cord, 7–11
   references, 12–13

INDEX

tissue damage and afferent barrage, 3–4
tissue damage and pain, 11–12
median nerve
  neuroma of palmar branch of, 110
  trapped at elbow, 72
microneurography, 30, 31
migraine, 36
morphine for malignant hand pain, 163–4
MRI scanning, 35, 39, 40, 153, 163
multiple sclerosis, 34, 35, 36, 37, 38, 39–40
muscle pain, 117
myelography, 35, 38, 40
  for brachial plexus avulsion, 153, *154*
myelopathy, cervical, 72

narcotics, 4, 94
nerve compression syndromes, 57
nerve grafting
  for avulsion pain, 79, 84
  for neuroma, 112
nerve transposition, 112
neuralgia
  postherpetic, 40–1, 140
  postsympathectomy, 15–16, 23–4
  trigeminal, 44
neurectomy, 108, 109
neurogenic pain, 139, 140–4, 148, 150
  and malignancy, 162
  from skin and from deep tissue, 29
neuromas
  and amputation, 4
  and cut nerve, 5, 6, 18, 83, 84
  and provoked pain, 116
  hypothesis, 18–19
  management, 100–13
  relocation of, 108, 112
  spindle, 112
  surgical procedures for, 89–90
neuropathic pains in limbs
  case histories, 28–31
  hot and cold patients, 32–3
  references, 33
neuropathies, entrapment vii, 69–83
neurophysiology
  and central lesions, 34–5
  and spinal disease, 37–8
neurostimulation techniques for intractable pain in hand and wrist, 139
  brachial plexus lesion pain, 143–4
  discussion, 142
  indications, 139–40
  references, 144
  results, 141–2
  summary, 144
  technique, 140–1
neurotisation, 79
neurotoxins, chronic use of, 31
neurotransmitters *see* Transmitters

nociceptor sensitisation hypothesis, 19–20, 31
non-steroidal anti-inflammatory agents (NSAID), 94
noradrenalin, 86

oedema, 143
oil massage, 91, 93
opioids, use of, 94
Osborne's band, 73
osteoarthritis viii, 59, *60*–1
  NSAID for, 94
  of apophyseal joints, 74
  of CMC joint, 62, 70
  of radio-scaphoid joint, 122
  of TMC joint, 122, 129–32
osteoclastoma, 64
osteoid osteoma, 64, 105
osteomyelitis of carpal bones, 61
osteoporosis, 41
  and causalgia, 86
  and rheumatoid arthritis, 59
  and Sudeck's dystrophy, 66
  and wrist fractures, 54
osteosarcoma, 64
osteotomies for malunions of distal radius, 133
overuse syndrome (also repetitive strain injury), 65–6

Paget's disease, 37, *64*
pain management programme, 96–7
painful hand, problems and solutions, 114
  carpometacarpal joint lesions, 126–7
  characteristics of pain, 117
  chronic compartment syndrome in first dorsal interosseous muscle, 133
  clinical manifestations, 114–17
  denervation of wrist joint, 132–3
  de Quervain's disease, 122–3
  distal radio-ulnar joint disorders, 127–9
  fractures of hook of hamate, 125–6
  interrogation and examination, 117–21
  lateral epicondylitis, 123–5
  references, 136–8
  reflex sympathetic dystrophy, 134–6
  trapeziometacarpal joint osteoarthritis, 129–32
painful peripheral nerves and peripheral nerve injuries, 69
  brachial plexus palsy, 75–81
  carpal tunnel syndrome, 69–72
  case histories, 81–3, 84–5, 90
  causalgia, 83–5, 86–8
  cervical spondylosis, 74–5
  drugs used, 94–5
  dystonia, 93
  functional paralysis, 95–6
  median nerve at elbow, 72
  pain management programme, 96–7
  painful, stiff hand, 90–3
  references, 98–9
  results, 88–9

RSD, 85–8
shoulder-hand syndrome, 93–4
summary protocol, 97–8
thoracic-outlet syndrome, 73–4
ulnar nerve compression, 72–3
painful wrist: problems and solutions, 48–9
  bony swellings around carpus, 58–9
  carpal instability, 50–1
  Colles' fracture, 54
  cysts and tumours, 62–4
  de Quervain's disease, 61–2
  distal radio-ulnar joint, 51
  fractures and dislocations, 54
  functional disorders, 65
  history and clinical examination, 67
  infective diseases, 61
  Kienbock's disease, 55–6
  nerve injury, 56–8
  osteoarthritis, 60–1, 62
  overuse syndrome, 65–6
  painful wrists in schoolgirls, 65
  references, 68
  rheumatoid arthritis, 58–60
  Secretan's disease, 65
  Sudeck's dystrophy, 66
  triangular fibro-cartilage, 53–4
  ulnar variance, 51–3
  writer's cramp, 65
palmar fascitis, 119
panarthrodesis, 50–1
paracetamol, 95
paralysis, functional, 95–6
Parkinson's disease, 36
peptides, 6, 9, 19
percutaneous cordotomy, 165–8
periosteal pain, 117
peripheral nerves
  and central nervous system, 6–12
  blocks, 134–6
  control of pain in, 142, 144
  injuries *see painful peripheral nerves*
  lesions, 139–40
  painful *see painful peripheral nerves*
peripheral pain, central causes of, 34–45
personality and pain tolerance, 117
Phalen's test, 57, 69
phantom limb pain vii, 11, 23, 42–3, 76, 140, 145, 146–7
  conclusions, 151–2
  incidence, 145–6
  pathophysiology, 147–8
  references, 160–1
  symptoms, 146
  treatment, 148–51
phenothiazines, 149
plasters, serial for crush injuries, 92
polyneuropathy and neurogenic pain, 140
posterior interphalangeal joints, denervation of, 133
postherpetic neuralgia, 40–1, 140

postsympathectomy neuralgia (PSN), 15–16, 23–4
pregnancy and carpal tunnel syndrome, 70
prostacyclin, 3
prostaglandins, 3, 19
proximal interphalangeal joints, treatment of painful, 93
psychological treatment for phantom limb pain, 148–9
psychologists, role of clinical vii, 95, 96–7, 98
purines, 19

radial tunnel syndrome, 123, 124
radiculopathy, 36, 38
radiofrequency generator for cordotomy, 166
radio-ulnar joint, 51
radius, shortening of, 51, *52*
Raynaud's disease, 14, 15, 22, 49
Raynaud's phenomenon, 15, 22
referred pain, 29, 42, 43, 116
reflex sympathetic dystrophy (RSD), 14–15, 16, 17, 44, 83
 and denervation of wrist joint, 133
 and peripheral nerves, 85–90, 140
 and personality, 84
 and shoulder-hand syndrome, 41, 94
 case history, 31
 sympathetic mechanisms in, 20–1, 23
 treatment, 85–87, 134–6, 142–3
reflex sympathetic overflow, 116
rehabilitation, 78
 and clinical psychology, 97
 and functional paralysis, 95, 96
 and management of painful, stiff hand, 90–1
 and painful neuroma, 107
 and RSD, 88, 136
 and shoulder-hand syndrome, 94
 and stimulation techniques, 144
 splints for, 81
relaxation techniques for pain relief, 81
repetitive strain injury, 65
resettlement, 78
rheumatoid arthritis, 14, 15
 and carpal tunnel syndrome, 57, 71, 72
 and causalgia, 83
 and RSD, 86
 and ulnar nerve compression, 73
 and wrist pain, 53–4, 59–60, 64
 modified Darrach procedure for, 128
 NSAID for, 94
 sympathetic mechanisms in, 21–2
rhizotomy vii, 143
RSD *see* reflex sympathetic dystrophy

scaphoid fracture, 54–5
scalenous anticus syndrome, 73
scleroderma, 93
Secretan's disease, 65
sensory world of hand, 1–3
shoulder-hand syndrome viii, 3, 35, 36, 41–2, 44, 93–4, 116
skin
 lesions, 8
 of painful, stiff hand, 91
 temperature, 86
sodium valproate, 95
somatogenic pain, 139
spinal cord disease, 37, 42, 43
 ischaemia, 38
 trauma, 39, 86
 tumour, 38
spindle neuroma, 112
splints
 for dystonia, 93
 for fracture of hook of hamate, 126
 for neuroma, 107
 for painful, stiff hand, 91–3
 for wrist, 123
 functional, for brachial plexus lesions, *80*, 81
spondylitis, ankylosing, 94
spondylosis, cervical, 37–8, 69, 74–5, 163–164
sprains
 of CMC joints, 126
stellate nerve blocks viii
 for malignant hand pain, 164
 for neuroma, 105, 107, 108
 for reflex sympathetic dystrophy, 87, 88, 134
stereotactic ablation for phantom limb pain, 150
steroids, 3, 120
 for carpal tunnel syndrome, 70
 for cervical spondylosis, 75
 for painful proximal interphalangeal joints, 93
 for phantom limb pain, 149
 for shoulder-hand syndrome, 94
 for stiff hand (painful), 90
 for tennis elbow, 124
strokes, 34, 35
 and shoulder-hand syndrome, 94
styloid process ununited, *58*, 59
Suave-Kapandji operation, 53
Sudeck's atrophy, 5, 58, 66, 83, 85, 87
 and malignant hand pain, 162
 and osteoporosis, 86
 and reflex sympathetic overflow, 116
 and shoulder-hand syndrome, 94
surgery
 and sympathetic maintained pain, 24
 DREZ *see* DREZ operation
 for carpal tunnel syndrome, 57
 for chronic compartment syndrome in first dorsal interosseous muscle, 133
 for carpometacarpal joint lesions, 126–7
 for denervation of wrist joint, 133
 for de Quervain's disease, 122–3
 for distal radio-ulnar joint, 127–9
 for Dupuytren's contracture, 93
 for fracture of hook of hamate, 125–6
 for injured nerve, 5–6
 for malignancy, 164
 for neuroma, 89–90, 107–110
 for osteoarthritis of basal joint of thumb, *131*, 132
 for osteoarthritis of carpometacarpal joint, 62
 for phantom limb pain, 149–50
 and reflex sympathetic dystrophy, 134, 135
sympathectomy viii, 4, 5, 14, 15, 16
 and dorsal spinal cord stimulation, 143
 and hyperalgesia, 32
 and neuralgia, 23
 and phantom limb pain, 150
sympathetic nervous system viii, 84, 86
sympathetic maintained pain hypothesis, 14, 15, 17–18, 20, 23
 blocks, 14, 15, 87–8, 134–5, 143
sympathetically dependent pain: physiology and clinical expression, 14
 herpes zoster, 15, 22–3
 neuroma hypothesis, 18–19
 nociceptor sensitisation hypothesis, 20
 postsympathectomy neuralgia, 15–16, 23–4
 Raynaud's disease, 15, 22
 references, 24–7
 reflex sympathetic dystrophy and causalgia, 14–15, 20–1
 rheumatoid arthritis, 15, 21–2
 SMP hypothesis, 17–18
 summary, 24
 vicious circle hypothesis, 16–17
synovial sarcoma, 64
synovitis, 64, 71, 72, 122, 123–4
syringomyelia, 38, 39, 70

temperature
 and hyperalgesia, 31, 32–3
 and Raynaud's disease, 22
 and thalamic syndrome, 35
tendons, multiple injuries to, 91
tennis elbow, 119, 122, 123–5
TENS *see* transcutaneous stimulation
tensynovitis, 66, 71–2, 122, 124, 25
thalamic stimulation, 141, 142, 143, 144
thalamic syndrome viii, 35–6, 43, 140, 142
thermography, 86
thoracic outlet syndrome, 73–4
thrombosis, deep venous and RSD, 86
tight fascia, 73
Tinel sign, 5, 69, 104

tissue damage
  and afferent barrage, 3–4, 9
  and pain, 11–12
tomography
  computed *see* computed tomography
  lateral, 125, 126, 127
transcutaneous stimulation (TENS) vii, 7
  for brachial plexus pain, 75–6, 77, 78, 82, 143
  for causalgia, 83, 88
  for chronic benign pain, 95
  for malignant hand pain, 163
  for painful neuroma, 107
  for phantom limb pain, 151, 152
  operation of, 85
transmitters, 19, 86, 160
trapezium, excision of, 62

trauma, 36
  and brachial plexus avulsion, 153
  and nociceptor sensitisation hypothesis, 19
  and reflex sympathetic dystrophy, 14
  and SMP, 17, 18
  spinal, 39, 86
triangular fibro-cartilage, 53–4
trigger finger, 119
triptafen, 77, 88, 95
tryptophan, 95
tumours, 36, 40
  and carpal tunnel syndrome, 70
  and reflex sympathetic dystrophy, 86
  cerebral, 42
  foramen magnum, 37
  glomus vii, 28
  pancoast, 162, 163, 164

  spinal, 38
  wrist, 62, 63, 64
  see also neuromas

ulnar nerve compression, 58, 72–3
  and thoracic outlet syndrome, 74
ulnar variance, 51–3

vertebral body malignancy, 163, 164
vicious circle hypothesis, 16–17

Watson's scaphoid shift test, 120
Wide dynamic neurons (WDR) 16 *et seq*
Wright's hyperabduction manoeuvre, 73
writer's cramp, 65